Theory, Assessment and Intervention in Language Disorders:

an integrative approach

ELIZABETH CARROW-WOOLFOLK

Consultant in Language/Learning Disorders

Grune & Stratton

An Imprint of the W. B. Saunders Company

Harcourt Brace Jovanovich, Inc.

Philadelphia, San Diego, London, Toronto, Montreal, Sydney, Tokyo

Library of Congress Cataloging-in-Publication Data

Carrow-Woolfolk, Elizabeth.
    Theory, assessment, and intervention in language dis-
orders: an integrative appraoch / Elizabeth Carrow-
Woolfolk.
        p.   cm.
    ISBN 0-8089-1918-0
    1. Language disorders.   2. Language acquisition.
3. Linguistics.
    I. Title.
    RC423.C28   1988
    616.85'—dc19   88-1646
                                                          CIP

Grune and Stratton
Philadelphia, PA 19106

Library of Congress catalog Number 88-1646

International Standard Book Number 0-8089-1918-0

Printed in the United States of America

88   89   90   10   9   8   7   6   5   4   3   2   1

"One cannot track language down, as a rabbit to its lair, because it has many tracks."

"The impatient or shallow student may find the way too arduous, for the road does wind uphill most of the way."

(BERRY, 1969, pp. 2, 4).

PREFACE

This book is the result of an effort to clarify for myself the many and varied positions regarding language and its disorders. An even more significant impetus for writing has been the desire to understand what language specialists do or what they say they do in assessment and intervention. The process by which theory is related to practice moves in two directions: theory is analyzed and traced to its logical practical consequences and practice is studied to determine the theoretical positions that are implied. Gradually the lines between theory and practice are discernable and different theoretical perspectives can be identified. Once the classification process is initiated, it becomes possible to identify the basic similarities and differences among theories.

Because theory by nature is abstract, it is often presented in a highly encoded form. As a result, it is comprehensible primarily to others whose concern is theoretical. However, the message conveyed in this book is that theory should permeate practice. For this to happen, theory should be presented in a straightforward manner using simple forms so that specialists and students at every level can comprehend it. For this reason, I have tried to minimize the use of technical and theoretical terminology in this book.

It has been interesting to me that there are actually few major issues on which theories differ. Apparent differences arise when theories are made to address issues that were not an original part of the theoretical construct. Of course, major theoretical differences can produce major practical differences. If the issues in which there are major differences are studied, it may be possible to negotiate a conciliation without major harm to the theory. Such a conciliation is beneficial to those involved with impaired language because an overall theoretical paradigm that integrates significant issues can serve to guide assessment and intervention procedures in a rational and valid way. I have begun this integrative process for myself and, in this book, I am sharing my thoughts with readers who may find a kernel of an idea upon which to continue the process.

I have attempted to present my position objectively because I believe that theories must be viewed with scientific detachment. In the way that empirical studies require adherence to measurement and quantification so theoretical positions should be based upon logic and be able to account for whatever facts are available from research. It happens that at times logic is impaired or facts are incorrect and so the presentation herein may be flawed. But if a seed is planted, I have succeeded.

The reader will notice that some issues in the book are discussed in several chapters. Each time a particular issue reappears, I consider it from a slightly different perspective and when dealing with theory, this modified repetition is important. I believe that positions are clarified if viewed within the framework of a number of theories and at different levels of theory and practice within the same theory.

For thirty years I have been obsessed with language and with integrating various aspects of it, as a graduate student, clinician, teacher, supervisor, administrator and now again as a student. Having observed the "rise and fall" of many theories, I, perhaps, do not get as wrapped up in current positions as do younger members of the profession. I do, however, take current ideas seriously and try to study carefully what new theorists propose. I always am rewarded with new insights into language and am awed at the speed with which these ideas are assimilated into our professional knowledge base. I also have observed the cycles and recurrences of ideas, packaged in new terminology and formats. Often the new terminology is much more descriptive than the old and the new labels provide clear distinction for old ideas. I do not believe, however, that *newer* is necessarily *better*.

Although many lament the gaps between theory and practice, I view the gap between theory application at the university level and practice at the school and clinic level to be of greater concern. The ideal of practice based on theory and its embodiment in a load of 100 children in a small room in a public school must, by virtue of circumstance, be difficult. Our task is to assist the practitioner to function effectively within his or her own context, with procedures that are specifically suited to his or her environment. Poorly-executed ideal procedures can be more detrimental to effective practice than functional non-ideal ones. Theoretical positions should remain at the level of theory until their value is demonstrated. School and clinic specialists should not need to feel guilty if they do not apply every new theory and related devices to assessment and intervention.

An encouraging sign of professional maturity is the respect for other positions that is discernable in recent literature. I consider this to be a healthy trend because few of us have a view from the top and so an approximation of a "true and valid" theory will result from communication among those that see different things or who interpret the same thing differently.

My early thoughts on theory integration were presented at a short course entitled *Language Intervention Programs: The Theory Behind Our Practice* at the annual convention of the American Speech, Language and Hearing Association in 1984 with colleagues Joan Lynch and Carol Waryas. In the course of preparing for the presentation, Jil and Carol helped to crystallize the theory classifications and served as gracious critics to my ideas. Joan Lynch and Betty Liles read the manuscript in various forms and offered suggestions for revision. I am grateful for their help.

I would like to thank Carlee Heit for her patience with the revision process, during which she produced numerous drafts of the manuscript.

The process of writing a book on theory has not been an easy one. I thank my husband, Bob, for sharing the burden.

I hope that these thoughts on theory and practice can become bridges that will link the various positions about language and thereby increase the communication among specialists. I believe that comparison and integration are powerful tools for understanding reality. Everyone needs to get into the communication process—the student, clinician, researcher, and theoretician. There is room for all points of view.

TABLE OF CONTENTS

INTRODUCTION

When faced with the complexities of human language, many theorists find it difficult, at best, to include all aspects of the human communication system within their theoretical framework. Most theorists simply carve out a piece to explain and describe, ignoring those aspects of language that do not fit into their specific schema. Some theorists have addressed the grammar of language and omitted its meaning; others have included in their theory the language process and omitted its context; still others have defined language only in terms of its use. Few theories incorporate language disorders into their description of language. Most of the existing theories are thus partial theories.

Because some specialists in the field of language disorders have no well-formed theory of language disorders of their own, they borrow a partial theory from another discipline whether or not the available data concerning disordered language can be accounted for by the theory. This borrowed theory is applied to language disorders with the implicit assumption that it explains the totality of language behavior (the nature of language, its acquisition, disorders of various types, etc.) even though the originator of the theory had not intended for it to be inclusive of all aspects of language. The facts are forced to fit into the original partial theories.

Other specialists in the field use an alternate approach. They try to explain all aspects of language disorders by using one theory to explain one aspect of the langauge process and another theory for another aspect. For example, one theory is used to explain the nature of language and its description, another is used for assessment and still another as a basis for intervention. Often the theories employed are mutually exclusive. The choice of theory is frequently one of convenience rather than logic and it is used until other theories become the vogue and are adopted by the academic discipline. Theories may even become a means by which members of subgroups within a profession identify themselves with each other, thereby eliminating others from their academic circle.

Theories that are used to describe and explain phenomena have different applications from those that are used as a basis for working with people. When theories are used as a basis for making decisions about matters affecting the effectiveness of intervention, the proper use of time and money and the attitudes of people, the professional cannot arbitrarily choose abstract theories that do not yield valid principles

> *Quote 1*
> As long as we lack a generally accepted system incorporating all the available psychological knowledge, any important factual discovery inevitable leads to the creation of a new theory to fit the newly observed facts.
>
> (VYGOTSKY, 1962, p. 10).

for making choices and decisions. In fact, the language-disorder professional must constantly test the effectiveness of a theory by the results yielded from its application.

Specialists in language disorders often find themselves in a quandary. They must provide assessment and intervention services based on partial theories or on partial descriptions selected from different theories, which in some cases are incompatible. They find that theories tend to be short-lived. *There is no unifying theory, model, or paradigm that has as its main focus the description of language disorders and the corresponding explanations of treatment paradigms.* There is no general framework into which all new or rediscovered knowledge can be placed.

Kuhn (1974) in his book entitled *The Structure of Scientific Revolutions*, describes the behavior of a profession or discipline without a paradigm. The practitioners of the discipline work from models acquired in graduate work and in subsequent exposure to the scientific and theoretical literature of the field, without quite knowing what characteristics have given the models the status of paradigms. Once various models or theories are adopted by a field, it is difficult to discover or characterize the common established bases of the field. Researchers and practitioners simply choose those theories that are compatible with their own views. The construction of a unifying or integrated paradigm does not take place and communication among professionals breaks down.

Developmental stages for the development of a paradigm for a given field are provided by Kuhn:

Stage 1: In the early days of a discipline, there is non-paradigmatic science—all facts are equally relevant.

> *Quote 2*
> If we are concerned with, for example, the nature of language, the mechanism of change and the nature of language disorders, there is, for each of these issues, a rich empiric and theoretic tradition for us to build from. Our particular challenge is to construct a choerent [sic] whole out of the available materials. If the "arm" of our theory requires air pressure and our "motor" is electrical, we have a theory that can't work.
>
> (JOHNSON, 1983, p. 55).

> *Quote 3*
> *We could be discussing language as an entity apart from the human beings who use it. Or we could be discussing some sort of physiological substitute, a hardware system that exists inside individuals. We could be using the term* **system** *to describe a set of observable behaviours, without making inferences about underlying structures . . . . **in yet another sense, to refer to some sort of software package, a "program" that an individual child or adult "has" which permits him to generate behaviors that are externally identifiable as "linguistic," "cognitive," or "social."***
> (BATES, BENIGNI, BRETHERTON, CAMAIONI, & VOLTERRA, 1977, p. 258).

Stage 2: As the discipline develops, it becomes multi-paradigmatic. Many paradigms (partial and complete) vie simultaneously for the attention of the scientific community.

Stage 3: Eventually, one paradigm may dominate for a while, then another.

Stage 4: Ultimately, an overall paradigm must encompass several subordinate paradigms.

The field of language disorders is somewhere between Stage 2 and Stage 3. If the profession is to function with maturity, there needs to be an integration of the theories and paradigms used as a basis of the work with the language disordered. Such an integration cannot be a mixture of discrete theories. It must be a cohesive whole made up of interrelated parts each of which fits logically and whenever possible, empirically with each of the other parts.

If assessment and intervention are practiced in isolation from theory, it is primarily because a cohesive paradigm that takes disordered language into account is not available. If the assessment of a language disorder and its effective intervention are to proceed in a valid and principled manner and to utilize effective procedures, a common theoretical base needs to be established for undergirding these activites. To generate a legitimate theory of language and its disorders, systematic and cumulative studies as well as logical scrutiny of specific issues need to be carried out.

A mature profession will be achieved when the practitioners of that profession have sufficient confidence in their own understanding and observations about the nature of their subject to use them as a framework for theory generation and for practice. If these practitioners continue to "look over their shoulder" for approval from other fields, their profession will not reach maturity. A number of years ago I expressed a theoretical position in an article I wrote and a reviewer wrote, "No one has ever said this before," implying that because it had not

> *Quote 4*
> *. . . we must subject current clinical models to rigorous tests against the most carefully specified and discriminated biologic, psychologic, and environmental conditions among our clients. Only such research will reveal the additional knowledge and clinical revisions that will enable our effective treatment of all human communication deficits.*
>
> (McLean, 1983, p. 125).

been said, I could not say it. We need to cut the strings of total dependency on child language and cognitive theories that do not account for disorders. We need to argue for those interpretations that do account for what *we* know and observe.

For a paradigm to be useful in work with language-disordered children, it needs to address all the questions about language.

It needs to explain:

1. The *structure and substance* of language. What is the knowledge individuals must acquire if they are to communicate by means of language and how is this knowledge acquired?
2. How language is *performed*. How do the various cognitive tasks interact in the development of meaning and in the process of performing language?
3. When and how language is *used*. Why is language used and under what social conditions does it vary?
4. *Who* develops and uses the language. What quality of organic system is involved? Is a particular system intact? What modifications need to be made in providing assistance?
5. How language is *modified*. Is the modification a process that takes place entirely within the child or does environment play a role? To what degree is the environment effective?

Such a paradigm also needs to account for data obtained from the observation of and research on language-disordered children: (1) language-disordered children are a heterogeneous group; (2) they change in profile with age; (3) simple exposure is ordinarily not sufficient for them to acquire language behaviors; (4) they have difficulty in generalizing new information; (5) in children, disorders of language frequently co-occur with disorders of cognition and learning; (6) their problem is most frequently found in the tools (speaking, reading) or in the process (memory, perception) for learning than in the content or ideas, etc.

In order to develop an overall paradigm, the scientist and theorist in the discipline of language disorders need to search for basic principles. The place to begin is with the paradigms that are presently used. Attempts should be made to understand their interpretation of reality as

> *Quote 5*
> *Because we can only investigate the neural bases of behaviors that we know how to describe and because the constructs with which we work shape both the questions that can be asked and the conclusions that can be drawn, the way that language, reading, and spelling are conceptualized will contrain our capacity to look for and to understand the neural mechanism that subserve these capabilities.*
>
> (KIRK, 1983, p. 4).

it applies to language acquistion, disorders, and assessment and the themes that run through the intervention practices. This should be done without preconceptions, with open and objective review of both old and new ideas, and with constant attempts at integrating them. The most important task is to bring what is known about disordered language into closer agreement with the applicable theories that have been generated by all disciplines. The alignment of experiment, observation, and theory will form the beginning of a paradigm. However, gathering evidence in isolation will not culminate in theory. Data must be gathered to test theory and integrated to form a paradigm.

Because a model or theory structures what questions are permissible and which intervention approaches are considered legitimate with reference to the theory's belief system, it is important that a model or theory selected by a profession reflect accurately the concerns of the profession. The professionals in the field of language disorders need to identify such a paradigm, recognizing that they may not agree with every part of it and may not be able to produce a full interpretation or rationalization of it. The emergence of a generally accepted paradigm will affect the structure of the field, its research, and ultimately the effectiveness of its activities—assessment and intervention. In fact, theory should permeate every aspect of clinical application. Kuhn predicts that the world will not change with a change of paradigm, but the researcher and clinician will work in a new and different world. Although they will perceive the same data as before, new insights from the data will emerge. Once the acceptance of a common paradigm has freed the researcher from the need to examine constantly the first principles of the field, she or he can concentrate on refining the questions about specific areas of concern knowing that the answers will contribute to the broad understanding of the field.

When the practitioner begins to base assessment and intervention on a comprehensive theory of language disorders, the decision-making processes as well as the assessment and intervention procedures will provide a challenge to her or him. Researchers will be interested in data from the clinicians to verify theoretical principles. Clinicians will look to theorists for the expansion of the clinician's understanding and so do a

> *Quote 6*
> *In general, the persistent manner in which intervention programs have reflected goals based upon linguistic and psycholinguistic information but procedures based upon operant conditioning can be traced, at least in part, to the fundamentally different purposes that motivated formulations of the original theories. Since behaviorism, as a psychological theory, emphasized **how** children learn language, the theoretical purposes were consistent with the procedural selection requirements of intervention.*
>
> (CRAIG, 1983, p. 108).

better job of working with disordered language. There will not be as much burn-out in the profession; clinicians will discover that the field of language disorder can provide interest and excitement for a lifetime.

A good beginning for the process of paradigm development is a review of the theories, models, and themes that have formed the bases of work with language-disordered children over the years. One of the purposes of this book is to attempt to describe the theoretical foundations upon which the parameters of the assessment and intervention of language disorders in children have been and are still based. Although there are numerous theories or models of cognition, of language, and of learning, I have chosen to describe and evaluate six, which I believe have had and still have direct influence on the treatment of language-disordered children. Rather than describe the characteristics of each theory or model in its entirety, I will emphasize those aspects that have had and still have direct bearing on language disorders. The theories will be presented as they apply to these disorders. Throughout the presentation, the similarities and differences among the theories and positions will be pointed out. To facilitate the description of the positions to be described, the term "theory" will be used to refer to the specific approaches, principles, and philosophies that have been used to define and describe language and the language system.

I will make no attempt to review new theories in the fields of Cognition, Learning, and Language Development unless they have already had an impact on work with language-impaired children. However, I sincerely hope that the framework presented here will be of some help in integrating new theories into an existing framework of language that includes language impairments as an integral part.

The review will include a brief description of each theory's classic and basic framework for understanding and describing language, how this construct has shaped the questions that the theory asks about language, and the conclusions drawn. The theory's orientation to language and its disorders will be presented in as simple a form as possible. The name given to each theory that is presented reflects, for the most part, its theoretical origins and its role in language disorders. These

> *Quote 7*
> *There is a balancing act to be played between the notions of sub-jectivity and objectivity. We have seen a change in clinical proce-dures, changes in terminology employed and something which both of these are related to—changes in theory construction. It is tempting to think of this sixth decade as one in which we are more objective about the assessment and treatment of com-municative disorders.*
>
> (PRUTTING, 1983, p. 255).

names do not necessarily coincide with the labels provided by the theorists themselves nor are they intended to reflect the labels given to academic discipline categories. The use of the name of the theory also does not imply that it is a complete explanation of that theory in its broader context. The description of each theory is partial, in so far as it reflects only those aspects of the theory that pertain to language disor-ders.

A second purpose of this book is to describe how the themes of each theory have permeated practices in assessment and intervention for language-disordered children. Each theory will be considered from the bases of the theoretical and practical contributions it has made to the field of language disorders and of the limitations it has in describing and accounting for the heterogeneity of problems in language.

A third focus of the book is on integration. I will attempt to recon-cile some of the differences among theories and to show how apparently disparate issues and ideas can be made to fit together.

Finally, I will try to present some thoughts and conclusions about the elements that are basic to a theory, which can serve as a foundation for describing language disorders in children and also about the integra-tion of assessment and intervention practices that are associated with these disorders.

Within each chapter the reader will find quotations from language theorists and specialists in language disorders. These have been chosen to illustrate the sources of theoretical thought that have guided the work with language disorders and to reflect the various positions that in-dividuals have taken in their approach to understanding disorders, as-sessment, and intervention. In some instances the quotations reflect research conclusions, but in most instances they are of a theoretical na-ture. In most cases, I have attempted to choose quotations from writings of specialists in language disorders who have applied general language theory to the discipline instead of using writings of the original theorist.

I have limited the inclusion of specifics in describing assessment or intervention approaches. There are many books that describe the "how to" and "how not to" but few that attempt to discover the rationale and logic and basic theoretical positions about language that undergird the practical suggestions. When the concrete domain is used as a guide, it is likely that differences among procedures are noticed. When commonalities are abstracted from specific approaches, most differences disappear or become unimportant. We are left with a few issues that are real and a few that exist only as semantic differences related to the basic nature of categorizing by different academic disciplines.

It is a comforting thought that most differences exist only in the mind of the perceiver. They persist only if the perceiver puts on blinders to the positions and contributions of others. I believe that there are few, if any, absolute statements we can make or positions we can take about language, its disorders, and practices in its assessment and intervention. Perhaps those of us whose major concern is language-disordered children need to practice the skills that we teach others, those of communication. If this is done, we may, together, be able to generate a theory of disorders that will help us do a better job of helping language-impaired children.

SECTION I

Applying Theories to Practice

The first five chapters of this book attempt to identify and describe the threads of thought about language that have been woven into the descriptions of language disorders and into the principles and methods of helping children with such problems. Although some of the theories are not presently held in high regard as having valid explanatory logic about language disorders, it is possible to find procedures and terminology in current use that are historically associated with them. For this reason, I have included them in this section.

This section of five chapters views the theories from different perspectives. Chapter 1 briefly describes six theories and their resulting influence on descriptions of language development, disorders, assessment, and intervention. Chapter 2 takes some of the issues regarding development, disorders, and practice and demonstrates the position of each theory regarding these issues. In Chapters 3 and 4 I have described the influence of the six theories on general assessment and intervention procedures, respectively, and have attempted to point out the major contributions and limitations of each theory to practices in language disorders. Chapter 5 attempts to identify the theoretical positions in the intervention methodologies and practices used in the field of language disorders. By analyzing language methodology into its basic components and sequences, it is possible to determine, to some degree, the point at which theory and practices differ.

1

LANGUAGE THEORIES AND LANGUAGE DISORDERS: An Overview

NEUROPSYCHOLOGICAL THEORY
  General Description
  Language Development
  Language Disorders
  Language Assessment and Intervention

BEHAVIORAL THEORY
  General Description
  Language Development
  Language Disorders
  Language Assessment and Intervention

INFORMATION PROCESS THEORY
  General Description
  Language Development
  Language Disorders
  Language Assessment and Intervention

LINGUISTIC THEORY
  General Description

Language Development
  Language Development
  Language Disorders
  Language Assessment and Intervention

COGNITIVE ORGANIZATION THEORY
  General Description
  Language Development
  Language Disorders
  Classification of Disorders
  Language Assessment and Intervention

PRAGMATIC THEORY
  General Description
  Language Development
  Language Disorders
  Language Assessment and Intervention

CHRONOLOGY AND RECIPROCAL
INFLUENCE OF THEORIES

THEORY, ASSESSMENT AND INTERVENTION
IN LANGUAGE DISORDERS: © 1988 by Grune & Stratton
AN INTEGRATIVE APPROACH

ISBN   0-8089-1918-0
All rights reserved.

There are numerous theories of language, but only a few of them have had an impact on the field of language disorders in children. A review of the literature in language disorders, both present and past, reveals themes of six major approaches to language: the neuropsychological, the information process, the behavioral, the cognitive organization, the linguistic, and the pragmatic theories. These categories are essentially distinctive and as such, each has played a special and unique role in the characterization, assessment, and intervention of language disorders in children.

This chapter presents an overview of these six theories, all of which have contributed to the development of the field of language disorders and have adherents today. Each theory is described according to its views on language development, language disorders, assessment and intervention. The theories will be described in general—not necessarily according to the views of one specific theorist. Only the most common views held by proponents of the theory will be presented, and wherever possible, the specialists in language disorders whose writings at a particular period were associated with a specific theory will be identified. The association of a particular specialist with a theory does not imply that the individual continues to hold the position described; indeed, that specialist may not have espoused that particular view at any other time except at the time of the writing of the referenced work. Their theoretical positions have contributed to the development of the field of language disorders and so it is important to include their work here regardless of whether the original authors still hold to the basic tenets of the theory. Some writers have formed bridges across theories. These have been pointed out whenever possible.

NEUROPSYCHOLOGICAL THEORY

General Description

The selection of the term *neuropsychological* to describe this theory does not imply that what is discussed in this section is the theoretical undergirding of the academic discipline of neuropsychology. The label was chosen because it best described the theories that relate the brain and language and, even more specifically, brain impairment and language disorder. The basis of this perspective is the neuroanatomy and pathophysiology of cognitive processes. The term *neurolinguistics* is used to describe that aspect of neuropsychology that deals specifically with the relation between the brain and linguistic form; the study of the neuropsychological system for using language is combined with the study of language structure. The peripheral mechanisms of sensation and perception are also included in the neuropsychologist's description of language.

> *Quote 1–1*
> *Just as adherence to physical fact is necessary in evaluating language theories, so too are formal linguistic facts ultimately required in constructing an adequate neurological theory.*
> (GRUBER & SEGALOWITZ, 1977, p. 15).

The earliest theoretical influence on the definition of language disorders in children came from the field of adult aphasia that developed rapidly after World War II. The literature in adult aphasia focused on the description and grouping of language behavior symptoms related to the parts of the brain that were impaired. When specialists noted that some children exhibited language behaviors that were similar to those in individuals with known brain injury, the category of childhood aphasia came into prominence (Myklebust, 1954; Eisenson, 1968, 1972). Because studies of the neural basis of language encompass the totality of neural systems and subsystems that contribute to the production and comprehension of oral and written language, the description of language of children according to the neuropsychological theory is similar to the description of the adult aphasic's semantic and syntactic systems within the framework of language reception and expression.

Although the study of the relationships between the brain and language is not new, there continue to be areas of innovative research that are constantly increasing knowledge in this area. An example of a recent neuropsychological issue that is important in understanding language disorders is that of hemispheric involvement in language (Millar & Whitaker, 1981). Studies have been carried out to identify which aspects of language behavior are controlled by the right brain and which by the left. This information will help in understanding the problems that co-occur with those of disordered language and will assist in the development of syndromes for groups within the major categories of disorder.

Psychoneurology and neurolinguistics are also related by theorists who analogize components of the brain and language to systems and models of artificial intelligence. These theorists use the concepts underlying computers for the analysis of complex systems used in cognition and language. Because of the study of artificial intelligence, there is beginning to be an integration of neurolinguistics theories with cognitive theories. Studies using artificial intelligence help to distinguish a performance notion from a competence notion by showing how a grammar may be represented for production (Arbib, 1982).

> *Quote 1–2*
> *We are, therefore, suggesting as a working hypothesis that the general, nonspecific states of maturation of the brain constitute prerequisites and limiting factors for language development*
> (LENNEBERG, 1967, p. 169).

Language Development

The idea that specific language functions are localized in the brain served as a basis for Lenneberg's (1966, 1967, 1975) thesis that the ability to acquire language is a neurobiological phenomenon and is relatively independent of intelligence or environment. These neurobiological endowments make communication uniquely possible for humans. According to Lenneberg, language, like other biological functions, unfolds according to a schedule, a consequence of the gradual differentiation and specialization of the brain. This schedule correlates with other maturational tasks and with the development of cerebral dominance (Lenneberg, 1966, 1967, 1975). The neurological structures must reach a state of readiness before input from the environment precipitates the language-synthesizing process.

Because language is considered a function of neurobiological development, the psychoneurologic theory places little emphasis on the role of the environment in the acquisition of language by children. The human models provide the form for language and serve to support its development but do not cause the onset or course of development.

Language Disorders

The basic premise of the neuropsychological theory of language disorders is that in such disorders the central nervous system, especially the cerebral cortex, is impaired. Waryas and Crowe (1982) wrote, "We must assume that language delay has a neurologic basis . . . we should view all language dysfunctions potentially as neurologic 'soft signs'" (p. 773). The degree and type of neurological impairment determine the degree and type of impairment of the language functions. The age of onset of a neurological problem also influences the type of language problem and/or the capacity for language learning and language recovery. The task of the specialist is to discover in general and in each individual child the relationship of cerebral pathology to impairments of language processes.

The primary focus in the classification of language disorders in the neuropsychological theory is that of differentiating disorders of language related to impairments of language areas of the brain from language disorders resulting from other causes such as hearing loss, emotional disturbance, or mental retardation. The causative factors are usually termed *pathologies* or conditions. Categorical distinctions are also made between the language functions that are impaired—comprehension, expression—but primarily in reference to the areas of the brain associated with these functions. This approach leads to the posi-

> *Quote 1–3*
> *We are not suggesting that syndromes of DLD [Developmental Language Disorder] precisely parallel the syndromes of acquired aphasia in adults. Nevertheless, since it would not be parsimonious to think that the organization of children's brain is fundamentally different from the organization of the adult brain, it is likely that similar symptoms reflect pathology in the same general systems in both children and adults.*
> (RAPIN & ALLEN, 1983, p. 165).

tion that the fundamental processes are separable from one another and therefore can be independently impaired (and independently improved). The description of the grammar of language was not originally an integral part of this theory, although recent literature in neurolinguistics attempts to differentiate between semantic and syntax problems on the basis of location of brain impairment.

Language Assessment and Intervention

The process of evaluating and studying children's language with the intent of differentiating language problems related to brain dysfunction from other types of language disorders was originally termed *differential diagnosis*. This designation has persisted in some circles. Specific concern in differential diagnosis is with the child's neurological system—the procedures of identifying the etiology as well as positive and negative signs of brain damage. The method of study is primarily by clinical observation of behaviors called *symptoms* and relating these to known brain damage. The early term for the rehabilitation process was *therapy*, implying the cure of pathology and/or the betterment of the condition. The role of the therapist was and still is considered incidental to the degree of disorder of the pathology or condition. Treatment effectiveness in young children is related to the maturational levels governing brain-behavior relationships. Attention is given to both receptive and expressive modalities.

The study of language disorders in children within the framework of neuropsychological functioning is described by Rapin and Allen (1983), who identified five syndromes of "Developmental Language Disorder" on the basis of the children's linguistic deficits. They suggested that although the syndromes do not precisely parallel those of acquired aphasia in adults, the similarity between the organization of the adult brain and the child brain makes it likely that similar symptoms reflect similar system pathology. Rapin and Allen believe that the study of children's syndromes and their comparison with those of adult

> *Quote 1–4*
> *Lacking the ability to directly modify the neurophysiologic struc-*
> *ture of the individual, why should one wish to know whether*
> *neurologic factors are causally indicated? First, it is necessary to*
> *realize that all learning, including that of language, must be con-*
> *sidered to involve neurologic structures and their development*
> *and organization. Specifically, input, output, association, and*
> *storage functions are required in some general sense, all of*
> *which are neurologically based. Knowledge of how the child*
> *functions in these respects has profound implications for therapy*
> *procedures, specifically in regard to the selection of input and*
> *output modalities, types of stimuli utilized, and the use of drill or*
> *other such structured tasks in therapy.*
> (WARYAS & CROWE, 1982, p. 774).

aphasics provide a basis for understanding the anatomic basis for the developmental language disorder syndrome.

BEHAVIORAL THEORY

General Description

Threads of behavioral theory or learning theory have run through language disorder theory since "language disorders" became an area of professional concern—about the same time or soon after the psychoneurologic theories about language evolved. The major theme has been that language behavior is learned when an individual (mother, caretaker, etc.) provides a stimulus, usually verbal, to which a child responds verbally and the child's response is reinforced. According to behavioral theory, the characteristics of the stimulus and reinforcement direct the level, speed, and adequacy of the language behavior that is learned by the child. Another factor that has been purported to influence learning is the degree of identification of the child with the caretaker (Mowrer, 1958, 1960). When one of the major elements essential to learning are impaired or absent, a language disorder occurs.

The foci of behavioral theory are the acts of talking and of receiving language. The adequacy of message reception is ascertained by observing the consequent behavior of the recipient. The adequacy of language production is based on the quality of surface forms only; the level of rule-based language behavior is not described.

Language Development

As just stated, behavioral theory describes language as a learned phenomenon; it develops because of and according to learning/training principles utilized by the environment. The child imitates the speech

> *Quote 1–5*
> The term "verbal behavior" has much to recommend it. Its etymological sanction is not too powerful, but it emphasizes the individual speaker and, whether recognized by the user or not, specific behavior shaped and maintained by mediated consequences.
>
> (SKINNER, 1957, p. 2).

models in the environment and is reinforced for the imitations that resemble the model. In general, language, as is all behavior, is thought to develop out of the interaction between the organism's behavior and the antecedents and consequences of that behavior (Sloane & MacAulay, 1968). The theory argues against innateness in language development, using as an argument that there are in fact nonlanguage children (Gray & Ryan, 1973). Because the learner's performance is shaped by the environment, he or she plays a passive role.

Behaviorism differs from cognitive and neuropsychological theories in that it refutes any association between language development and other cognitive and motor skills and strongly opposes a biological explanation of development (Staats, 1971).

Language Disorders

A characteristic of behavioral theory is that it does not address internal (mental) factors associated with language learning; consequently, the idea of "cause" is simply not a pertinent issue in the behavioral description of disordered language. Language is behavior; a child who does not *perform* is a nonlanguage child, and the nature of the problem (autism, aphasia, etc.) is irrelevant (Gray & Ryan, 1973). Failure to perform is a result of inappropriate training, either because the environment is deficient or because a disorder makes it difficult for the child to utilize the environment. Since all problems are treated the same, there is no need to classify disorders into types.

Language Assessment and Intervention

The essence of assessment, according to behavioral theory, is the clinician's judgment of the inadequacy of a child's language ability based on *performance* (what the child does), compared with what the child should be doing. The basic approach of this theory to intervention is that of *teaching* the nonlanguage child (using a basic stimulus-response [S-R] paradigm) to produce adequate language structure. Since all nonlanguage children are provided with essentially the same procedure, identification of the reasons for the lack of language are identified only if the child's specific problem interferes with teaching. Training, the key to behavioral theory, begins with a "baseline" description of performance. By schedules of reinforcement that assist the child in discrimination and generalization, the teacher helps the child acquire increasingly complex horizonal chains of surface structures.

The major factor in bringing about behavioral change is the environment and the environmental manipulation of antecedent and consequent events. The stimuli and reinforcement provided by the environment are the actual instruments of language improvement. As stated previously, the nature of the internal process of the child is not considered in this theory. Because the internal systems are ignored, the focus of intervention is on expressive rather than receptive language.

In the past decades, the essential characteristics of behavior theory have not changed in any significant way, although refinements have taken place. The theory continues to be utilized by some specialists with children who have language disorders, but is used mainly as a method of bringing about change rather than as an explanation of language development. The approach is particularly useful with severely impaired language-disordered children such as retarded and autistic children. It also appears that specialists who currently utilize behavioral approaches in intervention are attempting to integrate data from linguistic and pragmatic studies of children's language into that intervention. In other words, the content of intervention is being influenced by these other approaches (Miller & Yoder, 1974; McDonald, 1975).

INFORMATION PROCESS THEORY

General Description

Because of the difficulty in identifying developmental brain injury, brain impairment, or minimal cerebral dysfunction, and because of dissatisfaction with pure S-R theory, a theoretical direction taken by language-disorder specialists subsequent to behaviorism was toward an information processing description of behavioral involvement in language. A theory emerged that described the processes of language and their disorders without analysis of their relationship to the brain or to higher levels of cognitive processes. Although the single-path serial model of cognitive processing (sensation → perception → cognition → memory) has been in existence since the time of Aristotle, during the 1960s the model was integrated with the major functional psycholinguistic tasks—speaking and comprehending—by a theoretician who wished to provide validity to a modification of the S-R theory of Skinner. Osgood (Osgood & Miron, 1963; Osgood, 1967, 1968) proposed a mediating process between stimulus and response that led to a description of the input and output modalities involved in language and transmissions between these two within the cognitive system. The work by Kirk, McCarthy, and Kirk (1968) and by Wepman, Jones, Bock, and vanPelt (1960) expanded this theory by describing in detail a process by which the language code is received by the human cognitive system, translated to meaning, encoded back into the linguistic system, and uttered as speech. The emphasis in the expanded version, particularly as it was applied to language and learning disabilities, was not on describing language learning within the corresponding S-R framework, but on a description of a sequence of cognitive steps within the organism as it transmits a verbal stimulus from the sensory input level to the level of comprehension and when it formulates and executes verbal expression. This process was described in the form of a dimensional model. The theory described modality relationships (reading, aural comprehension) as integral but independent, and it differentiated between automatic and voluntary processes. This theory led to the development of standardized tests in many of the processing areas.

There is little or no description of the language code itself in the information process theory. Differentiation is made between sensation and perception, between perception and representation, between reception and expression, between language formulation and language repetition/execution, and between automatic and voluntary performance. However, the structure and use of language are ignored. The information process theory makes no attempt to explain higher level cognitive functions such as rule formulation, pattern analysis, inference, and so on. In this sense, then, this theory is still tied to behaviorism.

I originally selected the term, *cognitive process theory*, to label this theory, implying the inclusion of its basic descriptive elements within the general framework of cognition. Because this presention of theories includes one that I have termed *cognitive organization theory*, I decided to delete the word *cognitive* from one of them to prevent confusion. It is important to recognize that the separation of these two theories is not meant to imply that there is no overlap between them or that the pro-

---

Quote 1–6

. . . this kind of mediation-theory [nonrepresentational] **requires** *no symbolic processes; it is, indeed, merely an extension or complication of the Skinnerian single-stage model. But note also that it could quite easily* **become** *a representational mediation theory by changing the nature of element B—from an implicit linguistic response . . . to an implicit nonlinguistic response . . .*

It is one thing to claim that (learned) transitional dependencies provide an insufficient characterization of language performance; it is another thing to deny that they exist or have any psycholinguistic significance.

(OSGOOD, 1968, p. 496, 503).

> *Quote 1–7*
> *The developmental approach appears to be a more fruitful one. A child's performance is examined on a hierarchy of tasks in which each succeeding item is developmentally dependent on the skills required for the preceding tasks. To arrive at the hierarchical sequence, we need all of the following: (1) normative developmental data, (2) logical analysis of prelinguistic and linguistic tasks and (3) analysis of the performance requirements of these tasks. In the developmental approach, the level at which a child performs in relation to others is of less concern than how his performance on a specific task compares to that on succeeding, more complicated communication tasks.*
>
> (CARROW, 1972, p. 53).

cesses in the two theories are actually independent from one another. The separate description is a function of the original theorists' boundaries. What I call *information process theory* was originally a description that limited the higher level cognitive processes to what was called *mediation.* Although the cognitive organization theory (See page 17) includes perception and memory within its boundaries of description, the main focus is on higher level functions.

Language Development

The adequacy of language development in the information process model depends on the adequacy of each process in a system that includes a feedback loop—self-monitoring and monitoring by the environment. The premise is that the adequacy of each developmental process (e.g., comprehension) is dependent on the adequate development of the subprocess(es) (perception, memory) that precedes it in development and execution. Language develops in accordance to hierarchical steps, the basic simple processes forming the basis for higher level, complex behaviors.

Language Disorders

The information process theory characterizes language disorders in terms of impairments or developmental lags in one of the processes essential for comprehending or producing language. The type of disorder and its severity are determined by the level or modality at which the breakdown occurs. The theory of disorders is based on the concept of discrepant behavior—differences between skills (as compared with norms) that should be developing at about the same level within the individual.

Language disorders in the information process theory are classified by modality, process, and level. A child may have an auditory comprehension problem related to auditory memory or auditory perceptual deficits, or have a production disorder involving poor retrieval and/or semantic memory. The determination of the extent of disorder is related to the development period at which a processing problem occurs and its effect on the development of language functions at that period.

Aram and Nation (1975) described disordered language behaviors as related to language processing dysfunctions that appear as variable patterns of performance and are shaped by the developmental context in which they occur. The patterns of language disorder, according to Aram and Nation, arise from different points of disruption in the language processing system. The processing model used by Aram and Nation as a basis for assessment is based on the earlier models provided by Kirk et al. (1968), Wepman et al. (1960), and Carrow (1972).

Language Assessment and Intervention

Assessment procedures in the information process theory are primarily directed at identifying the child's processing strengths and weaknesses on a hierarchical scale of cognitive and linguistic skills. During the period when this theory originated, the children's problems were referred to as *deficits* or disabilities and the rehabilitation process considered to be one of *remediation* of a weakness or a replacement or substitution for the deficit. The assumption was and is still held by many specialists that if the weakness is strengthened, the language function will improve, or as an alternate to the strengthening of weaknesses, compensatory functions are developed. Both receptive and expressive modalities are considered important in the assessment and intervention processes.

_____ **LINGUISTIC THEORY**

General Description

Although linguistic theory has been continuously modified since Chomsky first described generative grammar in 1957 (Chomsky, 1957), several strains of thought have remained somewhat constant. According to linguistic theory, what is known in language is a system of abstract rules; the behavior called *language* is generated from this knowledge. The linguistic component of the human learning system is independent and distinctive from other cognitive functions. It operates according to principles that are unique to language. (A discussion of this uniqueness is described in Chapter 7, under the heading of modular theory.)

> *Quote 1–8*
> *The problem for the linguist, as well as for the child learning the language, is to determine from the data of performance the underlying system of rules that has been mastered by the speaker-hearer and that he puts to use in actual performance. Hence, in the technical sense, linguistic theory is mentalistic, since it is concerned with discovering a mental reality underlying actual behavior.*
>
> (CHOMSKY, 1965, p. 4).

Because some aspects of language acquisition appear to be innate and universal, the linguists conclude that language is biologically determined and evolves as a result of the unfolding of a language "device" in the child's system. The role of the environment is discounted. Because children appear to use creativity in language learning as well as unique strategies for acquiring rules, language cannot result from the child's passive observation and imitation of the adult language in the environment.

The focus of linguistic theory was originally on generative grammar, and the description of language was in the form of characterization of syntactic constituents. A later emphasis of linguistic theory was on semantic role analyses, particularly in child language (Bloom, 1970; Brown, 1973). Interest in semantic relations was a sign of the restoration of meaning in the description of language. This movement from an emphasis on syntax and the theory of innateness in development to an emphasis on semantics and the consequent concern with the cognitive role in language learning was a movement from a purely linguistic interpretation of language to a psycholinguistic one. It is the psycholinguistic position that will be of major concern in this book.

From the psycholinguistic viewpoint the component parts of language (Bloom & Lahey, 1978) are: (1) content—the meaning that is coded; (2) form—which represents the meaning, and (3) use—the

> *Quote 1–9*
> *Description in terms of a set of prevalent semantic relations may be little more than a technique of data reduction, a way of describing the meanings of early sentences short of listing them all. Even as a reduction technique it has a certain value. It reveals the fact that Stage I utterances, in all the language for which studies exist, concentrate on the same set of meanings, a set far short of the meanings that languages are able to express and, in adult usage, do express . . . . Besides serving to summarize data and to reveal uniformities it is possible, of course, that the semantic relations represent a psychological **functional** level in sentence comprehension and production but, of this, there is as yet no strong evidence.*
>
> (BROWN, 1973, p. 173).

> *Quote 1–10*
> *We can now rephrase the problem of linguistic abstraction. In acquiring the transformations that define language, children learn to relate deep and surface structures; but the deep structures of sentences are never displayed in the form of examples stimuli, responses, or anything else. They are abstract and, for one who does not already know the language, inaccessible. It is this simple linguistic fact, which every child faces and overcomes, that eliminates S–R theory as a serious explanation of language acquisition.*
>
> (MCNEILL, 1971, p. 18).

purpose of language in a particular context. According to Bloom and Lahey, language knowledge is the *integration* of content, form, and use. Bloom and Lahey's theory, because of its inclusion of "use" in the description of language, prepared the way for the resurgence of pragmatics into language theory and application. It also integrated meaning into the linguistic construct. I have included this theory within general linguistic theory because the focus of Bloom and Lahey's concern appeared to be on expressive language that they considered to be the linguistic aspect of their model.

Language Development

Language learning, according to the psycholinguist, is a form of induction. Children induce the relationship between their own resources and needs on the one hand and the integrated content, form, and use of the language in the environment on the other (Bloom & Lahey, 1978). The burden of acquisition is on the child's own system, which searches out structure in the language; therefore, the environment plays a limited role in acquisition. Some psycholinguists view the process as one in which raw data in the form of parents' speech feed into the child's language acquisition device. Others view the process as one in which the child actually "reaches out" to select those aspects of language from the environment that he or she needs in order to communicate. Therefore, children themselves develop language, using this exposure to speech as a trigger for the unfolding of the innate process. Structure is imposed on the input by the child, not derived from it.

Although the environment, in the form of teacher, is not considered as important as the child's own system, the order of acquisition of linguistic forms is related to the complexity of the linguistic input in terms of both its linguistic and cognitive structure as well as to the saliency of some forms over others. In other words, rather than considering language to be totally a result of biological unfolding of neural mechanisms as in the neurological theory, language is a function of the organism's linguistic mechanism's gradual decoding of the world of language events. Language rules are constructed by the knower's analysis of linguistic events. New language behaviors reflect self-regulated qualitative changes in the nature of internal abstract rules.

Language Disorders

If a child has language behaviors that are different from those of children his or her own chronological age, the child is said to have a language disorder. The problem arises because language-delayed children may be ill-equipped to discover linguistic rules. The focus is on the description of the language disorder itself not on the cause of the disorder.

Because etiology plays little or no role in the definition of language disorders in this theory, the disorders are not classified into causal categories. The classification of language disorders is based on behavioral differences, of content, form, and use in the language production of the child.

Language Assessment and Intervention

The object of assessment in linguistic theory is the description of linguistic behavior—the extent to which the child applies the rules of semantics, syntax, and pragmatics. The language that the child needs to learn is determined by comparing the child's language performance with that of normal guidelines, and not by judging adequacy related to underlying emotional, intellectual, or physiological factors. In other words (in order to understand disruptions of the system), the emphasis is on the description of what children do in language and what they have difficulty doing (Bloom & Lahey, 1978, p. 373). The major procedure used for determining deficiency is the analysis of a language sample. The language output is compared with normal developmental sequences

> *Quote 1–11*
> *Once the distribution of the forms in children's speech was observed and described in these earlier studies, it was possible to observe the semantic-syntactic meaning relation between the words . . . . Such distributional analyses were deeper semantic analysis in that they looked beyond the surface forms of the units that were combined. Using information from the children's behavior and the context, in addition to the words that were said, it was possible to make inferences about the underlying semantic-syntactic structure of their sentences.*
> (BLOOM & LAHEY, 1978, p. 46).

in language. Because the emphasis is on the analysis of language performance, the focus of intervention and assessment is on expressive
rather than receptive language.

Since, according to linguistic theory, language learning is primarily
a function of the child's own system, outside influences play a minimal
role in language change. The specialist can only facilitate induction. For
example, the specialist manipulates "the juxtaposition and proportional
frequency of exemplars, the perceptual saliency of key linguistic
elements, the clarity of meaning-in-context, and the match between the
focused-rule and the cognitive or linguistic resources of the child"
(Johnston, 1983, p. 54).

General Description

COGNITIVE ORGANIZATION THEORY

Although theories involving cognitive organization are not recent,
the application of such theories to language disorders emerged in
language-disorder literature during the 1970s. This theory (Kirk, 1983)
describes cognition as a constellation of perceptual, conceptual, affec-
tive, *and* linguistic elements among others; in other words, language is a
separate function but similar in structure to other cognitive attributes
and skills.

According to this theory the procedures and stages through which
language passes are basically the same as those of other cognitive tasks
and language is related to these tasks developmentally. A prominent
proponent of the cognitive organization viewpoint that considers
language as a separate but equal partner with other cognitive skills was
Piaget (1952, 1955; Piaget & Inhelder, 1958). He described the integral
relationship between language and other aspects of cognition in four
cumulative stages. He considered language as but one aspect of the
child's ability to represent and symbolize the world. The individual's
cognitive system is what permits him or her to construct internally what

---

Quote 1–12
. . . *Piaget has never been much concerned with individual differences among children. His interest, rather, has been in the
commonalities of development—in concepts that are mastered
by all children as they develop, precisely because such concepts
are necessary for any child's understanding of the world.*

*A fourth characteristic of the Piagetian approach is its emphasis
on the interrelation of different cognitive abilities . . . the continual
attempt is to specify the relations that hold across a range of
seemingly diverse tasks.*

(MILLER, 1982, pp. 163, 164).

is taken in from outside. Piaget proposed that the accomplishment of cognitive tasks such as object permanence, deferred imitation, cognitive awareness of time, space, action, and causality were basic to the development of language. Other theorists considered language to be built on these cognitive prerequisites (Sinclair-de Zwart, 1973).

Language and, consequently, language disorders were (and are) thought to be part of the cognitive function of mental representation. The acquisition of language takes place after considerable sensory-motor experiences have developed and the ability to symbolize has emerged. Sinclair-de Zwart (1969) said that language must be mapped onto the child's existing cognitive apparatus. She considered the psycholinguists (linguistic theory) to be preoccupied with the object of knowledge rather than with the "knower-symbolization-known" relationship.

Another aspect of this theory involves the identification of the role of cognitive factors in the "logic" of natural language—factors regarding the principles for organizing knowledge and procedural strategies for semantic interpretation (Fauconnier, 1985). Abstract cognitive organizational patterns are called *mental structures* by Piaget. Fauconnier (1985) uses the term *mental spaces* for domains used to consolidate certain kinds of cognitive information. Fauconnier's concept of mental spaces has been used to formulate a semantics for discourse (Dinsmore, 1987). These current theories add to the understanding of the relation between language and cognition.

Although the labels are similar, there are basic differences between information process theory and cognitive organization theory as interpreted in this book. Information process theory describes the pathway and events in the transmission of a verbal stimulus from its admission into the auditory system to understanding and from the initiation of an idea for communication to speech. It attempts to explain how deficits in the processing system can affect transmission. Cognitive organization theory describes the cognitive skills or knowledge (symbolization, induction, logic, inference) that are essential parts of the learning of any cognitive task, such as language reading, spelling, and so on. The theory considers these skills as developing in stages and similar for all cognitive learning.

In other words, the main issue on which the information process and cognitive organization theories differ with respect to language is the aspect of cognitive function that each describes. Cognitive organization theory describes learning language, whereas information process theory describes performing language. The focus in cognitive organization theory is the self-directed learning of the child and those higher level cognitive functions that permit this learning; in information process theory, the focus is on the internal transmission of verbal stimuli, the manner in which the listener converts the sounds into meaning by constructing an interpretation and then converts meaning into sound.

Language Development

The important development task in cognitive organization theory is learning to learn, which is comprised of three stages: (1) acquisition of complex relations (rules) and techniques of learning and skills for doing; (2) reorganization of the internal aspects of a system as new information is received (Piaget's accommodation); and (3) learning the approaches to problem solving (description, generalizing, inference, etc.) (Kirk, 1983). When the learner learns how to learn, efficient strategies are acquired and the store of available information is increased.

Essentially, learning cognitive tasks (including language) are based on the child's reorganization of internally represented data. New elements are admitted to the system unanalyzed and not understood— they form an internal data base that the child can analyze at his or her own rate. The child is not dependent on environmental influences but is sensitive to them. Although children follow the same general steps in their acquisition of cognitive tasks, the learning of the tasks may differ because each task makes different demands on the learner—what is learned is different. Mastery of one does not guarantee mastery of another. Skill is consolidated through practice; proficiency is marked by the shift to automaticity. The major responsibility in learning to learn is the child's.

Language Disorders

According to cognitive organization theory, difficulty in learning language is a cognitive problem related to difficulty in learning to learn. The basis of the disorder can be in any one of the common elements in learning to learn and can affect cognitive skills other than language. (Support for this position is argued from the multiple learning problems of many children with language disorders.) Recent research exploring the language-impaired child's level of functioning in nonlinguistic cognitive areas has continued to report cognitive deficits in these children (Camarata, Newhoff, & Rugg, 1981; Kamhi, 1981; Johnston & Weismer, 1983; Kamhi, Catts, Koenig & Lewis, 1984).

Classification of Disorders

This theory specifies that all language disorders are cognitive in nature. What appears to affect the development of language proficiency is the inadequacy of the child's own system to learn. Some disorders may relate to the store of information or data base (disorders of language

> *Quote 1–13*
> *This chapter brings together research findings that suggest that cognitive development, language development, learning to read and to spell can be viewed as instances of skill acquisiiton. Evidence is presented that cognitive development and the process of acquiring language skills involve problem-solving activity, the progressive reorganization of component parts of a task in terms of larger and larger working units, and the attainment of two kinds of knowledge: a growing understanding of complex relations and strategies for learning and doing.*
> (KIRK, 1983, p. 4).

knowledge), while others relate to the means of accessing the base and transmitting the knowledge (disorders of performance). The language deficiency therefore may affect the degree of competence that can be obtained and/or the manner in which the skill functions. Cognitive deficiency in other cognitive tasks may affect language and vice versa.

Miller (1981) considers both cognitive and language abilities, although independent, to be founded on common factors. Consequently, one of four conclusions can be made with respect to disorders:

1. Cognition (nonverbal) and language the same equals no disorder.
2. Language delayed in comparison with cognition equals language delay.
3. Language advanced over cognition equals efficiency of language experience.
4. Language atypical of cognition, gross asynchrony in one of linguistic processes, equals language disorder.

Language Assessment and Intervention

The evaluation of a child's problem includes assessing the knowledge the child has—a description of his or her cognitive and

> *Quote 1–14*
> *The more specific claim made in this study is that LI (language impaired) children have particular difficulty encoding information as opposed to storing and retrieving it. This difficulty can be attributed to the limited resources these children have in perceptual, attentional, and/or representational abilities for it is these abilities that determine how well information is encoded. Although it was not possible to rule out the possibility that other processing deficits affected LI children's performance, the data clearly indicated that these children do not encode information as well as normally developing children.*
> (NELSON, KAMHI, & APEL, 1987, p. 43).

language knowledge—and the strategies he or she uses in acquiring new cognitive information and language and the performance of the skill. It involves the evaluation of the language rules the child has discovered and the adequacy with which the rules are accessed and utilized.

The emphasis in intervention is threefold: increasing the child's quality and quantity of internal relations, improving the child's strategies of learning and discovering, and increasing the accuracy and speed of using the skill (e.g., language). Intervention involves making input available so that analysis and learning can take place. Input can be modified so that less complex and shorter units can be analyzed. Although the environmental stimuli are considered necessary, the emphasis in learning is placed on the organism.

PRAGMATIC THEORY

General Description

Pragmatic theory considers the basic function of language to be communication and its basic unit to be the speech act that occurs in context. The speech act includes the intention of the speaker and the desired effect on the listener. That which governs the adequacy of the speech act is the degree to which it communicates the intention of the speaker to the listener. Semantics and syntactics are derived ultimately from pragmatics (Bates, 1976a)—the manner in which they function in the speaker-listener dialogue determines their adequacy. The performance of a speech act is behavior governed by pragmatic rules and based on adequate semantic use.

An outgrowth of the emphasis on the development of communication skills has been the analysis of the language used in the interaction process. The analysis of grammatical use in terms of the demands dictated by the communicative function of the language (Liles, 1985) has taken two directions: (1) the analyses of single utterances affected by the specific context of the conversational turn-taking and (2) text analyses of groups of utterances and how meaning is maintained and organized across them (narrative, discourse, etc.).

Quote 1–15

The purpose of language is communication. The unit of human communication in language is the speech act, of the type called **illocutionary act***. The problem (or at least an important problem) of the theory of language is to describe how we get from the sounds to the illocutionary acts . . . . The rules enable us to get from the brute facts of the making of noises to the institutional facts of the performance of illocutionary acts of human communication.*

(SEARLE, 1975, p. 38).

Current pragmatic models characterize language in terms of communicative competence (Rice, 1986). The idea of competence implies behaviors judged within social and cultural systems as compared with the idea of language as mastery of structural forms. Although the interpersonal aspect of pragmatic theory is still the focus of the current interpretation of the theory, interpersonal communication is viewed within the broader perspective of the social and cultural milieus within which the communication takes place.

Muma (1986) emphasized another perspective of pragmatic theory that he labeled "functionalism." Viewed within the pragmatic interpretation of language, functionalism refers to intentions that are both the reason for and the product of language, that is, the intentions for communicating and the communication of intentions or content. Muma argued that the key to communicating intentions is the informativeness, not the form of the message.

Language Development

According to McLean and Snyder (1978), the child acquires language through interactions with the environment and from these interactions; these authors characterize the mutual reciprocity of the process as "transactional." The rules of interaction are developed as caretaker and child reciprocally vocalize in response to each other's vocalization—humans learn to speak in order to evoke a response (McLean & Snyder, 1978). In the interaction between caretakers and child, the caretakers are tuned to the linguistics needs of the child, and their speech to the child is characterized by features that are different from their speech to others (Berko-Gleason & Weintraub, 1978).

Pragmatic development is based on the child's acquisition of the semantic rules necessary to communicate an intent. The semantic rules, which involve the development of referential meaning, are established jointly through shared experiences. Thus, in pragmatic theory the environment is necessary for intention and motivation to be sustained.

> *Quote 1–16*
> . . . all of language is pragmatic to begin with. We choose our meanings to fit contexts and build our meanings onto those contexts in such a way that the two are inseparable, in the same way the "figure" is definable only in terms of "ground." According to this view, every act involved in the construction of meaning is itself a pragmatic act. The act of reference, the selection of lexical items to stand for one or more referents, and the combination of acts of reference into the core unit of semantics, the proposition, are all contextually based uses of language.
>
> (BATES, 1976b, p. 420).

From the viewpoint of functionalism (Muma, 1986), the realization of intentions constitutes the key motivation for acquiring language. Muma says that language learning begets language learning.

The environment helps in another way. It is the varying contexts, linguistic and environmental, within which structures are found that permit the language learner to abstract the rule governing that structure from other structures that are adjacent to it. The richer the environmental input, the more quickly can the abstraction process take place and the better defined are the rules of the structure.

Language Disorders

A language deficit in pragmatic theory is a breakdown in the complex transactional system that supports normal language (McLean & Snyder, 1978). The difficulty exhibits itself primarily in deficient knowledge of semantic rules which in turn cause a pragmatic problem which in turn causes a failure in social interaction (Lucas, 1980). The lack of appropriate responses on either the child's or the caretaker's part reduces expectations in both and therefore further reduces the child's purposive social language. Problems can occur in either the linguistic or supportive nonlinguistic aspects of communication. Because comprehension and expression are important to the communication exchange, both are important to the identification of a language disorder.

Language Assessment and Intervention

The major goal of assessment is to study the effectiveness of the child's interactions and success in using linguistic skills to manipulate his or her environment (Lucas, 1980). This is done through assessment of the child's semantic and pragmatic language in context—the manner in which he or she relates linguistic structures to a cognitive basis for social use (Lucas, 1980).

The goal of intervention is social communicative competence that includes linguistic and nonlinguistic behaviors. Since semantic learning

---

Quote 1–17

. . . the communicative system involves minimally two people interacting in both speaker and listener roles. The three components, the presuppositions about social and cognitive knowledge of the world, the linguistic rules (phonologic, syntactic, and semantic) and the pragmatic rules (linguistic and non-linguistic knowledge) represent the shared knowledge acquired in order to communicate.

(PRUTTING, 1982a, p. 130).

precedes pragmatic, the development of referential meaning is the first step in treatment. Reference is developed by focusing on concepts and lexicon in situations involving shared experiences between child and caretaker and among peers in a natural communicative setting. Social approval and successful communication is the natural reinforcer of adequate linguistic behavior. The communicative function is emphasized over that of form.

Since both comprehension and expression are an integral part of the speaker/listener dyad, both are included in the assessment and intervention processes.

CHRONOLOGY AND RECIPROCAL INFLUENCE OF THEORIES

The theories in this chapter have been presented in the general order of their emergence in the literature, but particularly the chronological order in which they impacted language disorders. I have hesitated to date each theory because it may imply to some readers that the theory is no longer used as a basis for practice with language-disordered children, and this is not true.

The following dates have been assigned to these theories in order to provide a perspective of the changes that have taken place in practice with language-disordered children and to show when the theories first influenced our work with these children (see McLean, 1983; Lund & Duchan, 1983, for historical notes):

1950	Neuropsychological
1960	Behavioristic
	Information Processing
1970	Linguistic (Semantic)
	Cognitive Organization
1980	Pragmatic

Although behaviorism preceded information processing from its theoretical position, the use of behaviorism in intervention with the language disordered followed information processing approaches.

Each of the six theories has its limitations for explaining language and its disorders. (These limitations will be described in Chapters 3 and 4). It is because of these limitations that the theories were partially rejected in favor of new ones that enriched the understanding about specific aspects of language. The new theories have influenced the older ones so that integration of ideas can be noted in definitions within each theory. However, not one of the theories encompasses the totality of language, a scope that is needed in work with the language disordered. A summary of the main positions of each theory relative to language development, disorders, assessment, and intervention is presented in Table 1–1.

TABLE 1–1.   SUMMARY OF SIX THEORIES OF LANGUAGE CLASSIFIED BY BASIC FOCUS, LANGUAGE DEVELOPMENT, LANGUAGE DISORDERS, ASSESSMENT, AND INTERVENTION

	NEUROPSYCHOLOGICAL THEORY	BEHAVIORAL THEORY	INFORMATION PROCESS THEORY
BASIC FOCUS	Language is derived from brain function. Specific language behaviors relate to specific areas of the brain.	Language is learned behavior resulting from antecedents and consequences of language behavior.	Language is described by a serial relation between input (sensation, perception, etc.), and output (encoding, imitation, etc.) processes.
LANGUAGE DEVELOPMENT	Language unfolds during the brain's maturational process.	The learners are taught language. It is trained and shaped by the environment.	Language develops as each component in the input and output serial process develops.
LANGUAGE DISORDERS	The degree and type of language impairment is related to the degree and type of brain dysfunction. Therefore, there are different kinds of language disorders.	The difference between the language behavior of a child and that of adult models constitutes a disorder. Variations in the nature, cause, and characteristics of disorders are irrelevant.	Deficits in the function of any of the processes in the sequence of decoding and encoding, impairs performance of subsequent processes. Different kinds of language disorders result and such differences are determined by comparison with age peers.
ASSESSMENT	The purpose of assessment is to describe and separate language deficits due to brain dysfunction from that due to other causes. This is termed *differential diagnosis*.	The purpose of assessment is to identify differences between what a child does and what he or she should be doing by adult standards.	Assessment involves the analysis of each process in the decoding and encoding sequence. Comparison is made between processes within the child and with other children by means of normative data.
INTERVENTION	Intervention is directed to the strengthening of or compensation for skills impaired in brain dysfunction by instruction using activities that require repetition.	Intervention uses a basic stimulus/ response/reinforcement paradigm to train behaviors that a child does not perform.	Intervention is directed to improve weak processes or compensate for them. Emphasis is placed on using child's learning style to instruct.

(Table 1-1 Continues)

TABLE 1–1.   SUMMARY OF SIX THEORIES OF LANGUAGE CLASSIFIED BY BASIC FOCUS, LANGUAGE DEVELOPMENT, LANGUAGE DISORDERS, ASSESSMENT, AND INTERVENTION *(Continued)*

	LINGUISTIC THEORY	COGNITIVE ORGANIZATION THEORY	PRAGMATIC THEORY
BASIC FOCUS	Language is a system of abstract rules from which an individual can generate an infinite number of utterances.	Language is one of many similar cognitive tasks that are instances of skill acquisition and are based on common cognitive knowledge and processes.	Language's primary function is communication, and its basic unit is the speech act that occurs in a context that helps to determine its form.
LANGUAGE DEVELOPMENT	Language rules are induced by a child whose own system controls the selection of rules and their internal construction. The process has universal characteristics.	The cognitive ability to learn rules and skilled behavior and to solve problems is responsible for the child's acquisition of language rules and his or her performance of language.	Language is acquired through interaction with the environment. The environment helps to shape the direction of acquisition.
LANGUAGE DISORDERS	Differences between a child and peers are judged on developmental indices. Problems are judged to be a result of a child's failure to induce rules. Cause of difference is not considered relevant to intervention.	Language deficits and related cognitive problems are a result of basic problems in the learning system. The impairment may be in the rule-learning area or in the area of performance and skill behavior.	Language disorders are a result of a breakdown in the interaction process in communication. This breakdown may be related to problems in the child's system or in the environment.
ASSESSMENT	Assessment involves detailed description of child's production of language structure by means of analysis of language samples and comparison with developmental data.	Assessment involves the evaluation of basic cognitive abilities (symbolic behavior, storage, retrieval, etc.) and the determination of their relation to the learning of cognitive skills, including language.	Assessment involves the description of the child's pragmatic skills observed in naturalistic settings.
INTERVENTION	Emphasis in intervention is on providing exemplars of target rules in a naturalistic setting and thereby facilitating rule induction.	Intervention is through teaching cognitive skills that may improve general learning. Modification of materials is provided to make rule induction easier and repetition is used for improving performance.	Intervention is provided in naturalistic settings for developing pragmatic skills. The environment is used to make target behaviors more salient.

2

COMPARISON OF THEORIES ON ISSUES IN DEVELOPMENT, ASSESSMENT, AND INTERVENTION

LANGUAGE DEVELOPMENT ISSUE

EXTERNAL VERSUS INTERNAL ASPECTS

CRITERIA FOR CLASSIFICATION OF LANGUAGE
DISORDERS

SEARCH FOR CAUSE IN ASSESSMENT

ORGANISM AND ENVIRONMENT IN ASSESSMENT
AND INTERVENTION

COMPREHENSION IN INTERVENTION

CONTENT OF INTERVENTION

REMEDIAL VERSUS DEVELOPMENTAL
INTERVENTION

STRUCTURED VERSUS NATURALISTIC
INTERVENTION

RULE DISCOVERY VERSUS PRACTICE IN
INTERVENTION

PROCESS VERSUS TASK IN INTERVENTION

ROLE OF THE LANGUAGE SPECIALIST IN
INTERVENTION

THEORETICAL OVERLAP

The specialist working with language-disordered children in the various clinical settings of the field is in the unenviable position of making decisions about assessment and intervention. This task can become difficult because there are many theories that seldom refer to applications from which to choose and because the instructional strategies referred to in the literature are usually not explicitly related to theory. Specialists might find that they are using techniques that are incompatible with each other or with the theory espoused. To further under-

THEORY, ASSESSMENT AND INTERVENTION
IN LANGUAGE DISORDERS: © 1988 by Grune & Stratton
AN INTEGRATIVE APPROACH

ISBN   0-8089-1918-0
All rights reserved.

stand the relationship between theories and assessment and intervention procedures, it may help to review the relationships between theory and specific issues on which assessment and intervention are based. This review covers issues presented in the previous chapter but uses a different organization. This chapter will look at issues such as content, environment, and comprehension and will explore how each of the six theories covered in Chapter 1 relates to each issue.

The use of illustrations to demonstrate the relationships among the theories with respect to the issues chosen does not imply a quantitative relationship that can be documented and measured. The figures illustrate the issue by a horizontal line with the two ends representing opposite positions along a continuum. The theories are then placed in relation to the positions they hold with respect to the issue, so the differences among the theories can be noted. With some variables, the theories may be explicit with respect to their position; with other issues a position is implied. In some cases, a theory makes no reference to the issue at all. In this latter situation, I have positioned the theory relative to the issue by induction from the theory's positions on related issues. The descriptions are to illustrate trends, not absolute classifications.

LANGUAGE DEVELOPMENT ISSUE

The explanation by a theory of the role that the environment plays in language acquisition as compared with the role that the organism plays influences the interpretation of the developmental process in language. At one end of the spectrum, in theories such as the neuropsychological and linguistic theories, the role of the child's organism is central; the child is viewed as having an executor integral to his or her system that receives, analyzes, stores, and organizes new elements and reorganizes the data that are already represented internally so that old and new data are combined. The acquisition of language is based on a child's activity. At the other end of the spectrum are theories such as the behavioral theory, in which the organism is passive. The environment bears the burden of responsibility in language learning. Illustration 1 shows the theoretical positions on language development by the degree of involvement of the organism and the environment in the *developmental* process.

ORGANISM	ORGANISM/ENVIRONMENT	ENVIRONMENT
NEUROPSYCHOLOGICAL		BEHAVIORAL
COGNITIVE ORGANIZATION	PRAGMATIC	
LINGUISTIC		
	INFORMATION PROCESS	

> *Quote 2–1*
> *My own suspicion is that a central part of what we call "learning" is actually better understood as the growth of cognitive structure along an internally directed course under the triggering and partially shaping effect of the environment.*
>
> *. . . much of our knowledge reflects our modes of cognition, and is therefore not limited to inductive generalization from experience, let alone any training that we may have received.*
> (CHOMSKY, 1980, pp. 33, 45).

From the organismic viewpoint, language development is viewed as an "unfolding" or emerging process that parallels the maturation of the brain. Lenneberg (1967) compared the emergence of language to that of other maturationally controlled behaviors that appear unrelated to special training procedures in the child's environment. The linguistic and cognitive organization positions resemble the neuropsychological position in that these theories consider the development of language to be primarily related to internal processes of the child as opposed to the effect of the environment; language is "acquired" by the child. The linguistic (nativist) position describes a unique process in which a child acquires language by using his or her *linguistic-specific* system by which the *rules of language* are induced and then stored and retrieved for the generation of language. The environment serves only as a trigger. Linguistic theorists describe the environmental role as a context with which a child actively interacts in acquisition of language rules of form, content, and use, but the context only provides a trigger to development—the environment does not shape it. Cognitive organization theory considers the acquisition of language to be similar to and to partake of strategies utilized by other cognitive behaviors; language acquisition is not considered to be a unique behavioral process.

The pragmatic and information process theories both consider the environment to be a critical factor in language development but in a different way. The information process theory describes a feedback mechanism by which the internal system sets up standards, evaluates, and judges performance. The feedback arises from others as well as self. The pragmatic theory has environment as its central factor in language

> *Quote 2–2*
> *The evidence is mounting that young children, in whatever culture, are spoken to in special ways, and that there are no cultures in which children learn language by mere exposure to it— by simply observing adults in discourse with one another, for instance.*
> (BERKO-GLEASON & WEINTRAUB, 1978, p. 214).

Quote 2–3
Language development is the result of the child's interaction with
the context—an active process whereby the relation between lin-
guistic categories (form) and non-linguistic categories (content
and use) are learned.
(BLOOM & LAHEY, 1978, p. 266).

development—the interaction between the speaker and a listener. It is the responses, reactions, and modifications of the listener that allow the language learner to "tune in" to the listener and guide him or her in identifying relevant structures and their corresponding rules; it is the association of the language structure with environmental events that help the language learner to discover the meanings of language, and it is the effect of delivering successful messages that serves to reinforce the use of specific forms as well as language in general.

Although some pragmatists describe the language learner's activity in selectively using the environmental context to "drive" the language process, similar to linguistic theory, this explanation of language development does not appear to derive directly from pragmatic theory as it does from linguistic theory. Linguistic theory's basic tenet is that the language learner learns a set of abstract rules. It can naturally follow that the learner simply induces these rules from exposure to many examples in the environment. The line from general theory to language acquisition is not so clear-cut in pragmatic theory. In the latter theory, the variable context—the environment—is an integral part of the process; perhaps the environment is thought to "teach" language. Evidence for the influence of the environment in pragmatic theory is provided by studies showing that the language of the caretaker has an effect on the language of the child (Bates, 1976a; 1977).

Behavioral theory places the larger portion of the burden in language development on the environment rather than on the organism. It views language as a behavior that is "trained" by the reinforcement of the environment to the child's response to an environmental stimulus. The responses are considered to be directly related to the stimuli.

Quote 2–4
This brings us to the problem of whether language behavior is
assumed to have been acquired by a process of learning or
whether it is viewed primarily as the result of an unfolding
process. If it is primarily the latter, then we must face every deficit
in language behavior as something built in by competence; on
the other hand, if we assume that language behavior is learned
and maintained through the variables of behavior theory, then we
are at least in a position to try to improve the behavior.
(SALZINGER, 1975, p. 186).

Different terms are used by the various theories to describe the developmental process of language. These terms clearly identify the position of the theories regarding this development. The terms are listed in Illustration 2.

TRAINED   TAUGHT/LEARNED   ACQUIRED   EMERGES/UNFOLDS

BEHAVIORAL   NEUROPSYCHOLOGICAL
        INFORMATION PROCESS
                PRAGMATIC   LINGUISTIC
                COGNITIVE ORGANIZATION

EXTERNAL VERSUS INTERNAL ASPECTS OF LANGUAGE

The six theories described here can be distributed with respect to whether they focus on external observable behavior or on internal "mentalist" behavior that is inferred by the external behavior. The behavioral theory clearly and explicitly excludes any process or condition of language that cannot be observed; the description of language is limited to the stimulus provided to an individual and the observable response of the individual. No attempt is made to determine what goes on in between. Linguistic theory is like behavioral theory in that it also focuses on behavior, but instead of concern with the input to the system, linguistic theory analyzes and describes utterances, surface structure, and production. Although language description by linguists includes a reference to content as well as to the induction process by which rules are learned, no attempt is made to describe or define the internal processes and strategies by which these take place.

Pragmatic theory is also primarily concerned with the external, social, and interactive processes needed for communication and with their linguistic counterparts. Comprehension plays a significant role in pragmatic theory because good communication requires accurate understanding of language as well as production. Revision processes are required in order to clarify messages and make sure they are understood. The notions of intention and purpose play a critical role in pragmatic theory, and both of these have internal connotations rather than external ones. However, there is no description or explanation of these internal processes.

The last three theories are primarily internal theories. Cognitive organization theory is concerned with learning and learning to learn and describes internal stages and sequences of development and acquisition of specific behaviors. Terms such as *problem-solving* and *rule acquisition* are viewed as essential steps to the process of learning a skill. The study of the cognitive organization of children is accomplished by observing and testing their behaviors. In this sense, cognitive organization theory is external. Information process theory, although having its origins in behavioral theory, does describe in its modified version the internal cognitive processes, stages, and modalities through which input is transmitted into the system and by which ideas are transmitted out of the system. Because information process theory does include the notions of input and response as well as feedback in its module, it can be said to be primarily internal but to have some external aspects. Neuropsychological theory is primarily internal but differs from the two cognitive theories in that the description is of anatomical and physiological conditions in the brain as opposed to descriptions of the cognitive functions of it (Illustration 3).

INTERNAL   **EXTERNAL**

NEUROPSYCHOLOGICAL   BEHAVIORAL
COGNITIVE ORGANIZATION   LINGUISTIC
INFORMATION PROCESS   PRAGMATIC

CRITERIA FOR CLASSIFICATION OF LANGUAGE DISORDERS

The basic criteria for making decisions regarding the presence or absence of a language disorder differ from theory to theory. The three major criteria are (1) differences in the child between language and other cognitive functions such as intelligence, (2) significant differences in the child's language functioning from the language functioning of other children within a specific environment, and (3) differences within the child with respect to the stages of mastery of other various linguistic abilities. To decide about disordered language by comparing a child's language functions with other cognitive functions within the child is compatible with the psychoneurological, information process, and cognitive organization theories because all of these theories integrate language and cognition. The implication in this approach is that all cognitive functions have a developmental timetable in relation to each other, and if one such as language is out of synchrony it indicates a specific disorder. These cognitive functions are seen to be related developmentally and, in some views, causally.

A decision of disordered language based on comparison with external criteria, age-related normative data in language is emphasized by the information process theory primarily. Standardized tests of language form the primary basis for classification.

Stage-related criteria and other developmental guideposts are used as a framework for disorder classification by pragmatic and linguistic theories. If a child's language stalls at a particular developmental stage in a sequence of stages or if the passage through the sequence is erratic, the child's language is considered to be different from normal and therefore disordered.

The behavioral theory considers any difference from mastery—the adult level of functioning—to be a difference that needs change in the direction of the adult model.

SEARCH FOR CAUSE IN ASSESSMENT

Historically, there has been disagreement regarding the need to identify the cause of a language disorder in assessment. The particular position held by a theory is related to the theory's view of the nature of language, its notion regarding the purpose of assessment, as well as the benefit of knowing the cause for management purposes.

Theories that describe language in terms of neuropsychological processes—the neuropsychological and the information process theories—have as one goal in assessment the discovery of the nature and cause of the disruption of language. In fact, the search for cause is one of the purposes of assessment insofar as this knowledge is purported to assist in understanding the child and his or her problems at the time of testing and in the future. If the nature of a disorder can be identified, its natural history can be predicted. The premise is that what may be the effects of the cause at one period of development may improve or disappear but what may be the effects at a later period need to be predicted and anticipated, and this can be best done by understanding the basic functioning of the child's cognitive system.

The neuropsychological theory considers the cause as the location of the brain dysfunction. The resulting effect on language is due to the role the particular part of the brain plays in normal language function. Knowledge of the cause assists in understanding problems that arise concurrently with those of language and that are related to the specific brain area that is impaired. This knowledge may also provide information as to what other areas can be used for compensatory purposes. The information process theory searches for cause because the transmission of language from input to expression is thought to occur in a serial fashion with each step serving as a prerequisite to subsequent steps. If the point of disruption of sequence can be found, the individual can be taught new routes or new methods of transmission.

The linguistic and behavioral theories consider the search for the cause of a language disorder to be irrelevant. These theorists suggest that what is done to change language behavior in intervention is the same regardless of cause and therefore there is no need to identify the cause. The child's disorder is described, its stage of development is pinpointed, and procedures are used to lead him or her through appropriate sequences in the ladder of development.

The cognitive organization and pragmatic theories do not explicitly refer to cause, but the cognitive organization theory would most probably resemble the neuropsychological and information process theories, describing language as it does in terms of stages of development of skills underlying specific cognitive tasks. One would assume that if any skill would not develop adequately, the subsequent skills and cognitive tasks dependent on these skills would be affected.

ORGANISM AND ENVIRONMENT IN ASSESSMENT AND INTERVENTION

Assessment and intervention are influenced by the theoretical position taken with respect to the child's role and the environment's role in language learning. Theories that describe language learning as resulting from *internal* activity on the part of the child—as being organic in nature—use an assessment approach that studies either the organism for evaluating the adequacy of the systems needed for learning (neuropsychological and cognitive organization) or the output of the system and makes inferences about the adequacy of the organism (linguistic). Intervention, according to these theories, does not use the environment as a primary instructional force; the clinician is viewed as a facilitator, one who "triggers" the system, who modifies environmental input so that less complex and shorter units can be analyzed by the child (the active learner), or who cues the analysis process by providing structures from which discoveries can be made easily.

The environmental position of the behaviorist considers *external* factors, the person(s) involved in a training function, to be the center of the language-learning process and the assessment/intervention process. The role of the environment (trainer) is not only as stimulator *par excellance* but as reinforcer of the child's (the passive learner) response. In fact, the reinforcement is seen as the significant element in bringing about change. The reinforcement role of the environment is also important in the pragmatic theory, but the type of reinforcement differs from that of behaviorism. In pragmatic theory, the reinforcement occurs naturally as a result of the effective linguistic communication that takes place in social interaction.

COMPREHENSION IN INTERVENTION

The choice of content with respect to expressive and receptive language is also influenced by theory. The behavioral and linguistic theories are both concerned primarily with production, whereas the pragmatic and information process theories are concerned with both input and output. The behavioral theory ignores comprehension, considering it to be unobservable and therefore unknowable. The linguistic theory does not consider comprehension to be a prerequisite of production and therefore not of highest priority in intervention.

The pragmatic and information process theories differ from each other in that the pragmatic theory focuses on comprehension and expression within a context of social interaction and the information process theory on the internal processes related to reception and expression. According to information process theory, comprehension precedes production developmentally and must also precede it in intervention. Production of forms is dependent on the comprehension of these same forms. In information process theory, the inclusion of comprehension in assessment and intervention is related to the role that comprehension development is considered to play in the development of expression. Theories that consider comprehension to predate expression include receptive language procedures in assessment and intervention (Illustration 4).

COMPREHENSION COMPREHENSION/PRODUCTION PRODUCTION
(RECEPTIVE)   (EXPRESSIVE)

COGNITIVE ORGANIZATION   BEHAVIORAL
            NEUROPSYCHOLOGICAL   LINGUISTIC
            INFORMATION PROCESS
            PRAGMATIC

Neuropsychological theory is also concerned with comprehension and expression, particularly as these relate to specific areas of the brain associated with these aspects of language. In neuropsychological theory the relationship between comprehension and expression disorders is not viewed necessarily as one of dependency but in terms of specific syndromes associated with injury to specific areas of the brain—either problem can occur in isolation from the other. Cognitive organization theory, being concerned with strategies, problem-solving, and other internal functions, leans more toward concern with understanding than with production.

It is interesting to note that although the behavioral and linguistic theories are similar in that both focus on the production aspect of language, they differ completely in what they suggest in the intervention process because of a difference in their view of language learning or acquisition and the role of the environment.

CONTENT OF INTERVENTION

The theory of language that the specialist accepts as valid influences the *content* areas or *components* of language that he or she evaluates in assessment and modifies in intervention. The components range from central cognitive aspects of language (inference, problem-solving) that are related to meaning to aspects dealing with the most peripheral surface structures such as phonology. Because behavior theory is concerned only with performance adequacy, the major focus of the theory is on phonology and syntax. At the other end of the scale is the cognitive organization theory, which is concerned with underlying conceptional development, relations, and the development of cognitive strategies. The other theories fall somewhere in between. Table 2–1 illustrates the major foci of the various theories. The types of skills or content included under the six component categories are as follows:

1. Concepts and cognitive strategies: problem-solving, propositionalizing, inference, rule-development, reconstruction of internal schemas to handle new information.
2. Processing skills: performance strategies, storage, access, retrieval, reproduction accuracy, automaticity.
3. Pragmatic behaviors: situations, intentions, transactions, context, messages.
4. Semantic knowledge: reference, association, connotation, case relations, meaning, cohesion.
5. Syntax use: modulations, refinement, sequence, grammatical rules, alternatives.
6. Phonological accuracy: articulation, phonemic sequencing.

Because each theory considers language as having specific components, it is these components that are addressed by the specialist who adheres to theory in clinical management. For example, according to linguistic theory, the specialist analyzes language production by means of a language sample; the sample provides information about the child's language form, content, and use. Using pragmatic theory as a base, the specialist observes within different contexts the language interaction of the child and the adequacy of his or her ability to express intentions, to maintain topics, and to take turns, as well as the effective and appro-

TABLE 2-1.   CONTENT OF INTERVENTION BY THEORY

THEORY	LANGUAGE COMPONENTS					
	I CONCEPTS/ COGNITIVE STRATEGIES	II PROCESSING SKILLS: PERCEPTION MEMORY, ETC.	III PRAGMATIC BEHAVIOR	IV SEMANTIC KNOWLEDGE	V SYNTAX/ MORPHOLOGY USE	VI PHONOLOGICAL ACCURACY
Behavioral					X	X
Neuropsychological		X		X	X	
Linguistic			X	X	X	X
Pragmatic			X	X	X	
Information Process		X		X	X	
Cognitive Organization	X	X		X		

priate use of forms for communicating. The cognitive organization theory guides the observer to evaluate general cognitive development, concepts, knowledge, method and rate of acquisition of new information, general rule behavior, and the language aspects of these. Thus, each theory leads the specialists into different content areas of intervention and assessment.

Theory dictates not only the content selected for assessment and intervention but also the order of importance of the content areas. The information process theory specifies that adequacy of perception and memory are essential to language so intervention should be directed to disorders of these processes prior to linguistic production. The cognitive organization theory stresses the cognitive bases of symbolization, representation, and concept formation as a foundation for language and so these should be taught prior to the linguistic forms that build on them. The *function* of language receives primary emphasis by the pragmatic theorist—the fact of communication is stressed over the form.

REMEDIAL VERSUS DEVELOPMENTAL INTERVENTION

The basic approach to intervention selected by a language specialist is primarily a function of theory. Such an approach provides the plan of where to start and in what sequence to move. The factor of content selection has already been discussed. Once content is selected, where does the specialist begin? Does he or she begin at a development level of language that precedes and undergirds the areas of deficiency and proceed in a natural language sequence, or does the specialist move right into the error level and remediate it regardless of developmental factors? Different theories have different approaches (Illustration 5).

REMEDIAL	REMEDIAL/DEVELOPMENTAL	DEVELOPMENTAL
BEHAVIORAL		LINGUISTIC
NEUROPSYCHOLOGICAL		PRAGMATIC
	COGNITIVE ORGANIZATION	
	INFORMATION PROCESS	

Gray and Ryan (1973) whose writings classify them in the behaviorial school, state ". . . the fact that language training is sought for children and the fact that the teaching of language has become such a social priority confirms the view that the developmental philosophy has been found wanting" (pp. 4–5). The opposite view (Bloom & Lahey, 1978) proposes that what happens at any point in development influences subsequent development and such dependencies cannot be ignored in progressing from one stage to another in language.

On one end of the spectrum, we find the behavioral and neuropsychological theories, which are concerned with retraining the behaviors that are disordered. Because the neuropsychological theory views disorders as they relate to malfunction of specific areas of the brain—distinguishing areas of comprehension versus expression, syntax versus semantics, speaking versus reading—a developmental approach would not logically follow.

According to Guess, Sailor, and Baer (1978), remedial logic supposes that older children who did not acquire specific language skills when they were young no longer possess the general abilities and deficits of young normal-language children and therefore are not suited to a developmental approach. The remedial approach, which is often associated with behaviorism, selects grammatical structures on the basis of environmental usefulness such as those that will enhance the child's control of environment. The remedial approach according to Guess et al. (1978) is particularly effective for the child with limited language.

Both linguistic and pragmatic theories, being concerned with the developmental aspect of the language and interactional behaviors observed in children, conclude that if normal children develop language in a specific order, the language-disordered child should follow that sequence in intervention.

Psycholinguists (Bloom & Lahey, 1978) believe that the universal built-in system of priorities in both conceptual and linguistic development indicates that there are factors that are responsible for sequential development and a resulting developmental dependency relationship among cognitive and linguistic tasks. They suggest that sequential dependencies in progressing from one language stage to another cannot be ignored.

STRUCTURED VERSUS NATURALISTIC INTERVENTION

The amount of structure that is used in intervention is related to theory. In a way, the degree of structure is related to the focus of intervention. Some theories place the focus of intervention on the clinician and the methods and techniques used by the clinician to teach the child language. These theories are the most structured. Other theories place the focus on the child—his or her style of learning, the strategies used by the child in solving the problem of language learning, the social interaction needed for the child to acquire and learn language. These theories have a moderate structure.

Intervention in a behavioristic setting is the most highly structured. In fact, structure defines behaviorism, specifying every element and every action in the environment. Behaviorism is predominantly clinician-centered. By nature of its focus in social interaction, pragmatic theory, a child-centered theory, requires the most naturalistic and informal environment. For children to learn the social use of language, learning must take place in a social setting. Linguistic theory, a language-centered theory, also requires some degree of informality. Since its basic tenet is the induction of language rules by the child, an environment with many exemplars of target rules is necessary for the induction to take place. The other two theories are somewhere in between, the degree of structure not necessarily derived from the theory.

Highly structured intervention is better accomplished in an individual setting, whereas informal, less structured intervention profits from a group setting in order to accomplish its goals.

RULE DISCOVERY VERSUS PRACTICE IN INTERVENTION

Approaches to intervention also differ in the strategies that are used to assist the child in mastering a specific linguistic task. Theories that consider language to be the acquiring of the knowledge of abstract rules (linguistic) will concentrate on that aspect of instruction, that is, they will assist the children to induce rules from examples of rule application. Theories that consider language either partially or completely as performance of skilled behavior (as in the use of strategies for accessing knowledge or for making language automatic) will include practice and drill in instruction. Illustation 6 shows how the theories may be grouped on the basis of strategies used in instruction.

PRACTICE	PRACTICE/RULE DISCOVERY	RULE DISCOVERY
BEHAVIORAL		LINGUISTIC
INFORMATION PROCESS	PRAGMATIC	
NEUROPSYCHOLOGICAL		
COGNITIVE ORGANIZATION		

Those theories that accommodate both rule knowledge and performance in language (cognitive organization) will have both rule discovery and practice as an integral part of intervention, the choice between these depending on a child's specific problem.

PROCESS VERSUS TASK IN INTERVENTION

An area of intervention related to the remedial/developmental issue is the one of process versus task. Process intervention refers to the selection of and intervention with cognitive processing skills that are considered to be basic to the development of specific language skills (information process and cognitive organization theories). Task intervention refers to the selection of a linguistic behavior (along a language developmental scale or not) that is different from normal and uses this behavior as a target to be mastered (behavioristic, linguistic). A possible grouping of theories on this basis is shown in Illustration 7.

PROCESS	PROCESS/TASK	TASK
INFORMATION PROCESS		BEHAVIORAL
COGNITIVE ORGANIZATION		LINGUISTIC
NEUROPSYCHOLOGICAL	PRAGMATIC	

The implication in process intervention is that there will be generalization from general learning process skills—problem-solving, inference—to a specific behavior and then to all types of similar cognitive behaviors. Clinical experience shows that the processes selected must be made applicable to important tasks in the child's environment for such an approach to be effective.

It should be noted that the behavior and linguistic theories use task orientation, even though they differ with respect to the remedial versus developmental approach, and with respect to the role of the organism in language acquisition. Both theories stress work with language production behavior.

ROLE OF THE LANGUAGE SPECIALIST IN INTERVENTION

Although the role of the language specialist varies depending on the type of problem, setting, and other factors, it is useful to distinguish the two extremes in intervention approach, that of direct teaching and that of facilitation. (This issue is discussed more comprehensively in Chapter 5.)

Direct teaching (Cole & Dale, 1986) is described as a structured planned instructional approach that uses primarily questions or imitation to elicit responses that are reinforced according to a specified schedule. The content is sequenced by ease of instruction, and the child is a passive participant.

Facilitation can be paired with what Cole and Dale (1986) call *interactive instruction* (although the two do not always go hand in hand). These require the specialist to use less structure both in context and procedures. The goals are to encourage the child to utilize his or her own system to induce the linguistic rules. The child's response to a specific target is usually delayed since it takes time to incorporate the new learning into existing constructs. The child is an active participant in the process. At the directed teaching extreme of the continuum is behaviorism and at the other extreme is linguistic theory (Illustration 8).

	INTERACTIVE	
DIRECTED TEACHING	**INSTRUCTION**	**FACILITATION**

BEHAVIORAL PROCESS   LINGUISTIC
   PSYCHONEUROLOGICAL   PRAGMATIC
      INFORMATION PROCESS   COGNITIVE ORGANIZATION

**THEORETICAL
OVERLAP**

In comparing theories on specific issues, it becomes apparent that there is considerable crossover among theories. This is an important realization for it states that different theories are rarely totally incompatible. The fact of overlap must be viewed, however, in terms of the rationale that explains specific positions. The application of two theories may be the same, but the reason for arriving at particular positions may be entirely different. The specialist who bases assessment and intervention practices on theory should understand the logic by which specific practices are evolved from the theory.

3

LANGUAGE THEORIES AND ASSESSMENT APPROACHES

NEUROPSYCHOLOGICAL THEORY
    Contributions
    Limitations

BEHAVIORAL THEORY
    Contributions
    Limitations

INFORMATION PROCESS THEORY
    Contributions
    Limitations

LINGUISTIC THEORY
    Contributions
    Limitations

COGNITIVE ORGANIZATION THEORY
    Contributions
    Limitations

PRAGMATIC THEORY
    Contributions
    Limitations

SIX THEORIES AND ASSESSMENT

The six theories described in Chapter 1 were presented in a chronological order based on the period when the theory had the greatest impact on the field of language disorders. A chronological presentation allows the specialist to view assessment historically, to recognize the contributions of each theory to the management process, and to understand the limitations that led to the evolution of subsequent approaches. Aspects of each of the six theoretical approaches to assessment can be found in current literature as well as in current practice, so in one sense the treatment of each theory has as much relevance today as it did in the past. The theory-based procedures that contributed to an understanding of language disorders were never discarded, at least by some specialists in the field. If assessment procedures are evaluated not so much on theory currency but on the basis of the contribution of

THEORY, ASSESSMENT AND INTERVENTION
IN LANGUAGE DISORDERS: © 1988 by Grune & Stratton
AN INTEGRATIVE APPROACH

ISBN 0-8089-1918-0

specific assessment concepts to the assessment process, specialists in language disorders will experience less confusion and contradiction in management practices.

This chapter will review each of the six theories described in the first chapter on the basis of their contributions to the language disorder assessment process as well as on the basis of their limitations to that process.

NEUROPSYCHOLOGICAL THEORY

One of the first approaches to assessment was differential diagnosis or categorical assessment. At the time of its prominence, it was considered to be a neuropsychological process. Assessment, according to this theory, is a process by which the major categories of disorders associated with language delay are differentiated on the basis of symptomatology. In the beginnings of differential diagnosis, the major categories were considered to be hearing loss, emotional disturbance, mental retardation, and aphasia. Recent categories include verbal auditory agnosia, autism, a predominantly expressive syndrome, and a semantic-pragmatic syndrome (Rapin & Allen, 1983).

The method of study of children in neuropsychological theory is by observing and describing a wide variety of behaviors—cognitive, motor, linguistic, visual, and auditory—and relating the findings to brain pathology. The study of both comprehension and expression is an integral part of the assessment, since the difference between them is neurologically indicated and performance difference in these processes is one of the main ways in which the categories of language disorders are differentiated. The assessment of intellectual functioning was an important part of the categorization process in the early days of the theory.

The major assumption in categorical assessment is that it is important from the standpoint of intervention to understand the reason why a child's language is delayed. Different kinds of disorders are associated with different kinds of language learning problems, and so the approach to intervention—group versus individual, direct versus indirect, cognitive versus linguistic—is dependent on the nature of the language delay and other problems associated with disorders of the various categories. According to this approach, the category in which a child is placed also influences the goals of intervention because certain types of disorders, such as autism, may not have the same probability for improvement as others. Such information is important to the specialist who needs to plan the length of intervention periods both within a session and over the entire treatment period. This approach considers treatment in areas related to language to be an important part of overall intervention and the role of the language specialist to be that of obtaining from assessment procedures an understanding of the total problem and of making referral for other services. Such activities are possible only if the nature and category of disorder can be identified by the language specialist.

Contributions

This approach to language disorders and the corresponding approach to assessment have provided the field of language disorders with an understanding of different categories of disorders. With information regarding the relationship between causes of language deficits and resulting language and nonlanguage symptoms, a description of and differentiation among the major categories of problems is possible. This analysis has led to a greater understanding of the relation between language and the brain, and between language and other cognitive behaviors. The approach draws attention to the complexity of children's language problems and to the variety of factors within the child that will influence placement, prognosis for language improvement, related intellectual problems, and so on. It helps the child and his or her parents to face realistically possible future problems related to a disorder.

Limitations

The major criticism of the categorical diagnosis approach has been that the emphasis on cause has made the search for the category in which to place a child the primary focus of assessment, to the neglect of the description of the language problem itself. Without such a description of language, planning for intervention is difficult at best.

Practices in assessment, using this approach, may lead to labeling children, even though the label may have no functional value for a child. Once a label is given, there is little likelihood that it will be reversed. Such labeling also obscures the differences between children within categories and the possibility that some children may have more than one problem.

Because categorical diagnosis requires evaluation of such a wide variety of abilities, specialists, working alone, may attempt to measure all the areas. This may result in uneven measurement—some objective and some subjective—for the various abilities and the use of selected procedures in fields for which the specialist has no preparation such as neurology or psychology.

Lastly, the categorical assessment approach does not evaluate the role of the environment in the child's disorder. Focus on a basic neuropsychological cause leads the examiner to observe *behaviors* that correspond to identified categories without concern for the manner in which the environment may have exacerbated the problem or helped to compensate for it.

Behavioral theory dictates what should and should not be evaluated in language assessment (Gray & Ryan, 1973). Because behavioral theory emphasizes that the teaching activity with language-disordered children be focused on expressive language (the product) only, there is no need for the examiner to study auditory or visual processing skills, cognition, or even the comprehension of language. Language comprehension is in the black box, therefore unknowable, therefore unteachable. Furthermore, according to this theory, there is no need for the examiner to determine the cause of the disorder because the language training that will be used is the same regardless of cause. The child is taught to do what he or she cannot do. The two basic questions the examiner asks are "What and how *is* the child speaking?" and "What and how *should* the child be speaking?"

The evaluator will need to have some understanding of language structure because there is a need to determine the areas where there is difference between what the child does and what he or she should be doing. However, the use of developmental stages in language is not essential to the assessment of the problem according to behavior theory, because the deficit area will be remediated regardless of what language structure precedes or follows it.

Instead of using standardized instruments for evaluation, the behaviorist prefers the use of criterion tests. These tests describe performance skills that experts believe children should have mastered at specific levels of development. The skills are presented in terms of task-oriented instructional objectives that are operationally defined. It is assumed that the items and their sequence on the criterion test are based on valid data or theory. The point at which the child performs successfully is termed the *baseline*, below which are the behaviors that a child has, and above which are those the child does not have.

Because reinforcement is an integral part of behavioral theory, it is important in the assessment of children with language disorders to determine what types of reinforcers will be effective with each child and the approximate schedule of reinforcement that will be needed.

Contributions

The primary contribution of behavioral theory to language disorder is in the area of intervention rather than assessment. However, the necessity of keeping careful and detailed records of those behaviors that a child can and cannot accomplish helps the specialist develop skills in observing and describing behaviors, particularly what the child does rather than what he or she can do. The practice of obtaining baseline behaviors during the assessment procedures has made it easier to record and evaluate change during subsequent intervention periods.

Limitations

Using the behavioral approach to assessment, the specialist ignores important aspects of language such as semantics, comprehension, and pragmatics. Meaning and comprehension are ignored because they cannot be observed, therefore they cannot be changed, and therefore they are not the subject for assessment. Evaluation of pragmatic behavior is also not part of the assessment procedure because it requires analysis of the environmental interaction between a speaker and listener. Although behaviorism considers the environment to play an important role in language, the role is a very specific one governed by defined requirements in stimulus and response behaviors. In other words, the emphasis is on form over content and use. In fact, the very essence of behavior theory is on behavioral change. Therefore, it is specifically directed to intervention rather than assessment. Learning about anything other than the actual language difference of the child is irrelevant.

INFORMATION PROCESS THEORY

Using the information process models described in Chapter 2 (Wepman et al., 1960; Osgood & Miron, 1963), specialists describe the language process in terms of input and output processes, auditory, visual, and tactile modalities, and reflex, perceptual, and representational levels. Assessment involves the measurement of the language-disordered child's functioning at each of the processes, modalities, and levels (Carrow, 1972).

The evaluation of many language-disordered children over a period of years has indicated that such children seldom perform equally well in all of the processing skills. According to information process theory, the concept of intra-child variability—the differences within children in the performance on various tasks, modalities, and processes—is considered as important as the difference between a child and his or her peers. The variability within children illustrates that seldom does a disorder in language occur "across the board" in all language tasks and that although a language-disordered child may display many areas of weakness, he or she may also have areas of language strength. According to

> *Quote 3–1*
> The input-integration-output construct can be used in many ways for both assessment and instruction. At the level of input, one attempts to determine what types of information the child can process via each sensory system. At the level of integration, the emphasis is on the study of meaning; at the level of output, efforts are made to determine which modes of response are available to the child.
>
> (JOHNSON, 1981, p. 19).

this theoretical position, information about the strengths and weaknesses (the profile) of the language-disordered child helps in planning the intervention program.

This theory clearly separates the input (receptive) functions of language from the output. The common bond between the two processes, as between auditory comprehension and expression, is at two levels, that of perceptual motor and that of meaning—the representational or integrational level. The stages that lead to comprehension, from the point where sequences of speech sounds are received to the point where these sounds are understood, differ from the stages that lead to expression, from the idea to the production of it. Although in essence comprehension and expression deal with the same knowledge, their performance may differ, dependent as they are on other accessing, storage, and processing devices. The focus on knowledge *and performance* leads to the possibility that comprehension and expression of language can be equally impaired since both have the same knowledge base—or unequally impaired with performance problems in one but not the other.

The role of cognitive processes such as memory and perception is important in the information process theory; the processes serve as a basis for the development of language skills. The role of the environment in the language processing cycle is by means of feedback, indicating the adequacy of the output. Assessment strategies include the measurement of all the processes that may relate to language and the

> *Quote 3–2*
> For some investigators, the main goal of speech and language assessment is to determine the child's level of performance and to compare it with norms on various tasks related to language. Others are more interested in studying, in a developmental sequence, the processes underlying language; their goal is to discover areas of ability and disability in each child and to relate the amount of disability at lower levels to those at higher more complex levels. If the former approach is taken exclusively, the examiner can employ only those measures for which norms have been established. This limits the areas of language that can be assessed and results in a collection of data having little internal relationship.
>
> (CARROW, 1972, p. 53).

attempt to integrate the findings in a way that will show this relationship in a specific child. In other words, the language assessment conclusion will, in addition to identifying the problem and its significance, describe the nature of the problem by a logic that traces the threads of disorder throughout the processing system.

During the period when the information process theory was popular, there was dissatisfaction with the subjective observations used in differential diagnosis. This dissatisfaction, along with interest in identifying specific processing skills used in language, led some specialists in the field to adopt a specific process analysis approach using standardized measures in the evaluation of language. Because norms were obtained for many of the processing tasks measured in assessment, this led to the development of standardized instruments for language akin to those used in measuring intelligence. Many of these tests are still in use.

Contributions

The major contributions of information process theory have been in the area of assessment rather than intervention. The task analysis approach used in information process theory highlights the interrelationship and dependencies that are said to exist among the various components of language—auditory perception, auditory memory, auditory comprehension, and others. Because of this position, researchers and other specialists have attempted to identify this interrelationship and, as a result, have provided the field with descriptions of different kinds of processing deficits that occur along with disordered language.

Insight is provided by the information process theory by its treatment of disorders not as a disease that individuals are born with, but as deficits within a constellation of skills, each of which exists along a continuum. In disordered language, some skills may be accelerated in comparison with others. The latter may be out of synchrony with the accelerated skills within the child and with those same skills in the child's age peers. This view that language behavior is made up of a variety of skills each of which has its own continuum, places the burden of judgment of disorder on the specialist who bases the decision on the degree of difference of the child's behavior from that of the special language environment in which the child lives and on the degree of difference of some skills from others within the child, particularly those that are related to general developmental and intellectual levels.

The establishment of a relationship among the various processes of language may assist in the early identification of language and learning disorders in children. It may be difficult, when assessing children prior to normal age of language onset, to identify those who will have a disorder of language. It is also difficult to identify preschool children who may later exhibit learning disabilities when they begin school. Early measurement of perceptual functions frequently provides a means of this identification. The frequent association between language/learning disorders and perceptual problems assists us in deciding that if the former occurs in a child, there is strong probability that the latter will also occur.

Information process theory implies that an understanding of the child's processing deficits is a help in understanding the child's best avenue for learning in general. This implication does not necessarily mean that the child's deficit can be changed (a view held by some theorists), but it does mean that the specialist, knowing the processing limitations of the child, can adapt the input in instruction and intervention to a level that the child can handle. A child should know his or her own learning strengths so as to use these strengths in study. Understanding the processing deficits could also help the specialist predict and prepare for the learning problems that might arise through the course of the child's language and academic life. A child might begin with a speech problem, then a language disorder becomes apparent, and later, when in school, the child has difficulty in reading, and so on. The specialist is responsible for recognizing that all of these problems may surface at some later period.

The use of standardized measures common in information process theory is a means of introducing objectivity into the assessment procedures. These tests help in preventing false conclusions in children whose language differences are not of a sufficient degree to be labeled language disorder. They also provide a place to begin in informal assessment by sampling from a wide variety of tasks. In other words, they assist in determining the broad nature of the problem, the significance or seriousness of the disorder, and in identifying assessment areas that need specific analysis.

Limitations

Information on the strengths and weaknesses in processing skills can be misapplied by the specialist if processing skills are used as the content in an intervention program. Even if processing skills can be improved, such improvement has been found to have limited effect on the child's learning of language or academic tasks. At the school level, there appears to be difficulty in matching test results in the processing skills to the curriculum.

The strong focus on standardized measurement of a child's processing skills that is part of the information processing theory leads, if used exclusive of other approaches, to inadequate and irrelevant assessment

> *Quote 3–3*
> *I challenge the emphasis or exclusive use of picture pointing, elicited imitation, and similar formats to evaluate language comprehension and production . . . . Speech-language clinicians must evaluate a child's communicative competence. To make this evaluation, we need to examine the types of stimulus presented to children in the classroom, on the playground, and in the home, and types of response that are required.*
> (LASKY, 1983, p. 47).

conclusions. The inadequacy arises when tests only are used, because such instruments tap a limited number of areas that need to be evaluated and do so in an artificial way. The implication is that the only abilities that need to be tested are those that these tests sample. What happens to those behaviors for which there is no test instrument? The use of one or two tests in assessment does not exhaust the possibilities of measuring the domains under study. Behavior is complex and dynamic and needs to be observed in various modes under varying conditions. If assessment is to look at strengths and weaknesses, the evaluator must study all relevant areas.

A second limitation in using tests only in assessment is the narrowness of scope in each instrument. An instrument for measuring semantics, for example, will have items that measure a broad range of semantic skills but will in no way be representative of all semantic skills in the language, much less of other aspects of language. Measurement by test will yield quantative rather than qualitative data; both are needed for adequate evaluation. Just as objectivity cannot be sacrificed for naturalistic data, neither can relevance be sacrificed for objectivity.

Lastly, the burden of collecting information on a broad range of cognitive functions may cause a specialist to neglect the in-depth study of language itself. Without the information that is obtained from the analysis of a child's productive language, the planning and execution of a good diagnostic program will be limited.

LINGUISTIC THEORY

The basic thrust of linguistic theory is that the language system is independent and different from other cognitive systems. As such, it emerges and operates according to principles that are universal and unique to that system, which in turn make the emergence of the linguistic components of language predictable and orderly. The assessment of language, according to this theory, therefore, does not need to include study of cognitive skills in isolation. These skills are studied only by observing how meaning and use interact within the child's productive system. Those aspects of cognition (meaning) and pragmatics (use) that

> *Quote 3–4*
> There are several principles of language sampling which are found in the literature and in the tradition of those who are doing language sample analysis to get a good, easy-to-analyze language sample . . .
>
> Better samples are obtained when the child is relaxed and interested in a familiar environment with a familiar interactant.
>
> There should be a long enough sample collected to include several occurrences of the behaviors which comprise the domain for the analysis.
>
> (LUND & DUCHAN, 1983, pp. 18, 19).

interact with expression (form) are considered to be *part* of the unique and distinct linguistic module of the system and not *external* to it.

According to this theory, because of the biologically determined nature of language emergence, language "happens" in stages that are basically orderly, regular, and predictable. The major task in assessing language is that of describing in detail the orderly progression of all aspects of language—the phonemic, morphemic, syntactic, semantic, and pragmatic—and the observable variables that modify this progression. The language aspects are studied by analysis of the language expression or output of the individual directly. The adequacy of the semantic and pragmatic aspects are inferred from the quality of the linguistic data from which the relation between form, meaning, and use can be observed. Assessment in language disorders therefore is directed exclusively to the analysis of language production data usually obtained by means of sampling. Because normal language stages are described from naturalistic data, information on the language-disordered child is obtained and analyzed in a similar fashion so that proper comparisons can be made.

Linguistic theory focuses on the rule-aspect of language, the operational knowledge from which the surface structure is generated. (Although Chomsky's original description of language differentiated between competence and performance, many subsequent linguists feel this distinction is artificial [Bever, 1970; Bloom & Lahey, 1978]). Because of the emphasis on rule behavior, assessment in language disorders functions on the basis that the observed differences in performance of specific children are related to problems in rule development. In other words, there is no differentiation between the knowledge of the rules and the performance of the language, therefore there are no performance problems to be differentiated from rule-based problems. The assessment goal is to search out and define those rules that have not been internalized by the child by analyzing the child's production. Linguistic theory is not concerned as to why the rules have not been induced by the child, but simply, as judged from the corpus of language

> *Quote 3–5*
>
> *It now seems safe to say that the examination of the semantic relations reflected in the early word combinations of language-disordered children has become common clinical practice.*
>
> *The relevant-component approach requires the construction of highly individualized probes designed to systematically examine potential patterns gleaned from relatively small samples of a child's speech. The use of clinician-constructed probes may be increasing as a result of the emphasis on nonstandardized assessment in recent literature.*
>
> (LEONARD, STECKOL, & PANTHER, 1983, pp. 25, 34).

taken from the child, which rules are apparently not in the child's rule system. (This aspect of the theory is reminiscent of behavioral theory.)

Movement away from a purely syntactic analysis of language in linguistic theory was led by Bloom in 1970. The influence of Bloom's semantic relations theory on the assessment of language in context has been significant. Her proposal that a child's meaning is not always clear from the study of surface structure only and that two- and three-word combinations can signal many different grammatical meanings when used in different contexts has led to the evaluation of the content of word combinations as children use them in actual situations. Following on Bloom's original description of semantic relations, Brown (1973) described the order of emergence of specific semantic relations in children's language. Brown's classification of early word combinations led language specialists to "fit" child language data into static semantic categories. Leonard, Steckol, and Panther (1983) suggested that natural probes into samples of children's language may yield a more accurate picture of their semantic relations in word combination than superficial classification of surface structure can do.

Because language is considered to be a biologically determined behavior, the role of the child is an active one and the role of the environment is minimal, serving to trigger or set in motion the mechanism that induces the rules and incorporates them into a system. In this aspect of language, the cognitive organization and linguistic theories have some similarity. However, because cognitive organization theory includes both knowledge and performance in its language description, this theory applies the *self-directed activity* to the explanation of self-regulated learning only—to the development of rule knowledge or the data base—and not to the performance or perfection of skill. Linguistic theory, on the contrary, considering language to be knowledge of rules, describes all of language acquisition in terms of self-regulated learning. Assessment in linguistic theory focuses accordingly on the child and his or her production, and not to any large extent on the forces in the environment or in the child that have affected the language development, either adversely or for the better.

Contributions

The impact of linguistic theory in the field of language disorders is almost indescribable. Among the many contributions to assessment made by this theory are a few that stand out over the others.

The emphasis on the internal language construction abilities of children has changed the foci of importance in language disorders from the specialist to the child. Instead of expending energies on assessment activities that involve the specialist, the assessment time is directed to the child: observing him or her, describing in detail the language used, and analyzing it for interactions in form, content, and use that appear to be present. Because the behavior of the naturally functioning system is the object of study, the information about language is obtained by naturalistic means and if possible in a naturalistic setting. This approach increases the possibility of obtaining valid information in assessment; the actual abilities of the child are mirrored in evaluation. The language system is viewed in action rather than passively.

As a result of linguistic theory, the language specialists' ability to understand, observe, describe, and analyze language structure in assessment has improved significantly over that which existed prior to the theory. The methods of language sampling, now refined and objectified, are used by specialists as a routine in assessment. The replacement of the *age* concept with the *stage* concept provides a realistic basis for describing language and for measuring improvement.

Of particular value in assessment has been the language developmental data in syntax and semantics that has been gathered by psycholinguists while in pursuit of knowledge about language acquisition. These data have given the language specialist guideposts for comparison of a child's language status. These guideposts in turn have provided a means for designing criterion-referenced test that are often used instead of norm-referenced tests.

A major contribution of linguistic theory to language assessment is its stress on the continuity between assessment and intervention. Assessment strategies using developmental sequences provide useful content for intervention. In fact, assessment is often considered as the first

> *Quote 3–6*
> *The purpose of criterion referenced testing is to specify the developmental status of the child . . . . Using the framework of the Piagetian theory of normal development, the clinician can identify the stage of development (i.e., the cognitive level of development) and the specific substage . . . . The clinician should structure the environment so that each youngster has repeated opportunities to demonstrate his or her level of cognitive development.*
> (TURTON, 1983, p. 66).

> *Quote 3–7*
> *Analysis of spontaneous speech has two primary advantages. The first is that research on normal language development has focused most intensively on spontaneous speech and that therefore there is a larger body of normative data. The second is that any testing situation must be to some extent artificial and constraining, whereas conversation with a child seems less so than interrogation typical of structured tests.*
>
> *The limitations on analysis of spontaneous speech are essentially two fold: First it is an inefficient use of time, and, second, only certain aspects of language development—primarily productive vocabulary and syntax—are observed.*
>
> (DALE, 1976, pp. 301, 304).

step in intervention, one in which the child's language behaviors are identified and described so that goals can be established for intervention. (This approach differs from the early approaches in which an evaluation was done for diagnostic purposes.) Furthermore, the analysis of rule-based behaviors encourages the use of function-based behaviors for intervening in language. This functional basis, the determination of where the child is and what he needs to learn the task, receives the emphasis.

Limitations

Because of the considerable variability among children in language development, it is difficult to generate norms for naturalistic language data and therefore difficult to confirm the presence of a language disorder. Nor do we have sufficient data to determine the range of variation in language skills within the normal population. Therefore, the use of a descriptive method of language analysis as recommended in linguistic theory may cause difficulty in differentiating between normal variability and a significant language problem in assessment. Children may be erroneously labeled as having a language disorder and be given special assistance when, in fact, their language behavior may be within normal limits and given time they could change language behaviors on their own. The use of sampling and other naturalistic approaches permits errors arising from variability in the child, in the tester, and in the method. The results obtained have not been found reliable, particularly for children above a specified meaning length of utterance (MLU). Data that are not reliable cannot be valid.

In linguistic theory, the assessment of language *behaviors* provides information relative to competencies that need assistance but nothing with respect to processes that are deficient. This theory ignores the basic problem that may be responsible for lack of competency. Lack of awareness of contributing factors may result in failure to identify

> *Quote 3–8*
> *The linguistically based theories all have one serious drawback in that they are concerned with the ideal child . . . . Social, motivational, and cultural variables are all ignored . . . . While performance is acknowledged to vary from child to child, such variability, whatever its cause, is ignored, often under the guise of "performance" differences, which are at best of peripheral interest. The result is a deliberate biasing of the theories toward accommodating one set of factors in language acquisition and ignoring almost all others.*
> (WARDHAUGH, 1976, p. 58).

serious problems in other areas that may inhibit further language acquisition and even may interfere with learning other language skills such as reading or spelling. One of the best ways of identifying language disorders in young children and predicting future learning disabilities is through perceptual testing. If this type of testing is not provided, the understanding of the scope of a child's problem will be limited. If there is no awareness of the underlying problem, a child may not develop strategies needed by his or her system to compensate for a deficiency.

The lack of importance placed on comprehension as compared with production puts children with certain kinds of language disorders at a disadvantage. Language-disordered children whose comprehension abilities are deficient but who have ease in echoing language often produce syntax and grammar at a level higher than their semantic level. Intervention directed at production does not ordinarily benefit the problem.

Lastly, emphasis on the linguistic aspects of language acquisition tends to downplay the role of the environment in learning. The context within which the surface structure is produced is as important as the production itself.

COGNITIVE ORGANIZATION THEORY

The manner in which cognitive organization theory views language in relation to other cognitive behaviors influences the assessment procedures in language disorders. This theory considers language to be one of many cognitive abilities or tasks that are independent but interrelated and similar in structure. The major cognitive abilities are similar in that they are dependent on the same learning skills for their development—problem-solving, pattern recognition, cumulative reorganization of internal information, rule-making, learning complex relations, and learning strategies of learning and doing. The major task of individuals in learning, from a Piagetian perspective, is to incorporate the world around them into their own activity and to modify the environment to their own ends.

The assessment of language disorders if executed within the framework of cognitive organization theory must evaluate the above cognitive skills as these relate to major cognitive tasks or abilities as well as to oral language. To put this theory into assessment practice, the specialist examines how the child solves language problems—how he or she discriminates, generalizes, and infers both with respect to surface grammatical structure as well as to word combinations that relate to complex meaning, and how he or she can make use of organization present in the input received. The specialist needs to evaluate the adequacy of the language rules and test the child's ability to make new rules. Thirdly, the specialist determines the child's ability to reorganize knowledge when he or she learns something new and to use the reorganized information in performing new language tasks. Fourth, the evaluator observes the child's ability to relate the different aspects of language to each other and the effect of change on one has on performance in the other; rule efficiency is compared with performance efficiency. Lastly, the specialist studies the manner in which the child organizes external data and the strategies and avenues the child uses to internalize it.

It is also important to this theory that the examiner study these same skills as they relate to other cognitive tasks in order to discover what learning problems exist, in addition to those of language the child may experience. In other words, is the disorder in an area that is common to learning a number of cognitive tasks or is it specific to language, its rules and strategies for performance?

Such an undertaking requires extensive testing (both formal and informal) and observation of a wide variety of cognitive behaviors and the ability on the part of the examiner to integrate findings so as to understand the dynamics of the child's language learning system. It is important therefore to examine the knowledge (the data base) the child has assimilated in various cognitive domains, the access to the data base (e.g., word retrieval), the execution or performance of the skilled behavior, and the learning strategies and skills he or she has in the capacity of a learner.

Contributions

The theory of cognitive organization puts in perspective the relationship between general cognition and language. Even specialists who do not agree with cognitive organization theory's description of the relationship recognize that cognition is important to the understanding of language. There is a need during assessment to look at cognitive prerequisites (if that is what is chosen to call them) in terms of knowledge or strategies.

A second important theoretical contribution is that of distinguishing between knowledge and performance (the term *performance* in this book is used to refer to the internal processing of a language input through the levels of perception, memory, comprehension, and storage and the processing of ideas into speech; the word *use* will be used to refer to the actual speaking of an individual, the speech act and its context) and the recognition that both are parts of cognitive tasks that must be learned. The knowledge—data base and rules—and the performance—access, retrieval, and strategies—are distinct aspects of the task. The former is related to acquisition and the latter to proficiency. In assessment, therefore, the theory recommends that both the accuracy of the rule base as well as the efficiency, latency, and fluidity of performance be evaluated.

Cognitive organization theory elucidates the common elements in different cognitive tasks as well as their uniqueness. It provides a framework for understanding how, for example, reading, spelling, and oral language behaviors differ but also what cognitive skills are basic to all of these tasks. This leads to an understanding of the multiple factors that can contribute to variable achievement and disorders and to a means of looking for these factors in assessment. In fact, one of the assessment methods is to compare performance strategies and rule knowledge in a number of cognitive tasks, especially those of reading, aural comprehension, spelling, and oral production and writing.

Lastly, the separation between the knowledge and performance aspects of cognition provides a rationale for understanding the similarities and differences between comprehension and production—both sharing in knowledge of linguistic rules of basic phonemic, morphemic, and syntactic units and semantics, but differing in the performance of them. This understanding helps to interpret the test findings in comprehensive versus expressive measures of language where the correlation between the input and output is high but not perfect and the correlation in the normal child is higher than in the language-disordered child. (See Carrow-Woolfolk [1985] for a review of the relationship between receptive and expressive test findings.) Support is therefore given to assessing both comprehension and expression.

Limitations

The basic disagreement of some specialists with the tenets of the cognitive organization theory is that it fails to account for the uniqueness of acquisition of the linguistic code. Chomsky (1980) and others have put forth the view that the principles that govern the emergence of language differ from those that govern other cognitive tasks. In other words, there is a distinct mechanism or device that guides the organism in the evolution of language, and this mechanism is of genetic origin. The mechanism is suited to acquiring language and it will do so almost regardless of the nature or amount of linguistic input into the system. The cognitive organization theory does not make such a distinction between language and other cognitive tasks.

A second criticism of this theory is that since language and cognition develop and are disordered differentially, they in fact are not dependent on—only supportive of—one another. A theory must at least attempt to explain these factors in order to be viable. Furthermore, because the relationship between language and cognition is not clear, the implications from the test results in both areas will also be unclear.

Such problems create difficulties for the examiner in studying children with speech and language disorders. These examiners may run the risk of attributing problems that are linguistic in nature to cognitive factors and of directing attention away from the analysis of linguistic expression itself. Some critics also believe that the most effective intervention is that directed toward the task itself (a problem in syntax or in semantics, etc.) instead of toward the underlying cognitive factors related to the problem.

PRAGMATIC THEORY

Pragmatic theory's shift from language to communication, from utterances to messages, has brought the purpose of communication and its social nature clearly into focus. For a message to serve its function, it must be received and received accurately; therefore it must be spoken according to communication rules that are accepted by society. The assessment of language from a pragmatic perspective increases the range of relevant behaviors that need to be evaluated by a hundredfold. Targets for assessment include the speaker, his or her intentions, knowledge, and use of linguistic rules, his or her knowledge and use of communication rules, the listener and context variations that have an effect on the speaker's coding of the message, and the manner in which the speaker responds to these variations. Context variables include the linguistic and situational contexts in addition to intentional and conversational ones. Geffner (1981) says that a pragmatic approach to assessment includes ". . . the interpretation of the child's utterance; the meaning intended by the child; the sensori-motor actions that precede, accompany and follow the utterance and the knowledge shared in the communication dyad" (p. 7).

> *Quote 3–9*
> Naturalistic language assessment is both interdisciplinary and developmental. Assessment is carried out in a natural play setting, involves interaction with peers, and includes parents as active participants. . . . This style and climate of interaction rests upon a belief that observational information is the essence of diagnosis, demanding a heightened responsiveness and awareness by the assessor.
>
> (TAENZER, CERMAK, & HANLON, 1981, p. 42).

Because much of the social interaction required in communication is of a generic sort and is required in other social activities, assessment in language disorders needs to address the level of interactive skills that should precede and undergird language. This necessitates a clear understanding of how social interaction and language relate to each other—to what extent they are dependent and independent. In other words, in addition to evaluating the child's knowledge of linguistic rules, assessment needs to study the child's motivation and needs to communicate and his or her ability to do so in real-life, interactive situations.

Some adherents of pragmatic theory consider semantics to be the core of adequate communication (Lucas, 1980). A child must know not only the referential meaning of words but also be able to identify figurative and idiomatic connotations. He or she must be able to perform linguistic routines associated with social rituals and be able to recognize inferred meaning in utterances in which individual words do not mean what they say. (In other words, the *meaning* in the mind of the user does not always correspond with the meaning of the surface structure used.) The effectiveness with which children communicate is also judged by the manner in which they use connective words when utterances are longer than a single sentence and in which they connect their own output to that which has preceded, spoken either by themselves or another speaker. Accuracy in surface structure is considered secondary to the communication of meaning, and meaning is judged on the basis of the precision, cohesiveness, and clarity with which the child communicates ideas. The assessment of pragmatic functions encompasses the comprehensive evaluation of the semantics within pragmatic boundaries.

Comprehension plays a significant role in pragmatic theory insofar as the effectiveness of language exchange between persons involves accuracy in understanding as well as in speaking. The ability to engage in a meaningful exchange depends on the ability to relate what one says to what has just been heard. If comprehension is not accurate, the corresponding production will also not be accurate in terms of the messages being transmitted. Assessment of comprehension is an integral part of pragmatic theory.

> *Quote 3–10*
> To summarize, we have presented three different types of analysis for determining the influence of the situation on a child's language. They are physical context analysis, speech event and frame analysis, and topic analysis. Each is flexible in terms of the elicitation procedure, the design of the transcript, and the analysis of the transcript, and each will differ depending upon what the particular child seems to be having difficulty with.
> (LUND & DUCHAN, 1983, p. 72).

Contributions

The paradigmatic shift to communication and pragmatics has caused the language specialist to recognize anew the importance to language of a child's interaction with the environment. Language is viewed not as a static but a dynamic process, one that can be evaluated accurately only if studied while in operation during the communicative process. Furthermore, this theory stipulates that the context needs to be included as part of the evaluation insofar as it contributes to the judgment of adequacy of the message. As a result, language evaluation can no longer be viewed as a measurement of static functions but as an assessment of a wide range of behaviors as they vary within the contexts in which they occur.

Pragmatic theory has brought a new perspective into the understanding of semantics. The broadened semantic notion includes not only what words mean (dictionary meaning) and what an individual means when he or she uses them, but also the effectiveness and accuracy with which the individual communicates the intended meaning to others by choice of words. This understanding has assisted specialists in identifying language problems that have hitherto gone unnoticed, and it has also made it possible to recognize and help the language problems of older children who in the past have been ignored for lack of ability to discover the specific linguistic areas in which they have difficulty. These considerations have generated fruitful insights into the nature of the language as it is used in communication. The field has blossomed in its study of narratives, discourse, turn-taking, and other subjects.

Indirectly, pragmatic theory gives an important role to reinforcement by recognizing that the most important means of ensuring continued development of language is to understand and respond to a child's communication. Increased accuracy in the performance of the speaker leads to increased comprehension of the message by the listener, which leads to further increases in the accuracy of performance. Thus, the environment plays a significant role in communication.

Lastly, pragmatic theory has focused the attention of the specialist on the role of social interaction in language. This has led to the analysis of prelanguage and extralinguistic interactive behaviors. Such analysis provides useful data on which to base intervention. It also provides a means of judging the communication of individuals who have no or little language but who may have or are able to develop interchange of some sort with others.

Limitations

The very breadth of pragmatic theory presents problems in its application to the assessment of disordered language. The task of evaluating the entire system of language as it is used uniquely and idiosyncratically by each individual and in each context is an overwhelming one both in terms of complexity and time. Generalizations about language performance are difficult to make, considering the number of intentional, social, contextual, and linguistic variables that need to be considered in the development of these generalizations. For these same reasons, it is difficult to gather data on the normal development of the various pragmatic tasks involved in communication. Without norms of some kind, decisions about disorders are difficult. Measurement of pragmatics is complex because the level and stability of pragmatic behaviors over time and context are personal and therefore variable. In assessment, implementation of this approach may lead to a subjective analysis of a wide variety of behaviors, probably those considered to be the most important by the individual language specialist. From this perspective, the decision about language disorders may lack accuracy, and the communication about disorders among professionals may be almost impossible.

There have been recent attempts to establish methodologies for validly and reliably using observational techniques in pragmatic studies (Klecan-Akers & Swank, in press). Dollaghan and Miller (1986) describe how observation can be quantified by: (1) specifying objectives of observation; (2) selecting and constructing an event taxonomy or coding system; (3) writing adequate recognition rules for events, thereby increasing observer reliability; (4) selecting a data recording system; and (5) structuring the observation context so that relevant data may be obtained. These procedures will assist the language assessment specialist once they have been studied within the language framework.

Prutting and Kirchner (1987) evaluated a pragmatic protocol developed by Prutting (1982b). This protocol was designed to represent 30 pragmatic aspects of language divided into three main categories: (1) verbal aspects (e.g., topic selection, turn-taking initiation, cohesion); (2) paralinguistic aspects (e.g., intelligibility, prosody); and (3) nonverbal aspects (e.g., body posture, gestures, eye gaze). Prutting and Kirchner found that the protocol generated four distinct profiles when used with

> *Quote 3–11*
> *Whereas the development of formalized pragmatic assessment instruments must await a clearer delineation of a normal developmental sequence, it is now possible to draw on empirical and theoretical literature to construct an organizational framework for analyzing performance in this area.*
> (ROTH & SPEKMAN, 1984a, p. 2).

language-disordered subjects. They also found individual differences in the distributions within the diagnostic categories. These authors concluded that the protocol seems to have clinical usefulness. They stated, with regard to their findings, "We offer our data as an early look at the way in which pragmatic deficits stratify across disordered populations" (Prutting & Kirchner, 1987, p. 105). Duncan and Perozzi (1987) compared the performance of children on Prutting's pragmatic protocol with ratings by clinical judges on a seven-point scale of communicative competence. The obtained Spearman rank-order coefficient of 0.75 was interpreted to support the concurrent validity of the protocol.

A second problem in assessing within the framework of pragmatic theory is the lack of clarity in the distinction between cognitive and linguistic functions and the consequent question about the language specialist's role in dealing with cognitive behaviors. Is it the language specialist's role to teach a child how to make inferences, for example, or how to engage in social interaction? If the answer is the former, how can a specialist handle the number of children with these problems and how does he or she distinguish which are disorders and which are characteristics of the child's personality or social background?

It also appears that pragmatic theory has a problem with integrating the concept of syntax (morphology) within its framework. The emphasis on the larger picture of language has led to relegating syntax to an unimportant role in communication. The implication is that once a child has an intention to communicate and does so in order to exchange ideas, the syntax necessary for communication-specific ideas will emerge. The relation between pragmatic and syntactic behaviors is considered unidirectional by this theory: pragmatic function precedes syntax. It is conceivable that for some structures for some children, syntax can precede pragmatics in much the same way that production can precede and be an aid to comprehension.

These comments are not meant to imply that pragmatics has not had a significant impact in the intervention of language-disordered children (Roth & Spekman, 1984b). On the contrary, the influence of pragmatics has just begun to be felt. We need, however, to continue our attempts at integrating all facets of language. There are numerous problems in this integration. Some of these will be discussed in subsequent chapters.

**SIX THEORIES AND
ASSESSMENT**

This chapter has provided a brief description of how the six theories included in this book impacted the assessment of language disorders in children. Each theory has been viewed from the standpoint of its contributions as well as from the criticisms that have been directed to the theory's assessment practices by those who oppose the approach. These criticisms are presented in terms of limitations. Table 3–1 provides a summary of the assessment procedures, contributions, and limitations of each theory.

TABLE 3–1. ASSESSMENT PRINCIPLES AND PROCEDURES DERIVED FROM SIX THEORIES AND THE CONTRIBUTIONS AND LIMITATIONS/CRITICISMS OF THESE PROCEDURES TO ASSESSMENT

THEORY	PROCEDURES AND CONTRIBUTIONS	LIMITATIONS AND CRITICISMS
Neuropsychological	1. Stresses importance of assessing child's neurological functioning. 2. Identifies patterns of language disorder by symptomatology similar to that in aphasia. 3. Categorizes neurological disorders into those of mental retardation, autism, and central auditory processing. 4. Emphasizes importance of measuring both comprehension and expression. 5. Provides means for educational placement.	1. Leads to emphasis on labeling. 2. Categories mask individual differences with class. 3. Does not include detailed language analysis. 4. Ignores role of environment in language and therefore in assessment.
Behavioral	1. Encourages task-oriented descriptions of language behavior. 2. Specifies language *differences* from adult norm in assessment. 3. Obtains baseline data for measuring change. 4. Classifies all language disorders into homogeneous category. 5. Studies the variables that serve to reinforce behavior for a child.	1. Ignores the analysis of any factors that may cause or maintain disorder. 2. Does not make use of developmental language data in assessment. 3. Does not consider comprehension problems as factors for assessment. 4. Considers language as independent from cognitive or motor skills, therefore does not include these in assessment.
Information Processing	1. Examines relationship between processing abilities and language. 2. Compares specific abilities within child to identify strengths and weaknesses. 3. Supports objectivity in measurement by standardizing test instruments. 4. Encourages the use of normative behavior. 5. Encourages early analysis of perceptual skills for prediction of later problems. 6. Measures both receptive and expressive language at all levels and through all modalities. 7. Provides a profile of disorder that includes perceptual, memory, and language performance—and intelligence.	1. Obtains data not always applicable to intervention. 2. Omits a detailed analysis of language. 3. Emphasizes processing skills causing imbalance in assessment. 4. Relies exclusively on standardized instruments. 5. Ignores the dynamic qualities of language. 6. Ignores the naturalistic aspects of assessment.

(Table 3–1 Continues)

TABLE 3–1.   ASSESSMENT PRINCIPLES AND PROCEDURES DERIVED FROM SIX THEORIES AND THE CONTRIBUTIONS AND LIMITATIONS/CRITICISMS OF THESE PROCEDURES TO ASSESSMENT (Continued)

THEORY	PROCEDURES AND CONTRIBUTIONS	LIMITATIONS AND CRITICISMS
Linguistic	1. Examines language in a naturalistic setting. 2. Describes language by analyzing samples of language behavior. 3. Uses normal developmental data for the analysis of syntax and semantics. 4. Searches for rule-based problems. 5. Emphasizes child-oriented assessment. 6. Stresses continuity between assessment and intervention. 7. Uses indices for comparison derived from language sample, e.g., MLU. 8. Emphasizes analysis of language production. 9. Uses stage rather than age for comparison.	1. Leads to difficulties in execution because of time constraints in certain settings. 2. Lacks indices of variability for developmental data. 3. Causes difficulty in distinguishing normal from disordered language. 4. Obtains indices from sampling data that are not reliable past early ages. 5. Gives less importance to comprehension than expression. 6. Fails to integrate linguistic data with cognitive status of child.
Cognitive Organization	1. Includes the assessment of cognitive skills as part of language evaluation. 2. Recognizes need to study both rule formation and performance skills in language. 3. Studies performance under constraints such as increased length and complexity of utterance and under stressful conditions. 4. Compares comprehension and expression in terms of knowledge commonalities and performance differences. 5. Studies the relation between cognition and language in the child. 6. Distinguishes cause of language disorder as a function of the linguistic or the cognitive system or the interaction between the two. 7. Studies all modalities—reading, writing, listening, and speaking—to explore similarities and differences in performance.	1. Leads to difficulties in execution because of time constraints in studying cognition and language. 2. Requires study of cognitive behavior not prepared for by language specialists. 3. Tends to be cause-oriented rather than task-oriented. 4. Fails to recognize language as a unique system and therefore limits the analysis of language. 5. Fails to recognize that aspects of the linguistic system appear to be independent of cognitive prerequisites.
Pragmatic	1. Studies language acts within the framework of context. 2. Considers language as dynamic and therefore examines it in action—the speech act. 3. Examines the adequacy of the relation between intentions and messages. 4. Studies semantics in relation to communicative effectiveness. 5. Studies social aspects of behavior in relation to language through examinations of prelinguistic and extralinguistic aspects. 6. Examines the interaction of child with environment and the role the interaction plays in language behavior. 7. Studies the effectiveness of language in executing pragmatic functions. 8. Examines pragmatic skills that undergird the use of language in interactive exchanges.	1. Lacks normative data on pragmatic skills. 2. Leads to difficulty in separating normal from disordered behavior. 3. Needed breadth of assessment difficult if not impossible in typical setting. 4. Exclusive emphasis on pragmatic skill deficiency may cause other problems to be overlooked. 5. Does not provide a way of integrating syntactic information in assessment.

4

LANGUAGE THEORIES AND INTERVENTION

NEUROPSYCHOLOGICAL THEORY
    Limitations for Intervention

BEHAVIORAL THEORY
    Limitations for Intervention

INFORMATION PROCESS THEORY
    Limitations for Intervention

LINGUISTIC THEORY
    Limitations for Intervention

COGNITIVE ORGANIZATION THEORY
    Limitations for Intervention

PRAGMATIC THEORY
    Limitations for Intervention

As language theory is translated into practical terms for use in intervention, its explanatory logic is dimmed. Questions of practicality and effectiveness are substituted for questions of validity, plausibility, and compatibility. As a result the examination of intervention approaches for the purpose of discovering their themes of theory is difficult, to say the least. The key issues that separate theories are usually distinguishable in textbook descriptions of intervention approaches, but because most intervention is pragmatic (used here to mean useful) specific differences among theories often disappear when intervention is actually carried out. The language specialist tends to use what works whether or not the theoretical undergirdings of the various methods are compatible, and whether the specialist verbally adheres to one theory over others. Unfortunately, the selection of methods from different theories is not made in a conscious and integrative manner. In fact, most specialists are not aware of the relation between theory and practice. For these reasons it is difficult to describe intervention approaches in terms of theory. What will be presented here is a logical analysis of the application of theory to practice as it has been generally described in the literature.

THEORY, ASSESSMENT AND INTERVENTION
IN LANGUAGE DISORDERS: © 1988 by Grune & Stratton
AN INTEGRATIVE APPROACH

ISBN 0-8089-1918-0
All rights reserved.

In this chapter, the contributions of each theory to intervention will be integrated with the discussion of the theory's implications for intervention. A section on the limitations of the theory-based interventions will follow each section.

NEUROPSYCHOLOGICAL THEORY

Since the basis of the neuropsychological theory's description of disordered language is the condition of the central nervous system, particularly the brain, intervention is directed to improving the function of that part of the brain that is damaged or developmentally immature and/or encouraging other parts of the brain to "take over" the function of the disordered part. Brain physiology describes the acquisition of behaviors or skills in terms of synapsis and pathways, and of the frequency of occurrence of behaviors required for some pathways and synapses to be selected over others to increase the facility for using the behaviors. In other words, repetition is required for the development of language and for teaching language to the disordered; frequent opportunities must be given for the individual with a disorder to establish new pathways or to strengthen those that are damaged or delayed. The most common method is by using pictures, structured stimuli (written or verbal), and events in a didactic manner.

The interpretation of language as a twofold process, expressive language located in Broca's area and receptive in Wernicke's area, causes a distinction in the intervention approach used for problems in one or the other area. If the disorder appears to be one of comprehension, the teaching strategies are directed toward improving the relationship between words and meaning. Specific verbal structures are used in conjunction with pictured events, objects, or persons until it is apparent that the language-disordered individual "understands." Pure imitation of verbal stimuli is not used because the individual with a comprehension problem is often able to imitate and use grammatically correct language, albeit the surface structure is empty. If the disorder is an expressive one, the language specialists provide repeated opportunities for the individual to use language structures that are simple and gradually changes to those that are complex. The goal is for the language-disordered person to generate and express language with facility.

Because all the modalities of language (reading, writing, auditory comprehension, and oral expression) are thought to be served by one central language area, the instructor uses reading to assist in auditory comprehension and writing to assist in expression. It is recognized that any one of these modalities can be selectively disordered. The others may be called on to serve as mediators for the one that is disordered.

The *content* of intervention is language itself with special emphasis in comprehension on semantics and in expression on syntax and grammar.

The environment in intervention is structured as are the actual instructional methods and materials. Because the subject's system is considered impaired, he or she needs structure in order to learn; he or she will not, according to this theory, deduce language from the environment by simply being exposed to it, even in a modified way. Modifications of the stimuli (loudness, time, rhythm) are means of emphasis so that the system will respond with greater facility.

Because damage to different areas of the brain result in different types and degrees of problems, the disorders are grouped into patterns of disability or symptom complexes. The core of each pattern relates to the level of intellectual functioning, to the primary disability (e.g., auditory receptive or expressive, motor), or to the degree of language impairment. Intervention procedures vary from pattern to pattern. According to Horner (1981), treatment effectiveness in children may depend on the degree to which it coincides with maturational phenomena governing brain-behavior relationships. Waryas and Crowe (1982) underscore the importance of stimulating, in early intervention, the neurologic organization for language learning so that the organizations become fixed in relation to the normal neurological sites for language acquisition. If intervention begins too late, neurological links may not be established because an important "safety valve" of neurological programming—cerebral plasticity—will be lost.

Limitations for Intervention

The major problem in the application of this theory is that the emphasis is on the description of the problems in language and those related to language, and not on intervention. Intervention is simply a means of "correcting" or improving the problem and so specific structured activities are developed to assist in each of the deficit areas. This approach implies that language is a static and passive, rather than dynamic and active behavior. Little consideration is given to situational or linguistic variables, to language exchange, to the extent, needs, and motivation of the speaker to communicate, or to communication itself. Thus, attention is given to teaching language skills that may have no functional use, and to the use of materials—e.g., pictures and sentences—that have no direct application to life. Therefore there is little generalization or carry-over to everyday communication needs.

The intervention approach that derives from concern with problems related to specific brain dysfunction and with the teaching of the skills associated with dysfunction, leads to teacher-oriented rather than child-oriented intervention. The specialist plays the significant role in intervention. Time is spent in giving instruction, information, or linguistic input to the child with less time given to the expansion of the child's language responses. The artificiality of the teaching environment may result in stilted and artificial language.

BEHAVIORAL THEORY

The major focus of behavioral theory is intervention. There is little if any concern for the cause(s) of a language disorder; nor is assessment an important task, except for identifying notable differences in language behavior. What is important is that, if change is to take place, the subject must learn to perform what he or she does not perform—that which others think he or she should perform—and for this learning to be effective, a well-defined and structured procedure needs to be provided.

Basically, behavioral theory is directed toward the modification of human behavior by means of what are considered to be critical elements of the learning process. The center of the teaching/learning paradigm is conditioning, which involves the sequence of stimulus-response-consequence. The consequence serves to increase or decrease the frequency of the response and thus is considered to be the pivot of the teaching strategies. Consequences that improve the frequency of response are called reinforcers.

Because stimulus, response, and reinforcement are essential parts of the teaching process, behavioral theory requires that their form be explicitly identified prior to the training program. The type (concrete-abstract, verbal-pictoral, etc.) and complexity of the stimuli need to be specified. Responses may take the form of nodding, pointing, gesturing, speaking, writing, and so on. The child may be expected to begin responding at his or her level and gradually move into more complex responses. Desired responses may need to be conditioned prior to initiating a language teaching program. Reinforcement, too, is described in very specific terms for each child. The type of reinforcement (verbal, tokens, etc.) and the schedule of delivery is decided on at the outset of the program. Thus, behavioral theory provides a means of charting change and monitoring the success of intervention.

Programming for teaching is an integral part of behavioral theory. Programming refers to the sequential presentation of discrete tasks that are minimally different and ordered according to complexity and related to the acquisition of a target behavior that has been previously identified. The programming structure is usually rigid and systematic, as each task that is taught is considered to be a prerequisite for learning subsequent tasks. A separate program may be constructed for each child. This program describes the nature of the stimulus, response, and reinforcement that is to be used.

In behavioral theory, the variable that sets the pace for the teacher is the criterion. The criterion is the standard against which the teacher makes decisions about the level of the child's mastery of each task. The criterion is most often defined by a specific number of correct responses (usually 10). The use of the criterion helps the teacher describe the child's progress in objective and precise terms and predicts the time needed to accomplish both specific and general goals. Judgment of goal acquisition is often in terms of frequency of occurrence of language items or particular grammatical forms (Bricker & Bricker, 1970, 1974; Kent, Klein, Falk, & Guenther, 1972).

Since this theory is directed toward changing behavior and uses the same techniques of behavioral modification for all behaviors, there is no need to group the language-disordered children according to cause. If children are grouped, teaching proceeds in a systematic manner using individualized reinforcement programs for each child. Each child must make a large number of responses for learning to take place.

A key aspect of behavioral theory that should serve as a model for all intervention is that of planning. Careful and specific planning of what to teach and how to teach is an integral part of each intervention lesson. The sequence of intervention events that are structured into behavioral theory form a pattern or rhythm with which children learn to be comfortable. The plan of the behaviorists also tells the specialist when to move on to the next step and how to integrate performance into spontaneous language.

Limitations for Intervention

One of the major problems in using strict behavioral theory principles in language intervention is the disregard by this theory of the meaning of language. Although there are children whose major language disorder can be described as one of production at the surface level of the structure, there are also many children whose problem lies at the level of association between the structure and meaning or at the meaning (cognitive) level itself. There is little or no evidence to demonstrate that the improvement of automatic performance of syntactic structures (in a situation devoid of meaning) brings about a corresponding change in semantics. To engage in intervention from a behaviorist point of view, one has to assume that language-disordered children do not have problems of semantics.

Strict adherence to behavioral methodology can make language interventions sterile and uninteresting to the child. It leaves no room for the child's need or lack of need to communicate or for consideration of environmental influences on the child's language. Because the input and expected response are artificially structured, the responses acquired by the child may also be artificial.

Often, the tokens of reinforcement do not have reinforcing value for the child. Just recently, a pharmacist, on learning that I was a speech pathologist, told me that he had been in speech therapy as a child. Then with actual glee, he related that whenever he made his "s" right (which he still did not do as an adult), he would get peanuts and the therapist never found out that he hated them.

The concept of language as essentially an interaction between a speaker and listener is absent from this theory. Also absent is the description of language in which the child regulates the input and restructures it internally to formulate rules. The primary involvement is on the part of the specialist.

INFORMATION PROCESS THEORY

The key to intervention in the information process theory is the hierarchical sequence that is said to exist developmentally and in language performance subsequent to mastery of language. This hierarchical sequence describes the dependency relation among perception, memory, representation, comprehension, imitation, formulation, and expression. Problems at the surface or higher level of the hierarchy (language comprehension or expression) are said to relate to and/or be caused by disorders at lower levels. The relationship is one in which cognitive skills are considered as integral parts of language, not only precursors to it. The relationship can be described as a spiral that begins and ends at the peripheral edges of cognitive behavior and that alternately and sequentially utilizes the component processes as they are needed.

The goal of the intervention program is twofold: to improve performance at the lower levels of the process so that higher level functions can be performed with greater ease and to assist the subject in learning compensatory behaviors, new ways of handling problems in those areas of language performance that are deficient. The premise for the first goal is that once the area of deficiency is strengthened and improved, the subsequent skills that are dependent on such an area will improve. For example, exercises for improving memory for digits are provided to increase the auditory memory, which in turn is believed to improve the memory requisites for language.

Closely tied to direct instruction for deficient areas are the procedures used for bypassing the deficiency. Advocates of the information process theory recommend "covering the bases," reaching the higher level functions by means of input to all the sensory levels: visual, auditory, tactile, and kinesthetic. This is called the *multisensory approach*. Knowledge about language therefore can be acquired even though the major channel through which language is ordinarily received is impaired.

Because language knowledge is thought to be ultimately independent of modalities of input and output but dependent on a common core in the various tasks (reading, writing, speaking, and listening), as well as in the processes of comprehension and expression, the intervention program uses these modalities and processes as means of supporting and influencing one another (as is done in neuropsychological theory). Language disorders and learning disabilities are seen as two sides of the same coin with oral language disorder being the one identified during preschool years and learning disability recognized when the language disorder and/or other processes in the hierarchy interfere with learning to read, write, spell, or understand word problems in math. Intervention, therefore, is not directed exclusively to oral expressive language.

In information process theory language is thought to be learned and therefore it can be taught. The instructional procedures are based on principles of learning, although not as strictly defined and controlled as in behaviorism. Whereas behaviorism concentrates as much or more on the response of the subject, information process theory stresses the importance of manipulation and modification of the stimulus. The hierarchy of language is thought to move from simple to complex and from concrete to abstract and so this sequence principle is used in presenting the verbal and associated stimuli and in accepting the response. In other words, the analysis of the language process follows a type of task analysis, a description of the process events and their prerequisites that take place in a language event; intervention follows the path of the task analysis.

An important responsibility of intervention in information process theory is to help the language-disordered child to compensate for his or her problems. To do this the child must know what his or her difficulties are and the factors that influence performance. For example, to identify that a child has difficulty in understanding jokes is important; to help the subject understand humor is also important, but most important of all is to explain to him or her the nature of the problem and how to respond in situations where other children are telling jokes. How can this child learn to identify and comprehend the punch line and how can he or she cover up if it is not comprehended? The subject must know his or her own learning style and modify the environment and approaches to learning accordingly. In these situations, the role of the language specialist is more broadly conceived than one that limits itself to oral language facilitation.

Limitations for Intervention

The establishment of a hierarchy of processing and linguistic skills in language development is of great interest at a theoretical level

> *Quote 4–1*
> *The conclusions reached is that specific abilities, as currently measured, may not be distinct from one another in language learning; do not appear to be prerequisites for language learning; and may not be improved in most children by current remedial programs. Most important, there is no evidence that the remedial programs designed to remediate these abilities improve general language functioning.*
>
> (BLOOM & LAHEY, 1978, p. 549).

and may even provide content for research. A theoretical hierarchy does not necessarily have empirical validity, however, and so should be used with caution as a basis for intervention. When a language specialist applies the theoretical hierarchical sequence to an individual, he or she may not take into account the many other variables, both internal and external, that may modify the sequence. Such sequential intervention programming is valuable in a general way, but not in terms of strict adherence to an order in teaching language to children.

Even though a specific processing and linguistic sequence might be shown to be accurate and developmentally valid, there is no evidence to support the position that an improvement in a skill that precedes another will bring about improvement in the second skill that is assumed to be developmentally dependent on the first. For example, efforts to improve auditory memory have not been found to bring about substantial change in language behavior. Therefore, isolated auditory processing skills do not appear to be valid content for intervention. Understanding the child's problems in processing may be of value in selecting instructional strategies to suit a child's learning style or in predicting future problems; it is not of value as content of intervention.

The emphasis on processing that is the core of information process theory may cause the specialist to neglect the central concern in the language-disordered child—the language itself. The major concern in intervention should be in bringing about change in language, and in order to do so, a complete analysis and description of the language and a plan that has language as its major focus are necessary.

Although there appears to be experiential and research support for the use of related language tasks such as reading and writing in strengthening and supporting oral language skills (and vice versa), this technique should be used with the recognition that the relation among the various language tasks has not been completely defined. There are, by nature of these tasks, modality and strategy differences in assessing and retrieving the rules of the language. Such differences should be taken into account when using one task to support another.

> *Quote 4–2*
> *The distinction between cognitive and semantic notions is necessary in order to place the nature of semantic notion training in focus. The goal of training cognitive prerequisites to semantic notions, as seen in the work of investigators such as Bricker and Bricker (1974), is quite different from that of training semantic notions. Although the latter is clearly dependent upon the prerequisite cognitive attainments, it is, nevertheless, primarily a linguistic enterprise.*
>
> (LEONARD, 1984, p. 153).

LINGUISTIC THEORY

In terms of intervention, linguistic theory concerns itself with form (syntax), content (meaning), and use (function) and the relation among these components. As noted in the previous chapter, assessment in linguistic theory looks at language production and infers problems in content or function on the basis of this output. In other words, the patterns of surface structure are studied to determine the type of disorder—form, content, or use. In intervention the emphasis is also placed on the surface linguistic data, although the content and use are integrated with the form. Even if the language deficiency may be a symptom of some other more basic problem, the linguist believes that remediation should be directed at the symptom, the difficulty which is creating the problem for the child. In this aspect, linguistic theory resembles behavioral theory.

The linguistic approach follows language developmental sequences in planning for intervention. The specialist parallels the order of emergence of linguistic forms in teaching these forms to the language-disordered child. Developmental sequence data are chosen above theoretical ideas or adult intuitions of complexity of specific structures, and so the intervention content is prioritized on a developmental basis. The provision of this developmental content to the field of language disorder is one of the major contributions of this theory to the field.

A major change in intervention practice for early language learning has been due to Bloom's (1970) focus on the relations between two-word combinations and meaning. Word combinations do not have static meaning derived from the meanings of the individual words, but variable meaning dependent on the context in which they are used. The thrust of intervention at this stage is no longer on developing the child's ability to produce two-word combinations, but on expanding the instances of semantic relations by adding new words to the basic structure so that the child's repertoire of structures can be used for varied purposes.

The emphasis in the linguistic approach is on production as opposed to comprehension, primarily because most of the developmental data available are on the production side of language. Data on the

> *Quote 4–3*
> *Part of my own definition of language intervention, for example, derives from the following assumptions: (1) that the human mind inherently seeks organizing principles, (2) that language behavior is generated from the knowledge of abstract rules, (3) that language rules are constructed by the knower based on an active analysis of linguistic events, (4) that new language behaviors reflect qualitative, self-regulated changes in the nature of abstract rules, and (5) owing to impairments of attention, memory, and auditory perception, some children are ill-equipped to discover linguistic rules.*
>
> (JOHNSTON, 1983, p. 55).

developmental sequences related to comprehension are not as complete as in production. Furthermore, linguistic theory questions the long-held assumptions that comprehension precedes production and therefore needs to be taught before production. Because intervention procedures in linguistic theory often present production units in the context of meaning, comprehension is indirectly included.

One of the basic tenets of linguistic theory is that what is learned in language is a system of rules. Consequently, the development of rule-behavior is viewed as the goal of intervention. The purpose of intervention is not to teach isolated structures to children having problems with those structures but to make it possible for the child to induce the rules governing those structures. Since the knowledge of rules of form, content, and use forms the definition of language in the linguistic approach, it is the acquisition of these rules that is the goal of intervention.

One of the most important influences linguistic theory has had on intervention is the notion of the role of the internal construction abilities of the child who induces the rules of language from his or her language environment. This self-regulation on the part of the child who actively internalizes language and incorporates it into a rule system has led the linguistic theorist to the description of the "facilitator" role of the specialist in intervention. Since the child's cognitive system is actively engaged in learning language, the role of the language specialist should be to provide the data the child needs for the induction of specific rules. The "facilitator" may modify the input data so as to make it easier to induce the rules, but the actual learning is essentially child-oriented and the process does not involve much of what is ordinarily considered as part of the teaching repertoire. Support for this approach is Bloom, Rocissano, and Hood's (1976) finding that tasks involving elicited speech produce responses that are fundamentally different from that which occurs in the child's usual situations. The theoretical position then is that given the proper input, the child's learning of language takes place almost irrespective of the environment. The specialist only "facilitates" the process.

Limitations for Intervention

As was mentioned in the previous chapter, concern with surface structure data only, even if they are analyzed in terms of form, content, and use, limits the specialist in understanding the child's problem and in providing the best approach to intervention. A child who has difficulty processing auditory information may not benefit from an intervention program that is primarily auditory—use of spoken instructions, directions, and verbal exchange. A child who processes visual/spatial information well may profit from the use of visual aids in intervention. Some modification of instructional methodology needs to be provided for children having specific sensory, perceptual, or motor difficulties. The data from extralanguage testing should not form the *content* of intervention but should be used in planning instruction.

The use of strategies for improving production only—modeling, imitation, expansion, and so on—will not, unless paired with events that indicate meaning, be of much value to the child who has a comprehension problem. Such a child usually has skill in echoing or in using strings of structures automatically, albeit in inappropriate situations. The theory of the relation of comprehension to expression may be unclear; the fact of the existence of children with problems of auditory comprehension is not.

In the application of linguistic theory to language disorders, there is need to reconcile, on the one hand, the position that language learning is self-regulated and therefore teaching should be only facilitative and, on the other hand, the consideration that the language-disordered child may have difficulty in the induction or self-regulating process. Linguistic approaches to intervention stress the facilitator role of the specialist because the child is thought to have the major role in learning. In other words, the specialist provides a situation in which the child receives input modified to a limited degreee by amount or saliency. The assumption is that a language-disordered child will induce the rules of language in a manner similar to that of the normal child given a semicontrolled situation and provided with selected and moderately organized input. The role of the specialist is limited except to provide the appropriate situation. However, the possibility that the child's inductive system may be defective and that this in turn may dictate a different route of language internalization does not appear to be addressed. If the child has

---

Quote 4–4

In mentalism, the clinician functions as a "facilitator," highlighting salient language subcomponents and their interrelationships and increasing the frequency with which the child has opportunities for experiencing these language events.

(CRAIG, 1983, p. 113).

not learned language adequately in the natural environment, why should one assume that he or she will do so when given more of the same? The fact of disorder should be taken into account in the application of any theory to practice.

Finally, exclusive attention to teaching rules in intervention implies that all language is knowledge of rules and that performance problems do not exist. If one is convinced of the validity of this position, teaching the rules of language only is the appropriate goal of intervention. If so, such areas as word finding and retrieval and production efficiency would have no place in the content of intervention.

COGNITIVE ORGANIZATION THEORY

Because one of the basic elements of cognitive organization theory is the adequacy of the child's skills in learning how to learn, the goal of intervention is directed toward the improvement of these skills. As pointed out previously, the linguistic and cognitive organization theories are similar with respect to the role of the child's system in self-regulation, reorganization of input, and acquisition of rules. What may differ from the standpoint of intervention is that the linguistic approach modifies the language input so that the child's defective system may more easily induce the rules of language; the cognitive organization approach also directs its attention to the level of efficiency of the child's system. The child is assisted in solving language problems, inferring and generalizing language rules, reorganizing new linguistic input, using strategies of language retrieval, improving efficiency of performance, and other skills.

This approach to language intervention relates the learning of general cognitive skills to linguistic ones insofar as they are considered to be part of the same basic process. If, for example, the child's inference skills in language are considered inadequate for his or her needs, intervention will consider both nonverbal and verbal aspects of inference in intervention since they are both part of the problem-solving ability of the child. In other words, inference is considered to be a general cognitive ability. Verbalizing inference simply adds an element to the general task. A child's problem may be in inferring *or* in verbaliz-

---

Quote 4–5
Ideal cognitive skills training programs would include practice in the specific task-appropriate strategies (skills training); instruction in the orchestration, overseeing, and monitoring of these skills (self-regulation training); and information concerning the significance of those activities and their range of utility (awareness training).

(BROWN & PALENCSAR, 1982, p. 14).

> *Quote 4–6*
> One must go beyond accuracy to automaticity. In human ac-
> tivities that require high levels of proficiency and skill, a con-
> siderable amount of time must be spent in practicing the skills
> leading to master.
>
> (SAMUELS & EISENBERG, 1981, p. 63).

ing the inference. The same may be true for other tasks such as
reorganization of the system when new information in introduced, rule
formation, retrieval, and so on. All can have both nonverbal and verbal
aspects, and this theory considers it to be important to distinguish these
in the child. Is the problem a general cognitive problem or one that is in
the addition of the verbal element to the cognitive task? The answer influences the type of intervention chosen—work with the cognitive
problems or with their linguistic correspondents.

Cognitive organization theory also distinguishes between learning
the rules and executing the behavior. This theory considers both as being
kinds of knowledge—the knowledge of knowing and the knowledge of
doing. This distinction then separates the knowledge of the rules from
performance of them. The intervention activities for teaching the
knowledge of the rules follows the same basic procedures of that of linguistic theory—modifying the input so that the problem-solving and induction can proceed with greater facility. However, if a child's language
disorder lies with execution or performance, retrieval, speed, facility, or
accuracy rather than with rules, the intervention procedure takes a different turn, one of increasing the efficiency, accuracy, and automaticity
of performance by means of practice, cuing, or other methods of helping
the child "do" language better.

Although not expressly stated by the theory, this approach would
consider both comprehension and expression as essential parts of intervention, comprehension as a means of identifying adequacy of the rules
and improving content, and expression as a means of producing accurate
rules plus performing efficiently. If comprehension and expression are
equal, the disorder might be one of inadequacy of rule knowledge and
intervention would be directed to that problem. If the expressive
problem is greater than the receptive (with the comprehension essential
within normal limits), the disorder may be one of performance and intervention would be geared toward improving performance efficiency.

Limitations for Intervention

A theory of cognitive organization provides a general framework
for understanding the cognitive system, and as such it assists the
specialist in describing the commonalities and distinguishing among the

various components of cognition. When such a theory is applied to language, there is a need to recognize that some aspects of general cognitive skills such as problem-solving and rule formulation may differ in significant ways among the various cognitive tasks, particularly language. Perhaps more to the point, does language differ at any level from other cognitive tasks, and if it does where does its linguistic noncognitive aspects stop and its cognitive aspects begin? Excursions into cognition in intervention should therefore be taken in a formal manner, one that clearly specifies the relationship between language and cognition in the particular skill or task that is being considered for intervention.

The use of theoretical principles from cognitive organization theory for intervention requires that the language specialist have an ample background in theory and studies of cognition. Such use may also have implications for the role and scope of the language specialist involved in intervention with language disorders.

PRAGMATIC THEORY

Pragmatic theory has had considerable impact on intervention content and procedures in language. The basic concepts that have influenced intervention are those of message, interaction, and context.

The concept of message implies that the intent of the speaker in a speaker/listener relationship needs to be accomplished and that the speaker's meaning needs to be transferred. However, as mentioned previously, the meaning of the message is not always a sum of the meanings of the morphemes in an utterance. The literal interpretation of the words may not be what the speaker intends. The listener needs to recognize factors that contribute to the interpretation of the message, such as shared information between speaker and listener, environmental situations that have preceded or co-occur with the message, utterances that have preceded the message, as well as factors related to the particular speaker and listener. According to pragmatic theory, intervention programs should assist children in understanding and producing

> *Quote 4–7*
> *Our intervention goals however have always been toward shaping social growth of the individual with a communicative handicap, even in the past when we concentrated primarily on phonology syntax, and semantics. We have always been in the business of social change and the promotion of human welfare as a consequence of altering communicative behavior. The pragmatic shift brings this issue closer to the surface and gently reminds us of our raison d'etre.*
> (PRUTTING, 1982a, p. 132).

messages instead of concentrating only on the comprehension and production of grammatical forms in sentences. Children need to be made aware of the many variables that influence the meaning of an utterance and how to interpret each variable's contribution to the meaning.

The use of the concept of *message* in intervention has led to intervention techniques that emphasize the reinforcing value of successful communication. Such techniques provide situations where a child must rely completely on verbal communication for delivering instructions, descriptions, and so on. For example, barriers may be placed between the child and the listener(s) so that no information is available to the listener(s) except what the child is providing. The demands of the communication interchange require exact and explicit messages. If the message is received incorrectly because the message has been inadequate, the speaker recognizes the need for accuracy and completeness and self-corrects. If the message is received accurately, the speaker's performance is reinforced.

A second concept that pragmatic theory has stressed in intervention protocols is social interaction or transaction. This concept is broader than that of message, involving as it does the social relations between individuals and among groups. Good communication involves functioning within a set of rules set up by a particular society. These rules involve the particular roles of speakers and listeners with respect to age, position, and other factors; the rules pertain to specific linguistic routines to accompany specific social acts; and the rules govern appropriate behavior with respect to taking turns in conversation or discourse as well as to listening and reacting. Intervention, if it is to be concerned with good communication, must include these rules of linguistic interaction as part of its responsibility. Developmental data regarding the above topics have helped to order intervention sequences for these pragmatic skills and have assisted the specialist in providing an environment that is conducive to good communication.

A third concept of pragmatic theory that has influenced intervention is that of context or setting. If the context (which includes physical environment as well as persons) influences the messages given and received, then context should be included as an integral part of planning the intervention procedures. Restricting intervention to a single room and person will limit the child's ability to generalize and to understand the variables that affect messages. Some communication theorists believe that intervention should be carried out in a naturalistic setting and in a social context, with as little interference as possible on the part of the specialist other than providing a topic that will elicit the desired language. This appraoch means that intervention takes place in a group setting and the intervention is in the form of providing opportunities for children to alternate between being speaker and listener. Other specialists integrate some direct teaching of target language behaviors

> *Quote 4–8*
> . . . *clinician behavior can be conceptualized pragmatically as a "role-bracketing dynamic." The clinician close-brackets a previous child turn by meeting the constraints established by that message and then establishes a new set of constraints or open brackets a message to which the child must relate subsequently.*
> (CRAIG, 1983, p. 115).

within this naturalistic setting, thereby adding structure to the process. It should be pointed out, however, that the concept of structure in pragmatics is not analogous to the idea of structure in syntax and semantics. These latter two components of language can be isolated both theoretically and in practice for the purpose of study. Pragmatics by its very nature is an integral domain requiring the context for the exploration and function of language. In fact, the concerns of pragmatics have evolved into a concern for communicative competence that integrates form, content, and use in appropriate and *effective* communication (Schiefelbusch, 1986).

In addition to modifying intervention procedures, pragmatic theory has significantly expanded the content of intervention for language-disordered children and consequently has changed the kinds of things specialists do. A list of these might include interactive skills, topic setting, turn-taking, discourse, language routines, or cohesion in narratives. This broadening of intervention content applies to all ages although the greatest impact has been with children over 8 years of age, because by this age, most of the syntactic and grammatical structure has been mastered, but problems in semantics and pragmatics continue to be evident.

Although the broadening of the content of intervention has had a major impact on *what* is taught, the most important contribution of pragmatics has been in modifying the procedures used in intervention. Pragmatic procedures are valid for intervention in modifying syntax, semantics, or cognitive behaviors, as well as in modifying pragmatic behaviors. The belief of pragmatics that all language intervention should be functional and therefore interactive in order to achieve language change is its most significant departure from traditional intervention.

Limitations for Intervention

One of the major problems in the use of pragmatic theory in intervention is the lack of normative data for the tasks described as pragmatic functions. The lack of information regarding the point along the continuum of language development, where each of the pragmatic skills begins, and the lack of variability data regarding performance of normal language children for these skills makes the selection process for children with problems a difficult if not impossible task. In addition to difficulty in separating children with pragmatic disorders from those not having problems is that of recognizing, without normative information, what to expect of children once in intervention, how fast or how much they should be able to learn at a specific age level.

Related to this problem is that of the selection of pragmatic skills for intervention. Lack of knowledge of how these skills interact with one another developmentally makes it difficult for the specialist to plan the order in which the skills should be taught. Questions such as, "Where does intervention begin?" "Which pragmatic skills should I teach first?" are added to, "How do I know if the child's performance is a disorder or if it is within normal limits?"

Because many of the pragmatic behaviors in language are related to and, in some instances, dependent on cognitive behaviors and skills, it may not be clear to the specialist whether the child's problem is one of cognition or one of language. One could suggest, for instance, that the ability to use cohesion in narratives is a cognitive skill rather than a linguistic one. To what extent and under what conditions should a language specialist teach cognitive skills? If some of the disorders in pragmatics are due to cognitive problems, what effect does working on language skills have? The concepts of pragmatics and the corresponding focus on interaction are valid for looking at language development. The focus on the environment, however, may cause us to neglect the problems that may occur within the individual and that interaction intervention alone cannot improve effectively. This concern can be addressed, perhaps, by the position of the pragmatists that the cognitive, linguistic, and social domains are so integrated within the individual that change in one will automatically produce change in the other, particularly if the intervention script is one that involves the three domains.

Pragmatic theory is often linked with naturalistic settings and group intervention, although this linkage may not be a logical one. Some language specialists interpret the idea of naturalistic setting to mean that all or most intervention should take place in an informal group situation—a child should be placed with his or her peers. However, the assumption that the most natural setting for communication is a group setting is false. Most of daily communication takes place between two persons. Even in the child's "group" environments—a classroom, a playground—the interaction is usually between two children. These, too, are naturalistic.

Even if informal group interaction were theoretically sound, good intervention would be difficult to conduct unless the goal of intervention is purely group interaction. Each child's needs and consequent plan for intervention may differ. It would take a well-organized and clever specialist to provide effective intervention in an informal setting. This is not to say that the intervention setting should be in a room with a specialist and child. One can provide the most naturalistic setting possible for the most *effective* intervention. This approach may mean some degree of structure is necessary in order for change to take place within a definable time. Furthermore, the specialist should be able to monitor the change and record it.

Perhaps the future direction that needs to be taken in pragmatics is the application of theory to practice. Once specific descriptions of procedures using pragmatic theory are available, the value of pragmatic theory can be realized. Presently there appears to be considerable agreement with respect to the tenets of the theory but considerable diversity in translating the theory into intervention processes.

SIX THEORIES AND INTERVENTION

This chapter has provided a brief description of how the six theories included in this book impacted the intervention of language disorders in children. Each theory has been viewed from the standpoint of its contributions as well as from the criticisms that have been directed to the theory's intervention practices by those who oppose the approach. These criticisms are presented in terms of limitations. Table 4–1 provides a summary of the intervention procedures, contributions, and limitations of each theory.

TABLE 4–1. INTERVENTION PRINCIPLES AND PROCEDURES DERIVED FROM SIX THEORIES AND THE CONTRIBUTIONS AND LIMITATIONS/CRITICISMS OF THESE PROCEDURES TO INTERVENTION

THEORY	PRINCIPLES, PROCEDURES, AND CONTRIBUTIONS	LIMITATIONS AND CRITICISMS
Neuropsychological	1. Bases therapy on improving brain function that is damaged or developmentally immature. 2. Trains other parts of the brain to take over function of damaged part. 3. Relates improvement to facilitation of synapsis and requires frequency of occurence of behaviors. 4. Uses repetition provided by examples of pictures or objects. 5. Uses different procedures with different localization of disorder—comprehensive or expressive, oral or written. 6. Uses structured procedures to maintain attention and avoid distraction.	1. Lacks evidence available for neurological bases for improvement. 2. Gives little attention to situational variables. 3. Uses teacher-oriented didactic instruction that is not functional. 4. Does not provide naturalistic topic and exchange formats.
Behavioral	1. Modifies language by stimulus-response-consequence paradigm. 2. Considers consequences the pivot of training—to increase or decrease frequency of response. 3. Involves structure in each element of the paradigm. 4. Highlights programming through sequential presentation of minimally different discrete tasks. 5. Considers each task to be a prerequisite for subsequent tasks. 6. Uses criterion as standard against which teacher makes decisions about progress—usually in numbered trials and successes. 7. Uses same procedure for all children.	1. Uses artificial format that yield artificial language. 2. Ignores comprehension and the meaning of language. 3. Disregards functional language in interactive settings. 4. Sets behavioral rather than rule-induction goals.

(Table 4–1 Continues.)

TABLE 4–1. *(Continued.)* **INTERVENTION PRINCIPLES AND PROCEDURES DERIVED FROM SIX THEORIES AND THE CONTRIBUTIONS AND LIMITATIONS/CRITICISMS OF THESE PROCEDURES TO INTERVENTION**

THEORY	PRINCIPLES, PROCEDURES, AND CONTRIBUTIONS	LIMITATIONS AND CRITICISMS
Information Process	1. Directs teaching to problems at lower level of hierarchy and proceeds in a progressive sequence. 2. Considers hierarchy to represent perceptual, memory, and representational interaction with language. 3. Considers multi-sensory input as means of bypassing disordered faculties. 4. Presents stimuli that follow simple to complex, concrete to abstract guides. 5. Uses comprehension improvement as a prerequisite to expressive teaching because expression is dependent on comprehension. 6. Treats language and learning problems as if they are two sides of the same coin. 7. Teaches compensatory method as integral to system.	1. Uses a hierarchical system that may not be a valid description of language processing. 2. Neglects factors outside the system that influence the relation among its parts. 3. Lacks attention to language itself due to concern with processing. 4. Trains isolated processing skills that have little or no carry-over to language.
Linguistic	1. Uses the interaction of form, content, and use as input. 2. Facilitates rule-induction for expressive language improvement. 3. Directs intervention at expression, the symptom, rather than the cause. 4. Measures improvement in developmental stages following growth patterns of normal language. 5. Provides data for child's constructive system to internalize language in naturalistic settings. 6. Expands semantic relations instead of combining words.	1. Ignores cause that may later produce additional problems. 2. Overlooks disordered system that may not induce rules normally or follow development stages of language. 3. Ignores the language performance system. 4. Does not give sufficient attention to comprehension.
Cognitive Organization	1. Teaches cognitive prerequisites to language before teaching language. 2. Works on common cognitive skills (pattern-analysis, categorization) for learning how to learn. 3. Considers that language is learned in the same way as other tasks. 4. Applies different procedures to rule-induction problems as to performance disorders. 5. Considers practice to be an important component in improving performance. 6. Treats comprehension and/or expression as either disorder of knowledge or as performance disorder and applies intervention accordingly.	1. Does not consider language as unique in learning. 2. Applies general learning procedures of instruction instead of specific language methods. 3. Suggests that language is always dependent on specific cognitive precursors. 4. Does not recognize that language can be the means of learning specific cognitive skills.
Pragmatic	1. Uses messages and texts that carry information as the best means of intervention. 2. Teaches skills of social interaction in language as well as language itself. 3. Considers functional language use to stimulate the desire for accuracy in production. 4. Considers good communication to have reinforcing value. 5. Emphasizes both understanding and producing messages. 6. Considers the best teaching environment is the natural environment. 7. Uses pragmatics as both content and method of intervention.	1. Lacks documentation for developmental sequences in pragmatic skills. 2. Lack knowledge in normal variability in pragmatic tasks. 3. Does not clarify relation between pragmatics and cognition. 4. Fails to consider that pragmatics is so broad that it moves into boundaries of all learning. 5. Does not clearly define naturalistic setting.

5

THEORIES AND INSTRUCTIONAL TECHNIQUES AND PROCEDURES

BASES FOR COMPARING INTERVENTION
APPROACHES

INPUT-ORIENTED APPROACHES
  Type I Approach
  Type II Approach
  Type III Approach

RESPONSE-ORIENTED APPROACHES

Type IV Approach
Type V Approach

INPUT-RESPONSE CYCLE APPROACH
  Type VI Approach

FACILITATION

LANGUAGE INTERVENTION—THE MIDDLE
GROUND

As a theory is filtered through the many factors that modify it before reaching the intervention stage—the individual specialist and his or her training and personality, the environment where intervention is practiced, the particular problem and needs of the child, the age of the child—the theory has less and less influence on the ultimate procedure used. The previous chapter discussed the influence of theory on the general intervention direction taken by the language specialist. At that level, the level of general approach, the theory is still a strong directive. Language theory also influences content, whether the specialist chooses to work on comprehension or expression, on cognitive or linguistic skills, on syntax, semantics, or pragmatic skills. However, at the next level of application, the level of instructional *procedures* and *techniques*, the effect of theory is scarcely apparent. What specialists frequently do in the intervention setting is what they have seen others do, what language programs direct them to do, or whatever works.

THEORY, ASSESSMENT AND INTERVENTION
IN LANGUAGE DISORDERS: © 1988 by Grune & Stratton
AN INTEGRATIVE APPROACH

ISBN   0-8089-1918-0
All rights reserved.

Quote 5–1
Intervention cannot continue to combine goals and procedures across paradigms. A theoretical mismatch between goals and procedures is problematic since goal-setting [assessment] and goal-attainment [intervention] are interlocking systems . . . . The clinician must cope with this inconsistency by uncomfortably vascillating back and forth between paradigms.
(CRAIG, 1983, p. 109).

This chapter will analyze the instructional procedures and techniques used in language intervention and indicate, where applicable, the theory (or theories) with which the procedure or technique is compatible. I have attempted to abstract the principles of methodology so as to clarify their similarities and differences. No specific procedure or approach will be identified.

BASES FOR COMPARING INTERVENTION APPROACHES

In an attempt to ferret out those factors that are similar among procedures and techniques and those that differ, I found it helpful to organize them on the basis of three dimensions: (1) the variables on which they differ (or are similar), (2) the degree of structure used with each of these variables, and (3) the approach mode the procedures follow (see Fig. 5–1). There appear to be six major variables in intervention that can be modified and that distinguish theories. The modification most often is one of type and amount of structure. The variables are discussed in the following sections.

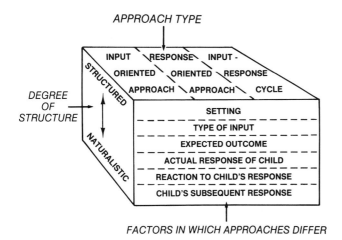

FIGURE 5–1. A three-dimensional description of approaches to intervention describing the degree of structure and other factors in which approaches differ.

1. The Setting. This term refers to the environment in which intervention takes place: informal setting (home or clinic/school, informal situation/play), formal setting (in a clinic, using chairs and a table), and group or individual, etc. If intervention is at home, in an informal situation or play, and uses a natural group, the setting is said to be *naturalistic*. As change is made in the setting by intervening in the direction of greater control over the context, it becomes less naturalistic and more structured or formal.

2. The Input. (I have chosen the word *input* to avoid the use of the term *stimulus*, as in behaviorism.) Input in this sense refers to what the child receives and/or the context in which he or she receives it. Intervention by its very nature implies that something is done by someone to bring about some change in language. The "something" may be only providing a situation in which the child receives a large amount of verbal stimulation. Or it may be using a modified verbal stimulation—changes in frequency, type, or length. Or it may be the means by which specific input is highlighted or made salient. The input may consist of a verbal stimulus paired with its semantic meaning and/or with an event, so that form, content, and use are integrated in the learning process. This, too, may be provided in a naturalistic or structured manner.

3. The Expected Outcome. This variable describes what the specialist wants the child to do—the specialist's objective. It may be that the specialist wants the child to induce rules from the verbal input with which the child is bombarded. In this instance, the specialist may not be concerned with immediate production of a particular grammatical form. In a more structured approach, the language specialist may expect a specific verbal response or imitation.

4. The Child's Response. This variable describes what the child actually does. In approaches where the child is expected to formulate a rule internally, he or she may not respond overtly to any specific verbal stimulus, but rather continue to verbalize in general. Where specific structured input is provided, the child may be expected to respond with specific words or sentences, by imitating the input, by answering a question, by completing a partial sentence, by describing a picture, and so on. The goal in this more structured method may also be rule induction, but greater structure and opportunities for specific responses are provided for this to take place. Even within structural situations, there are differences that arise from the role, passive or active, the child plays in intervention (Leonard, 1984).

5. The Reaction of the Environment to the Response. In this variable as in the previous ones, there may be different degrees of structure that the specialists use in reaction to the child's response (or non-response). This reaction may range from a general increase in the amount of verbal stimulation or a communicative response to what a child has said to a highly structured specified reinforcement that is part of a preplanned reinforcement schedule. Within these extremes are various reactions—showing approval of what has transpired, or simply reacting to the child's response as if it is a message and responding to the child's message with understanding or noncomprehension.

6. Child's Secondary Response. In instances where the intervention is carried on in an interactive way and the child's message is either understood or not, the child may respond again modifying those aspects of the message that are not clear.

By considering the degree of emphasis placed by different procedures on the specific items in the above range of variables and the degree of structure within each item, I found it useful to group the descriptions of intervention provided in the literature into three general approaches. Within each general approach I have placed types of intervention that are similar in their basic intervention philosophy. These types are not discrete approaches; instead, they represent points along a continuum of structure and input/output emphasis. This division is an arbitrary one but one that I believe assists in understanding the similarities and differences in intervention. The three approaches are listed below.

1. Input-Oriented Approaches. This term refers to approaches that place emphasis on what the specialist does in order for the child to acquire (induce) language.

2. Response-Oriented Approaches. These approaches seem to emphasize what the child does in response to the input of the specialist.

3. Input-Response Cycle Approach. This approach combines the first two but also provides for a sequence of communicative events to take place as part of the acquisition process.

Although the focus of this discussion of intervention methods will be on the learning of linguistic tasks, the same principles apply to teaching cognitive or pragmatic ones.

INPUT-ORIENTED APPROACHES

The input in intervention is what the specialist does both specifically and generally in order to achieve his or her goals. The degree of input modification, the structure of the modification, the degree of structure in the context in which the input takes place, and the nature of the input itself (cognitive, linguistic, etc.) are features that partially differentiate theories *within* this category.

Type I Approach

At the least environmentally structured and least input-modified end of the continuum is the totally naturalistic setting in which children are placed with other children (and perhaps a language specialist) and encouraged to interact naturally so that the input of each member of the group serves as a stimulus to the others. The theoretical support for this approach comes from the need of the child to have input serve as a trigger for setting into motion his or her own self-regulating language system (linguistic theory). The group situation is believed to be the most naturalistic, the most nurturing, and the most reminiscent of what mothers do during development. It is considered by some to be the most effective means of providing for the child's needs (Taenzer, Cermak, & Hanlon, 1981; Fey, 1986). Although the ultimate goal is improvement of the child's production, the response by the child to the language stimulation of a specific target rule is usually delayed (perhaps for days or weeks) because of the frequency of occurrence of the target that the child needs in order to master the rules. In a naturalistic situation exemplars of the target rules may not occur frequently by chance, so time needs to be provided for the child's rule induction. The child's correct production of the target is therefore delayed with respect to the input stimulation. (This procedure, which has primarily linguistic origins and which therefore is strongly associated with improving the *production* of language, is reminiscent of procedures recommended by Winitz [1973, 1976] for training in comprehension.)

This approach can be considered loosely scripted. A script is a conceptualization of how an event in a particular lesson or situation will unfold. Included in the script are the characters involved in carrying out a particular function and the flow of action between the parts of the event. They can be thought of as general plans for carrying out an episode. A weak script does not specify order of occurrence, whereas a strong script does (see Schank & Abelson, 1977; Nelson, 1986a; Duchan, 1986b). The specialist allows the child to direct the intervention session through the child's selection of toys, games, and so on, and consequently frequent shifts will occur in the topic or activity. There is minimal overt planning for elicitation of specific linguistic constructions.

For the purposes of this book, I will refer to this approach as type I and will illustrate it as follows:

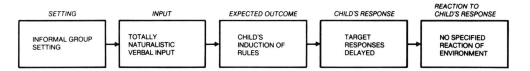

The naturalistic approach lends itself to the utilization of a variety of intervention agents (Craig, 1983). Since the purpose of this procedure is to stimulate language, the participation of parents, teachers, siblings, and peers can be incorporated into the program. The provision of communication opportunities of a wide variety will also serve as a means of generalizing language skills and thereby multiply the effects of the clinician's time with the child.

Type II Approach

Some structure is introduced when the specialist manages the topics of children's interaction by his or her selection of toys, experiences, and other stimulating materials. The structure changes may be only in the environmental—not in the linguistic—input. The children are allowed to interact naturally with one another—to explore and discover, to play and communicate. The child's environment is manipulated so that the child needs to ask, demand, question, and so on.

Another change in the degree of structure may be introduced by choosing specific linguistic strings to serve as an input to the children and providing these in a systematic manner. The specialist manipulates the environment and consequently the input so as to emphasize certain linguistic structures over others. The linguistic input is used in conjunction with events, things, or general situations that have meaning for the child. I will refer to this approach as type II and illustrate it as follows:

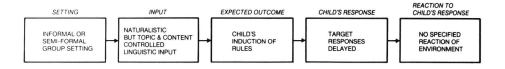

Note that the differences between types I and II are in the setting and input. In order to control the input, some structure is added to the setting. As soon as there is direct manipulation of environmental input, the theoretical position begins to move away from an "innate" constructionist position to one that gives at least a small role to the environment in guiding acquisition.

Type III Approach

At the next level, the specialist modifies the linguistic input itself, rather than only selecting specific exemplars as is done in type II. Even some theories that consider language acquisition to be a function of the child's self-regulated inductive processes, for example, the linguistic theory, can accept some modification of the natural linguistic input to the child in the environment. This approach will be labeled type III and is illustrated:

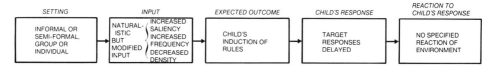

This method of modifying the input while retaining the integrity of the stimulus can be accomplished by increasing the *saliency* of the critical element of the input—emphasizing those characteristics of which the child needs to be made aware. Increasing the saliency does not change the basic structure of the language in a linguistic stimulus. It relies on the increase in the child's attention to and recognition of the information made available to him or her and on the corresponding ability of the child to use the information for changing his or her language behavior. The modification of the linguistic input by increasing the linguistic saliency also requires that the environmental structure change from a totally naturalistic one to one that is somewhat controlled by the specialist.

Another way of modifying the input in addition to increasing its saliency is to *organize* it in a manner that will facilitate discovery on the part of the child. The organization may involve repeatedly sequencing the elements of the input in such a form so as to draw attention to a particular target structure. The location of a target in words or sentences in variable contexts provides the emphasis needed for the child to induce the rule. The presentation of verbal input together with situational and conceptual meanings aids in semantic development while at the same time providing rule exemplars.

Quote 5–2
For such children, the interventionist serves as a facilitator whose activities present a body of linguistic data that is abnormally easy to analyze. To acheive this accessibility, he or she manipulates variables, such as the juxtaposition and proportional frequency of exemplars, the perceptual salience of key linguistic elements, the clarity of meaning-in-context, and the match between the focused-rule and the cognitive or linguistic resources of the child.

(JOHNSTON, 1983, p. 54).

One example of a type III input-oriented approach is the modeling approach originally developed by Bandura and Harris (1966). (The modeling approach, which takes many forms, is often structured rather than purely naturalistic. For this reason I have also included it in the Type IV approach.) The child listens to numerous different inputs, all of which include the language behavior being taught, within well-formed sentences or phrases. The child is expected to induce the underlying structure—not imitate the various examples provided by the input. The actual use by the child may come in a speech event that temporally follows the original modeling situation but after some delay. (Success with modeling procedures has been reported by Leonard, 1975; Courtright & Courtright, 1976, 1979; Muma, 1978.)

In the three intervention types that depend on the system of the child to internalize, reconstruct, and formulate linguistic rules and that minimize the role of the specialist, one in which the specialist provides the stimuli to trigger the child's system, there is no expectancy regarding the immediate response of the child. In fact, this approach recognizes the time needed to develop rules from input, and therefore the child's language is not predicted to change until well after specific stimuli have been presented. In other words, time must be provided for the child to restructure before incorporating new material into his or her system. Therefore, the child does not need to respond immediately, nor is the child encouraged to do so. In the input-oriented approaches, the specialist is truly a facilitator—there is no direct teaching involved or any attempt to manipulate the child's response system. The specialist simply tries to make it easier for the child to use his or her own system to learn.

Intervention procedures that are completely input-oriented and require no specific response on the part of the child usually produce no awareness on the part of the child regarding his or her own language. In the response-oriented approaches to be described in the next section, there begins to be an awareness on the part of the child that the specialist is attempting to modify the child's response. The child at that point begins to use his or her metalinguistic skills to monitor and change his or her own language patterns. It should be noted that as the specialist increases the degree of modification of the input, the approach moves away from the purely naturalistic to a more didactic one. There is also movement away from a child's control over his or her own selection and induction of language to direction and guidance from the environment.

RESPONSE-ORIENTED APPROACHES

The response-oriented approaches to be described in this section differ from the totally naturalistic ones that have little or no linguistic or

> *Quote 5–3*
> *The following sequence of interventions is implemented in the context of stimulating interest centers.*
>
> - *The facilitator imitates and participates in the child's sensory exploration.*
> - *The facilitator provides tactile and affective stimulation.*
> - *The facilitator initiates sensory exploration.*
> - *Exploratory experiences are accompanied by simple oral language contacts by the facilitator.*
> - *The facilitator attracts attention to a dimension of the environment by creating a change or disturbance while encouraging the child's verbal interaction.*
> - *The facilitator mirrors what the child is doing by describing what is figural to the child.*
> - *The facilitator assumes the role of playmate for the child and leads the interaction while describing the here and now activities.*
> - *The facilitator creates an added verbal dimension for the child to consider during the interaction.*
> - *The facilitator poses a dilemma asking for the child's help to resolve a problem.*
> - *The facilitator draws attention to physical, temporal, and spatial relationships.*
> - *The facilitator presents contradictory responses in dialogue with the child to create disequilibrium.*
> - *The facilitator provides support and encourages the child's verbal interaction when the child engages in conflict.*
>
> (Taenzer, Cermak, & Hanlon, 1981, p. 45).

situational structure. There are differences in the degree of structure of the input, expected response, and reinforcement and differences in the degree of activity on the part of the child. Because the plans in response-oriented approaches are specific relative to the expected responses of children, they are said to be tightly scripted. Even within the category of tightly scripted approaches, however, there are different degrees of structure that are utilized. The most structured in all variables is found in behavioral theory.

Response-oriented approaches imply that language disorders may be either rule-based or performance-based. Response-oriented approaches are those that rely on the premise that, although language is induced by a child, the defective system needs the input to be modified in such a manner so as to provide many experiences with a target within varied contexts and/or to allow the system to respond in less complex response units if necessary. This approach is also based on the premise

> *Quote 5–4*
> *The type of approach used to facilitate delayed language should be different from the approach used to remediate the unsystematic and/or nonsequential language acquisition.*
>
> (Lucas, 1980, p. 75).

that learning occurs gradually, and so response expectancies should be graded. Initially, the expected response may be one of pointing, matching, or selecting. In other words, the input units provided and the responses required allow the child to internalize and perform the rules at a rate and in units that the child's system can handle. A response approach also recognizes that concentrated practice is needed for performance to become automatic. It is not enough to induce a rule; performance must become easy, efficient, and automatic.

The input units in the response approach may be syntactic, semantic or pragmatic, the pairing of surface structure with events, or whatever other skill is needed. The internal structure of the linguistic input may be modified in the direction of simplification. Because of the need to control the input and the response, the context for teaching may be semiformal and/or semistructured. And because a specific response is elicited and expected, there is no delay in the child's response; it follows immediately after the input.

It should be noted that instruction in both the input-oriented and response-oriented approaches are teacher-directed. The teacher direction in the input-oriented approach is covert; it takes the form of establishing general goals for each child and provides broad input bombardment of a naturalistic nature in order to stimulate the child's own language acquisition skills. Teacher direction in response-oriented approaches is overt, directed toward specific goals using specific, graded activities and requiring a large number of graded responses from the child. The assumption in the response-oriented approach is that the child's own system either is not inducing the rules adequately or cannot easily learn to perform language efficiently, accurately, and automatically. Therefore, no amount of input and facilitation will cause language to improve if there is not also some structure in both the input and response to assist the child in learning. Allowance for a graded response may be necessary in intervention for productive language because it may be difficult for the child to retrieve and handle productively all the grammatical aspects of an utterance in addition to the targeted form or lexical item.

Type IV Approach

The type IV approach is a response-oriented approach in which the specialist modifies the linguistic input and permits a graded response from the child. One method of grading the input and therefore controlling the response is expansion; the child's own output is used as a basis for the specialist's input to the child. The child's output is modified slightly and modeled back to the child in the direction of increased grammaticality, or the specialist verbalizes the child's intent prior to the child's act. Other ways of using the child's output for the specialist's elaboration are expatiation which elaborates or broadens the topic, and alternation, which deals with the underlying logic of an utterance (Muma & Pierce, 1981). Expatiation allows the child to control the discourse topic, while the adult comments on it. This approach also ensures that the adult remains within the semantic knowledge boundaries of the child. Nelson (1975) suggests a form of expatiation called *recasting* in which the adult listens to the child's utterance and then reformulates it using different syntactic forms while retaining the semantic aspects. She suggests that this approach has a positive effect on the development of certain syntactic forms.

The following are techniques initiated by the specialist (although the child's own language may be used) that reduce the complexity of the input and the consequent response of the child or may allow for creative responses (Muma, 1978):

1. Completion—in which sentences or other units derived from a child are presented to the child with something missing and the child is asked to complete the input in varied ways;
2. Replacement—in which the child replaces portions of a structure;
3. Combination—in which a child is asked to combine two or more sentences in different ways, etc.

Support for the child's responses, a method of providing a crutch when a child cannot respond without help, is also suggested by Muma (1978). This support may be in the form of parallel talking, cueing (verbal or contextual prompts), or buffering—allowing the child to "back up" a form he or she does not know with one he or she does, as in "Daddy, he go."

Support for assisting the child in sequencing the content of a story or narrative can be provided by pictures illustrating the content sequence. Support for semantic expansion of words can be accomplished by requesting that the child describe fully all characteristics of objects, by requesting classification of objects and words, and so on. The input and expected response in semantic development differs from that in syntax development. Semantic development relies heavily on the pairing of *events* and *objects* in the environment with linguistic forms and the use of this pairing as input.

In general the type IV approach provides acceptance or nonacceptance of the child's behavior, language, or communication by subtle or explicit reactions to the child's attempts. Acceptance that includes new information provides a bridge for continuing the communication (Wells, 1981). If the acceptance is supported by prompts for more information to be provided by the child, it is referred to as "turnabout" (Kaye & Chainey, 1981). Nonacceptance techniques may take a form that is ultimately helpful to the child instead of causing a communication breakdown. If a clinician intentionally misunderstands a child's inaccurate production of a target, the child may try to revise in order to improve communication (Weiner & Ostrowski, 1979). Others (Weitzner-Lin & Duchan, 1982) suggest that a "puzzled look" or "expectant waiting" may be a sufficient stimulus for revision.

The type IV response-oriented approach described above is illustrated as follows:

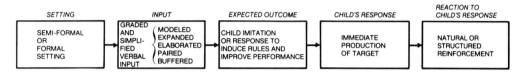

Within the same type of approach are other methodologies for increasing ease in response. These involve methods that provide means of improving access to and retrieval of words and structures as is done by association, chunking (grouping certain units together), and imitation, which if used sparingly can allow internalization of wholes to be later separated into units by the child. (Bruner [1974] suggests the memorization allows internalization of the rules that a child can use later in a narrative of his or her own.) Winitz (1983) cautions that if the form that is presented to the child is at the level of the child's language and the child's language is at the two-word level, it is difficult to maintain a realistic communicative experience. He suggests that short grammatically correct sentences be used as stimulus although only two words are expected from the child. He also suggests that since the response-oriented approach stresses expression, care must be taken not to force production of specific language forms in a way that is not comparable to the manner in which children normally begin to use language.

In working with adolescents, the method of instruction is often structured in both the input and response modalities, and in many instances the written language form is used. Materials are structured so that the adolescent can learn systematically using self-study methods.

It is possible for the child to be an active learner in the type IV approach if the language specialist allows the child to participate in topic selection and if those language forms are selected for intervention that have particular meaning for the child or are based on the child's needs. The addition of structure does not mean that the child must be passive.

Type V Approach

Another type of approach in the response-oriented group is that of behaviorism. It differs significantly in the degree of structure and in specificity from the type IV approach. Very specific verbal stimulus materials are provided and equally specific responses are expected. Only those responses that satisfy the specifications are reinforced. When the input is specific and considered to be a stimulus and the expected response is specified also, and when there is a scheduled program of reinforcement and this sequence occurs in a planned manner in a structured environment, the approach is called behavioral modification. I will classify this approach as type V.

A modification of the behavioral approach that "teaches" in the child's natural environment and is defined as a naturalistic approach is called by its proponents, *incidental teaching* (Warren & Kaiser, 1986b). Although behavioristic in principle, it draws from the other types of intervention previously presented. The interactions in this approach between the adult and child arise naturally in an unstructured situation as opposed to what happens in traditional behavioral modification where the stimulus originates with the adult. In fact, the child controls the instances in which the teaching occurs by initiating the interaction in the process of trying to obtain something from the environment. (The environment can be arranged beforehand to increase the likelihood that the child will initiate requests.) The child thus provides the topic and the opportunity for the adult to transmit new information. The adult uses increasingly specific prompts to ensure the use of the preselected target. Modeling, shaping, and contingent reinforcement are utilized to provide multiple exemplars and multiple opportunities for practice. Warren and Kaiser (1986b) suggest that incidental teaching reinforces the child's communicative attempts as well as encourages the use of specific forms and providing for cross-modal transfer, the spontaneous production of previously heard utterances through processes associated with generalized imitation.

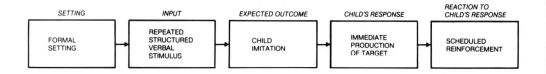

SETTING	INPUT	EXPECTED OUTCOME	CHILD'S RESPONSE	REACTION TO CHILD'S RESPONSE
FORMAL SETTING	REPEATED STRUCTURED VERBAL STIMULUS	CHILD IMITATION	IMMEDIATE PRODUCTION OF TARGET	SCHEDULED REINFORCEMENT

INPUT-RESPONSE CYCLE APPROACH

Type VI Approach

An approach that utilizes both the input and response modes in interaction with others, I have termed the *input-response cycle approach*. It is also referred to as the *interactive approach* (Cole & Dale, 1986). Although on the surface it appears to resemble types I and II approaches, the interactive approach is more tightly scripted than the former two. A plan for interaction is specified with regard to pragmatic and linguistic goals that in turn require specific delineation of the cognitive content and topic. Essential to this approach is actual communicative exchanges involving a cycle of inputs to the child and the child's response.

Perhaps central to the difference between the interaction and the naturalistic approaches is that the naturalistic approach implies carrying out intervention in a naturalistic environment—with a group of children at play in the home. The interactive approach focuses on the "natural" communicative interactions between the child and others in the environment. The emphasis is not on *where* but on *how* (Craig, 1983). Interactive intervention may be naturalistic but not necessarily so.

An effective way of using response as an input in an interactive way is to allow a child to initiate language as an input to other children. The specialist asks a child to be teacher and to explain how to accomplish a specific task, for example, how to get to a specific place. The child's role of providing input to other children's responses has a twofold effect. A self-originated verbal response to one's own ideas is a level above responding to someone else's input with respect to complexity and mastery of specific forms or procedures. The child must be careful to explain fully so that the other children will get the correct message. There will be self-monitoring as the instructions are given and natural reinforcement if the task is accomplished successfully. Most classroom teachers will agree that their knowledge of something they thought they knew was increased during the process of teaching it.

Some specialists recommend placing barriers between the child serving as the "teacher-child" and the other children so that the listeners will not have visual access to objects or pictures that the "teacher-child" has. This tactic makes it necessary for the child giving directions or describing an event to increase the informativeness of his or her utterances and therefore to be exact in his or her choice of words. The greater the demands for accuracy placed on the system, the more effective the system will be in accomplishing the task. (Anyone who has tried to communicate in a foreign language over an international long distance call can attest to the improved ease in eliciting vocabulary and syntax that results from the demands made by the necessity to inform.)

This input-response cycle approach, which has its origins in pragmatic theory, uses the messages of real-life situations as the input to the child to which the child must respond by understanding and returning messages of his or her own. If the child's message is understood, his or her communication is naturally reinforced (Friel-Patti & Lougeay-Mottinger, 1986). If, however, the message is not understood, the child must modify his or her utterance—"fix the breakdown"—until it is clear to the listener (Duchan, 1986a). As the child concentrates on the delivery of a message, he or she tends to concentrate on those elements that will ensure the accomplishment of his or her purpose. The grammatical aspects of the message will be important to the child insofar as they clarify the meaning. Teaching or at least generalizing grammatical structures in this way is considered to be more effective than teaching them in isolation. Craig (1983) says that in this type of approach, "conversational and structural development are distinguishable but functionally inseparable . . ." (p. 103). This approach I have labelled as type VI.

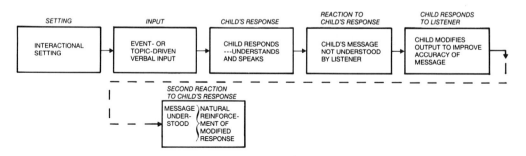

The input-response cycle is particularly effective when the goal of intervention is semantic rather than syntactic. This is especially true in developing or refining complex concepts and their corresponding vocabulary. The stimulus, which is originated by either the specialist or other children, produces not simply a one-to-one comprehension but demands responses that require cognitive processing, problem-solving, association, and causal reasoning. Exchanges that are cognitively oriented need structuring both linguistically and with reference to the topic. Carefully selected questions (such as *why* or *how* questions) provide a means for eliciting responses that require the involvement of cognitive processes and therefore the use of semantically rich language.

Play has been suggested as a format for intervention of this type (Craig, 1983). Through the use of play, according to Craig, the specialist can provide a variety of experiences within which the child can learn the tasks that are targeted, experiences that appear natural and have the potential to recur. The focus on discourse in play allows a reciprocal interchange between the specialist and child and encourages the child to learn, indirectly and naturally rather than artificially, that central function of language, social communication.

Controlled storytelling as described by Lee, Koenigsknecht, and Mulhern (1975) bridges the latter two approaches. The stories that attempt to replicate naturalistic events, conversations, and settings are

> *Quote 5–5*
> An interactive model provides the clinician with a dynamic context for teaching language to young children. Language treatment based on play and daily life experience with an adult who provides modeling and expansion of the child's forms and meanings is similar to normal language processes.
> (KUNGE, LOCKHART, DIDOW, & CATERSON, 1983, p. 81).

controlled with respect to theme, characters, and events as well as to grammatical target forms; the latter are included a number of times in the story. Spontaneous responses are accepted and specific responses expected on request.

A procedure built on the structures imposed by events that occur in the child's environment (Nelson, 1986b) is also a good example of the type VI approach (see Chapter 10 for a description of this theory). Event structure includes the actors, actions, plot, sequences, and verbal interactions that are part of daily experiences such as eating and bathing. Nelson's hypothesis is that these events are represented in children's memories and the representations serve as the data for thinking and talking. Intervention based on event structure theory provides not only the verbal material for interaction but natural events in which the interactions may take place.

FACILITATION

It is impossible to identify the "true" meaning of the term *facilitation* from reading the current literature in language disorders. Early literature (Patterson & Cobb, 1971, 1973) described the concept of facilitating and inhibiting stimuli within the context of ongoing interaction. These authors referred to events with high sequential probabilities as facilitating stimuli and events associated with low sequential probabilities as inhibiting stimuli. Hubbell (1977), in exploring ways of facilitating spontaneous talking, reported data indicating that approval, physical positive behavior, and compliant behavior serve to inhibit spontaneous talking. In summarizing the work of Hetenyi (1974) and Seitz (1975), Hubbell (1977) concluded that verbal interaction is more important than verbal stimulation in children's language development. Hubbell defines facilitation as "interacting with the child by following the child's lead in play and talking, using verbal techniques such as labeling, expansion, and parallel talking" (p. 225). Hubbell cautions that the data be interpreted within the boundaries of the goal of spontaneous talking at the early stages of language development. Others, says Hubbell, such as children with specific processing problems, may not be able to benefit from a facilitative approach.

Presently the term *facilitation* is used to describe all types of procedures from the naturalistic ones to those that emphasize response elicitation and feedback. Perhaps facilitation is not being used as a descriptive term for a specific way of carrying out intervention as much as a term to use instead of others for what we have been doing all along. The current opinion appears to be that as long as we do not use the terms *stimulus*, *schedule of reinforcement*, *operant*, and others like them, we are on safe ground. In some instances, after careful descriptions of language acquisition as a self-generated and self-directed process that requires only a trigger from the environment, and after describing the role of the specialist as a facilitator who simply manipulates the environment in a manner that the child's system can more easily induce the rules, intervention is said to be a process of eliciting responses from the child, reinforcing them, and providing feedback to the child. I do not disagree entirely with the latter approach to intervention; I only caution that it is necessary to clarify terms and specify behaviors rather than to camouflage and elevate them by using currently acceptable terminology. In other words, there needs to be consistency from theory to practice.

LANGUAGE INTERVENTION—THE MIDDLE GROUND

Some of the literature in language intervention has described intervention in terms of two major approaches, each representing opposite theoretical positions. On one side is the position that behaviors emerge or are acquired relatively exclusively by the executor within the child who selects and induces from the environment the rules of language. The interventionist's role is to provide the trigger or to facilitate what is happening in the child (linguistic position). At the other extreme is a system that ignores internal factors, instead using a rigid system of providing linguistic stimuli and reinforcing the response so that language behaviors can be learned (behavioral position). These two approaches are referred to as *interactive language instruction* and *direct language instruction* by Cole and Dale (1986), who have described the characteristics of each approach.

As illustrated in this chapter, the truth of the manner in which intervention is actually carried out is probably somewhere in between. Perhaps also is the truth as to how it *should* be carried out. The definitions of language on which these two positions (Cole & Dale, 1986)

Quote 5–6
Direct-language instruction and interactive instruction appear to give comparable effects in facilitating language skills in language-handicapped preschool children. Neither program appears to be superior overall, for either specific aspects of language development or for subgroups of children identified by degree of language delay or cognitive ability . . .

. . . it is also possible that a merging of the two models [direct instruction and interactive instruction] would be more effective than the exclusive use of either. A concept or language structure might be presented initially using direct instruction for rapid acquisition and later extended using interactive methods for generalization to a variety of contexts.

(COLE & DALE, 1986, p. 215).

are based are definitions of two of the language theories described in this book. In subsequent chapters, I will suggest how these and other theories of language can be expanded to account for the various facets of language and its disorders. Once we have a clearer notion of language and its disorders, we will have a more accurate framework within which to describe intervention.

Perhaps an even better way to think of the truth of intervention than as a middle ground is to recognize that one type of intervention may be better suited and valid for one type of child than another (see Table 5–1 for a summary of the intervention approach types). Type I intervention approach, the completely naturalistic one, may be suited for children who have normal inductive processes, but who are delayed in language development for whatever reason; these children may need additional experience with exemplars. Types II and III intervention approaches may be for children whose attention or inductive processes do not function with precision and who need help in drawing attention to specific rules. Both of these approaches are facilitative.

There are some children who do not induce well at all and need "crutches" to learn in a somewhat artificial manner what most children learn from exposure. Others may have performance problems rather than rule-based problems. Even when they know the rules, they may have difficulty producing language efficiently and automatically. These children may profit from the directness of a type IV intervention approach.

Type V, the behaviorist approach, may be suitable for children whose behavior and level of performance is sufficiently impaired that complete structure and conditioning is the only way to bring about change in language. Craig (1983) suggests that a combination of operant conditioning and structural and conversational goals may be the most tenable procedure for low-functioning broadly impaired individuals.

All children can profit from use of the type VI approach, the interactive approach. This method works well for generalization and stabilization and more closely replicates the natural language-learning environment of children. The interactive approach should be included as a part of every intervention progam as the basic framework from which procedures evolve and as the goal toward which the procedures are directed.

The use of the interactive or pragmatic approach in intervention needs to take into account the specific needs of language-impaired children. Problems may arise in basing the entire intervention process on the assumption that language-disordered children learn in the same way as children without such problems. Recent literature emphasizes the nurturant-naturalistic approach to intervention (Taenzer, Cermak, & Hanlon, 1981; McLean & Snyder-McLean, 1984; Fey, 1986) that replicates the context in which normal children develop language.

TABLE 5–1.   DESCRIPTION OF VARIABLES CLASSIFIED BY SIX INTERVENTION TYPES ASSOCIATED WITH INTERVENTION APPROACHES

VARIABLES	APPROACH TYPES					
	NATURALISTIC ◄─────────────────────────────────► STRUCTURED					
	INPUT-ORIENTED			RESPONSE-ORIENTED		INPUT-RESPONCE CYCLE
	TYPE I	TYPE II	TYPE III	TYPE IV	TYPE V	TYPE VI
Setting	Informal group	Informal or semiformal, group	Informal or semiformal group or individual	Semiformal or formal setting, group or individual	Formal setting	Interactional setting either naturalistic or formal
Input	Totally naturalistic	Naturalistic but topic and content controlled linguistic input	Naturalistic but modified input to increase saliency and frequency	Graded and simplified verbal input modeled, expanded, etc.	Repeated structured verbal stimuli	Event- or topic-driven verbal input message
Expected Outcome	Child's induction of linguistic rules	Child's induction of linguistic rules	Child's induction of linguistic rules	Child imitates or responds to induce rules and improve performance	Child imitates	Child develops communicative competence
Child's Response	Target responses delayed	Target responses delayed	Target responses delayed	Immediate production of target	Immediate production of target	Child responds, understands message, and speaks
Reaction to Child's Response	No specified reaction—continuation of activity, or communication	No specified reaction of environment, continuation of activity, or communication	No specified reaction of environment, continuation of activity, or communication	Natural or structured reinforcement	Scheduled reinforcement	Child's message not understood by listener
Child's Response to Listener	No specified reaction—continuation of activity, or communication	No specified reaction of environment, continuation of activity, or communication	No specified reaction of environment, continuation of activity, or communication	None specified	None specified	Child modifies output to improve accuracy of message
Second Reaction to Child's Response	No specified reaction—continuation of activity, or communication	No specified reaction of environment, continuation of activity or communication	No specified reaction of environment, continuation of activity, or communication	None specified	None specified	Message understood—natural reinforcement of modified response

Connell (1987), however, found that two teaching procedures, imitation and modeling, had opposite relative effects on a group of language-impaired children compared with children who were learning language normally. The language-impaired children showed better generalization of an invented morpheme when the instruction used imitation than when the instruction used modeling. The reverse was true for the children with normal language. Connell concluded that language-impaired children benefit more from teaching strategies that are adapted to their unique learning style than from those fashioned after the style of children who learn language normally. Perhaps discussions in subsequent chapters of this book can help to identify some aspects of language that need special consideration in working with language-impaired children.

The approaches to intervention will also vary with the child's stage of language development. Children at the level of emerging language may profit from naturalistic, developmental, and interactive methods. As children's language becomes more complex, some structure, at least in the environment, may need to be introduced. Children who have acquired most of the language rules and use them with efficiency may have "fossilized" errors or residuals of previous problems in language. A direct approach would probably be more efficient than a naturalistic one, although the principles of interaction and meaningfulness would need to be adhered to.

The important and critical task is to match the approach to the needs of the child. I have seen a situation where what is now called *productive language intervention* was used with a child who echoed language without understanding the language of either himself or others. The child just kept imitating the input. Why would anyone work on production when the obvious need of the child was to understand?

The needs of the child may vary with the particular task that he or she is learning. It may be helpful to switch instructional strategies, working in a naturalistic mode in the beginning of intervention and then, at the level of establishing an effortless and automatic performance, changing to more structured techniques. Or the reverse may be appropriate: we may need to switch from tight scripts to loose ones. In subsequent chapters, I will argue for a broad interpretation of language and language disorders. If our definitions and theory of language include performing as well as knowing behaviors, conceptual as well as linguistic components, the instructional methods we use and find effective will more accurately match our theory.

SECTION II

Integrating Theoretical Issues

The review of theories in the first five chapters has illustrated that each theory has made and still makes significant contributions to the field of language disorders, but in the application of theories to assessment and intervention, none can stand alone. If it were possible to integrate specific theoretical issues in a manner that is logical, a better framework for working with language-disordered children might be generated. Integration does not mean combining parts of different theories to resemble a theoretical potpourri. Integration must entail a cohesive weaving of parts supported by logic and capable of accounting for the totality of the communication system.

Rather than attempting to integrate the entire spectrum of language theory at one time, however, language specialists need to focus attention on subparts of a cohesive paradigm and do so in detail and in depth, mustering whatever empirical evidence is available to support their positions. Close examination of specific issues may help to integrate apparent disparities among divergent theories, bring theory and practice into closer agreement, and contribute to the development of an umbrella paradigm.

The following six chapters describe specific issues that are of significance in work with the language-disordered child and on which theories often differ. Each chapter will describe the issue and attempt either an integration of different viewpoints or an acceptance of a specific viewpoint. The effect of an integration or of a particular position on assessment and intervention will be described.

In Chapter 6 I argue for the distinction between knowledge and performance and support this distinction with data from language-disorder literature. Chapter 7 attempts to describe the components of language and speculates how these components may be organized in relation to each other. The role of auditory processing in language and its disorders is presented in Chapter 8.

Chapter 9 points out the importance of understanding the role comprehension plays in language and consequently in the intervention of language with disordered children. The positions regarding language development, the interactive and the constructionist, are reviewed in Chapter 10. An attempt at pointing out commonalities and differences between oral and written language makes up Chapter 11.

6

INTEGRATING THEORIES: THE ISSUE OF KNOWLEDGE AND PERFORMANCE

A theoretical issue that deserves careful attention because of the implications to clinical practice is the issue of the knowledge/performance distinction in language. This issue will be discussed here and my position regarding this issue will be presented. An attempt will be made to integrate the various theoretical positions describing language knowledge and language performance.

THE KNOWLEDGE/ PERFORMANCE DISTINCTION

Some Historic Interpretations

Although some language specialists take for granted the distinction between language knowledge and language performance, others believe that such a distinction is artificial. Illustrative of the position that there is

THEORY, ASSESSMENT AND INTERVENTION
IN LANGUAGE DISORDERS: © 1988 by Grune & Stratton
AN INTEGRATIVE APPROACH

ISBN   0-8089-1918-0
All rights reserved.

and should be a distinction between knowledge and performance is Kean's statement (1982): "It is taken here as an obvious and necessary assumption of the study of human linguistic capacity that a human being with normal mature command of his native language both knows something (his native language) and can use that knowledge to produce and comprehend sentences" (p. 176). Chomsky's (1980) claim supports that of Kean; he has stated that in theory one could know a language without having the capacity to use the internally-represented knowledge and also that a person might increase his or her capacity while gaining no new knowledge. Fodor (1983) believed it obvious that knowledge does not become behavior by virtue of its content, but that mechanisms exist that will bring the behavior and the propositional structures that are cognized into conformity.

Bever (1970), on the other hand, rejects the claim that a linguistic grammar is in any sense "internal to such linguistic performances as talking and listening" (p. 344). Bever further suggests that such a distinction has no functional value in understanding children's language.

Figure 6–1 shows useful distinctions in knowledge/performance classification of language behavior. Basically, linguistic theory describes

KNOWLEDGE	What is known	• Language rules—grammer, semantic and pragmatic • Language meaning—concepts and ideas associated with linguistic forms • Non-linguistic content
	Act or process of knowing	• Discovery • Rule Formation • Pattern Analysis • Rule Access • Representation, etc.
PERFORMANCE	What is performed	• Speaking (signing) • Comprehension (auditory) • Writing • Reading
	Act or process of performing	• Attention • Preception • Memory • Parsing • Recognition • Recall • Retrieval • Formulation, etc.

FIGURE 6–1. Useful distinctions in knowledge/performance classification of language behavior.

> *Quote 6–1*
> *In collecting my thoughts about competence and performance, I began with a strong suspicion that these words mean different things to different people, and that much of the disagreement that this distinction has inspired in recent years could be understood if we thought in terms of people who believed they were talking about the same thing but really weren't.*
> (MILLER, 1975, p. 201).

the *knowledge* of the linguistic rules governing syntax, semantics, and pragmatics as language. The information process and cognitive organization theories describe, in addition to that of language knowledge, the internal processes involved in *performing* language (as opposed to the behavior of speaking, the speech act), in which a learner through his or her own action develops strategies for processing language and then can actually speak; the knowledge is of doing as well as of rules. If we theorize that language is knowing something, knowing how to do it, and being able to do it efficiently, language behavior can be described as being generated from the *knowledge* of abstract rules and executed by *performance* strategies. This integrative view might describe language knowledge as (1) the rules that form the syntactic construction of phonological or semantic patterns, and (2) the system of object-references and thematic relations (Chomsky, 1980). This knowledge forms the data base of the language. The integrative view might then describe language performance as the means and strategies by which the input is analyzed and stored and the data base is searched, accessed, retrieved, and passed through the input-output system (see Fig. 6–2).

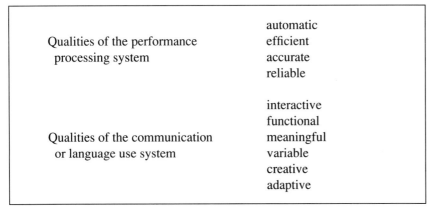

Qualities of the performance processing system	automatic efficient accurate reliable
Qualities of the communication or language use system	interactive functional meaningful variable creative adaptive

FIGURE 6–2. Qualities of the performance and communication systems.

> *Quote 6–2*
> *In the language-disordered child, it is not sufficient to describe only the linguistic behavior of structure, and through it, semantics and use; the constituent skills involved in acquiring and using language are important to the definition of disorder.*
> (CARROW-WOOLFOLK & LYNCH, 1982, p. 203).

If there is evidence for a knowledge/performance distinction, the importance to the field of language disorders of establishing support for it cannot be overestimated. The logical corollary of such a distinction is that deviant language may not be exclusively related to impairment of linguistic knowledge (rules) or for that matter to impairment of linguistic capacity (performance). If language comprehension and production are determined to some extent by linguistic performance strategies as well as by language knowledge, language disorders may be a function of deficits in linguistic knowledge *or* deficits in linguistic performance. If this is found to be a defensible position, the procedures involved in language assessment and intervention should reflect the role of the cognitive system in performing language as well as its role in rule acquisition. In other words, the analysis of language disorders and their management should reflect the complexity and number of the processes that undergird language.

A language model that distinguishes between knowledge and performance is useful in explaining or describing the four domains of language—reading, writing, listening, and speaking—as well as explaining the similarity and differences in language knowledge and performance among individuals with disordered language, such as those having hearing impairment, and individuals who are bilingual (Carrow-Woolfolk & Lynch, 1982).

This chapter seeks to establish the logical validity of a distinction between language knowledge and language performance and to suggest procedure differences in language assessment and intervention that may evolve from the consideration of knowledge and performance as separate neuropsychological behaviors.

Terminology and Points of View

Although in psychological measurement literature, the term *performance* has referred to nonverbal behaviors (i.e., WISC Picture Arrangement and Picture Completion [Wechsler, 1974]) as opposed to verbal behaviors (i.e., WISC Repeating Digits and Vocabulary), the term *performance* in psycholinguistic literature has a different interpretation. Psycholinguists have distinguished between competence and performance. This distinction was originally hypothesized in generative

> *Quote 6–3*
> *The present framework permits the introduction of constructs such as compensatory strategies and task constraints for defining developmental language disorders. These are performance rather than competence issues, but constitute an elaboration of Chomsky's description of performance beyond memory and attention factors. The theoretical framework for understanding developmental language disorders presented in this paper suggests that they are more profitably viewed as a disorder of performance rather than competence.*
> (KIRCHNER & SKARAKIS-DOYLE, 1983, p. 230).

grammar, to wit, that *competence* was a set of highly restricted generative language rules or abstract mental structures that an individual operates on when he or she *performs* the language (Chomsky, 1965). In this context, errors made in the application of the rules were considered errors in performance; these errors were due to the limitations in performance imposed by the organization and limits of an individual's memory.

A later period in psycholinguistic theory found psycholinguists disagreeing with Chomsky's conception of competence and performance. Bever (1970), commenting on the artificiality of the distinction, suggested that the focus on knowledge that distinguishes it from the manner in which the knowledge is used ignores the fact that developmentally, the child's knowledge of linguistic structure is partially determined by his or her performance of language—by those processes that are involved in its acquisition. Bever further rejected the claim that a linguistic grammar is in any sense internal to such linguistic behaviors as comprehension and expression. In fact, he appeared to be suggesting that the behavior strategies that make the perception and production of sentences efficient are part of competence.

Bloom and Lahey (1978), while in essence agreeing with Bever, replaced the term language *performance* with that of language *use*. They stated that "knowledge about the use of language is knowledge about knowledge and a part of competence" (p. 60). The use of language, according to Bloom and Lahey, includes not only the nonvariant rules that govern specific use but also those that vary with linguistic and nonlin-

> *Quote 6–4*
> *The integration of content/form/use makes up language competence or knowledge. Such knowledge can be conceived of as a plan for the behaviors involved in speaking and understanding messages . . . At the same time that the plan directs the individual's behavior, it is, itself, evolving and changing as a result of those behaviors. Children learn language as they use language, both to produce and understand messages.*
> (BLOOM & LAHEY, 1978, p. 23).

guistic context. This position was taken earlier by Labov (1969), who stated that the variable rules, resulting from fluctuations in actual production and comprehension, are distributed in regular ways, and by Cedergren and Sankoff (1974), who considered such regularities of variations as part of competence.

This interpretation of performance (as a performance act, the interpretation that considers performance as an integral and not distinctive part of linguistic knowledge and interprets the term within the context of language *use* as per Bloom and Lahey) appears to be beyond that of Chomsky's original definition of the performance process, which referred to the effects of behaviors such as perception and memory. Chomsky apparently was describing internal processing means and strategies by which language knowledge is stored and then analyzed, searched, accessed, retrieved, and passed through the input-output channels. Bloom and Lahey's term *use* was expanded to include the idiosyncratic concatenations of grammatical forms selected by the individual to communicate intended ideas and the situational and contextual restraints on the utterance of messages. The conclusions of Bloom and Lahey based on their interpretation of the term *use* argue against the need for a knowledge-performance distinction. According to their view, the language competence of individuals should include not only knowledge of language rules, the adequacy of which are dependent on the processes used for acquiring them, and not only behavioral strategies for performing language, but also the idiosyncratic variations in their language use that result from factors within and external to themselves and that contribute to the manner in which they speak and understand.

In the documentation of language behaviors of the normal developing child, the position of Bloom and Lahey, Labov, and Cedergren and Sankoff is defensible. The description of the developmental stages of children's language should be based on what children do, and the variations among children, whatever the reasons for the differences, should be part of the distributional characteristics of the language. The synergy of language should be the focus of study of normal language. Perhaps in studies of normal children, the position is acceptable because the processing systems through which children perform language are considered to be essentially normal. A normal child's language is judged and described on the basis of the language behavior itself. One need only study the speech act to determine the nature of the child's competence. This position is not as defensible when applied to language-disordered children. In terms of interaction, it does make a difference if a child's language problem is related to the child's linguistic rule system, to his or her strategies for accessing the rules and to the cognitive underpinnings of meaning, or to the mechanisms by which nonverbal events (sound) are translated into linguistic ones. This information may not be apparent in the corpus of a child's spontaneous speech.

> *Quote 6–5*
> *While the grammatical rules make possible the extrapolation of new sentences from old ones, the system of behavioral strategies make more efficient the* **perception** *and* **production** *of sentences.*
> (BEVER, 1970, p. 312).

In working with language-disordered children we may need a theoretical perspective that takes both aspects of language into account, one that views knowledge and the performance process as separate components of language. Achieving this perspective would entail an integration of the linguistic and cognitive descriptions of language. The linguistic theorist describes language as the knowledge of linguistic rules governing syntax, semantics, and pragmatics that a child, on exposure to the rules, acquires through induction, self-regulation, and organization. The cognitive theorists, in addition, describe the process of performing language, in which a young learner through an active process develops rules and strategies for comprehending and producing language and then learns to produce language in an accurate and efficient manner. If we theorize that language is knowing something and doing something, then knowing language behavior can be described as being generated from the knowledge of abstract rules and the doing involves the execution of language by performance strategies. In this book when the term *performance* is used, it refers to the internal performance processes just described.

Empirical Support for a Distinction

A first argument in support of a knowledge/performance distinction is found in aphasia literature. Empirical and clinical studies of adult aphasics have demonstrated the selective disruption of processes in which language difficulty occurs in one input system such as reading, but not in another, such as aural comprehension. An example is a study by Goodenough, Zurif, and Weintraub (1977), who compared the recognition by Brocas aphasics of oral versus written presentation of grammatical articles (determiners). Three subjects clearly recognized an inappropriately used article in written but not oral form. Unless we hypothesize that there are separate language knowledge bases for the different domains of language, the difference in responses to oral and written linguistic events in these aphasics must be attributed to differences in language performance or site of lesion and not to differences in language knowledge.

If we question whether both the oral and the written performances were undergirded by the same knowledge base in this study, we find the evidence in favor of a single knowledge system. In second-language learning, in which the performance system is demonstrably intact in the native language, a defective rule system in the second language is evident in *both* oral and written language. A single rule system governs both input and output modalities and both oral and written domains. The problems in the second language derive from inadequate knowledge of the rules of that language, not from performance inadequacies.

Another argument for the knowledge/performance distinction is the occurrence of performance without knowledge and vice versa in some types of language disorders. Some level of performance is evident in the autistic child's ability to recall and repeat entire linguistic phrases in a grammatically correct fashion without "apparent" generative knowledge of the semantic or syntactic rules of the language. It appears that some autistic children receive, discriminate, and store language units and then utter these language units in grossly appropriate situations (Carrow-Woolfolk & Lynch, 1982). These children appear to have performance without knowledge. The apraxic child, on the other hand, may have knowledge without performance. McNeil and Kimelman (1986) state that there is evidence to support the premise that aphasics are language competent; their problem is one of language performance.

A third factor that may support the knowledge/performance distinction is the frequent occurrence of cognitive processing deficits in language-disordered children. The research literature describes numerous cognitive behaviors that may or may not be linguistic-specific and that are unrelated to linguistic knowledge itself, in which language-disordered children differ from normal language children. For example, studies by Tallal and Stark (1983) and Tallal and Piercy (1978) have demonstrated that some language-impaired children develop abnormally in their response to temporal and spectral cues and the rate they occur normally within speech. They found that the more deficient the language-impaired children are in this ability to process rapidly changing sensory information, the greater is their delay in receptive language. Although Tallal and her colleagues do not conclude that a causal relationship exists between the processing problems and language disorders, they recognize that both problems frequently co-exist. We might hypothesize that some language disorders may be related to some kinds of processing capacity deficits so that when the latter is constrained the former is impaired, thereby implying the existence of separate functions for knowledge and performance.

A fourth argument in support of a knowledge/performance distinction is that of the (apparent) relationship of the comprehensibility of an utterance to the type and degree of embeddedness of sentences. Using essentially the same grammatical structures in two sentences, the separate units of which can be understood by the average native speaker of the language, we can produce, by embedding, one sentence that is much

> *Quote 6–6*
> *All of us know from direct experience that occasionally this knowledge [which allows a person to produce and understand an unlimited number of sentences] becomes inaccessible to us, as when we fail to recall a particular word (that is just "on the tip of the tongue"), or when we are guilty of a solecism ("You must review your subscription by the fifth of the month in which you expire") or when we misunderstand a perfectly well-formed sentence ("The horse raced past the barn fell down"). There is thus a distinction to be made between the knowledge that makes it possible for us to speak and understand a language and the way in which we employ this knowledge in producing and comprehending actual utterances.*
>
> (HALLE, 1978, pp. xii-xiii).

more difficult to understand than another. The ability to decode embedded sentences would not appear to be related to the listener's knowledge of language rules but rather to his or her cognitive ability to identify and store temporarily the semantic units of each embedded portion of the utterance. Consequently, the ability to comprehend can be related to performance factors as well as to language knowledge.

Split-brain studies, as well as those related to dichotic listening, illustrate that the responses by an individual to linguistic stimuli vary with the ear or the side of the brain receiving the stimulus. If these process-dependent factors can influence the response to linguistic input, the performance system does appear to have a responsibility in language behavior that is separate from the operational knowledge of the rules of the language.

A last argument is the occurrence of speech errors in the expression of normal speakers. As Fromkin (1972) says, many transformations occur between the act of ideation and the final act of speaking. The fact that these normal speakers have "slips of the tongue" indicates that what we know and how we perform are not always in synchrony. The act of "performing" speech sometimes is at variance with the plans for execution.

MULTIFACETED ASPECTS OF KNOWLEDGE AND PERFORMANCE

The claim of a distinction between knowledge and performance carries with it an obligation to identify more clearly the elements involved in language knowledge and in language performance. To assume that this is a simple process is naive. Three questions that need to be addressed are: (1) Are there levels and kinds of language knowledge? (2) What are the shared knowledge/performance aspects of comprehension and expression? and (3) Where does performance stop and knowledge begin or vice versa?

Kirk (1983) differentiated between the act or process of knowing and that which is known by this process. The act or process of knowing includes such behaviors as attention, perception, memory, thinking, and problem-solving (planfulness, thinking, and automatization) and is essential to the development of most cognitive skills. For each specific domain of learning, Kirk suggested that two types of knowledge are acquired: (1) the learner learns how to learn the skills of that domain, including efficient strategies for discovering and using higher order structures, organizational principles, and sets of rules and for accessing the data base; and (2) the learner develops and expands a data base or store of available information proper to each domain. Kean (1982) described this data base in language as the *grammar* and because the grammar is a characterization of what it is to know a language, independent of the mechanisms of use of that language, it will contain in itself no access mechanisms. In the case of the various modalities of language (reading, writing, speaking, and listening), the data base may be the same; however, some of the particular skills necessary for accessing the base may differ.

As Bellugi, Poizner, and Zurif (1982) have stated, there are linguistic-specific and channel-specific aspects of language. The channel-specific aspects may include some of the basic cognitive operations such as perception and memory and some parts of the skills and strategies for using that modality to access language. The linguistic-specific aspects may include other processing strategies of discovery, access, and use, as well as the data base or knowledge of the rules. The linguistic-specific aspects would be the elements common to all linguistic components: reading, writing, speaking, and listening. The data base for language may also include the concepts that form language meaning, the relation of the concepts to the linguistic structure system, and the rules that govern that relationship between concepts and structure and the use of the language.

The term *channel-specific* (or modality-specific) is not meant to imply that all perceptual/cognitive operations are independent of language. There appear to be psychological operations, particularly in the auditory channel, that are unique to the tasks involved in converting nonlinguistic to linguistic phenomena (during the comprehension and expression of utterances). There are also certain characteristics of language behavior that appear to be the function of cognitive factors common to nonlinguistic operations and that may in fact be extrinsic to language (Caplan, 1982). Integration theories suggest that sensory modalities are separate from one another and originally specific, only becoming integrated during development by association with a common response such as language (Chapanis, 1977). Goodglass, Barton, and Kaplan (1968) suggested that intervening between stimulus presentation and meaning may be a modality-nonspecific process (a supramodal process). (The extent to which the aspects of the linguistic task may be modular-discrete and operating on unique sets of principles or non-modular and sharing in principles governing all cognitive behavior will be discussed in the next chapter.)

We find then that the concepts of language knowledge and language performance are not simple and unidimensional. The concept of language knowledge may include cognitive aspects as well as linguistic ones in the information storage systems. Some aspects of knowledge are proper to a specific domain (such as reading); other knowledge is common to all language domains. Some performance functions (the act or process of knowing language) are common to all sensory channels (linguistic-specific), but others (type of memory, perception) are unique to a single channel (channel-specific).

KNOWLEDGE/ PEFORMANCE AND COMPREHENSION/ PRODUCTION

An important issue to those who are concerned about the language-impaired is that of the relationship between comprehension and expression. What implication does the knowledge/performance distinction have on that relationship? To what extent do comprehension and expression share knowledge and how and at what level do they differ?

On the one hand, it may be proposed that there is an equivalence between comprehension and production in the area of language knowledge, as well as in some of the procedures in carrying out aspects of sentence processing. At some point these processes may also differ; Garrett (1982) suggested that they "differ incontrovertible at their 'extremities', if nothing more" (p. 209).

In terms of their equivalence, Frazier (1982) and Fodor and Frazier (1980) proposed that there is a common body of grammatical knowledge that might be accessed and utilized in both tasks. This shared knowledge may be, for example, in the form of information about the well-formedness constraints of the language; the information can be accessed in both comprehension and expression tasks. Furthermore,

> *Quote 6–7*
> *The evidence is, of course, scattered and of mixed character. Perhaps it is enough that it strongly suggests, even if it does not prove, a very similar organizational principle for comprehension and production systems—namely, that the decomposition of the processing system reflects the decomposition of language structure in linguistic rule systems. On this view, the architecture of the processing system for production and that for comprehension provides another instance of motivated convergence in the two systems.*
> (GARRETT, 1982, p. 223).

Frazier suggested that there may be a common set of procedures to *retrieve* grammatical information, to schedule the flow of information, and to monitor and direct the processors at specific points in the process.

In describing their theory of *incremental procedural grammar* for sentence formulation, Kempen and Hoenkamp (1987) compared perception and production. They concluded that syntactic parsing, which they consider to be part of the language perception (comprehension) process, is remarkably similar to syntactic formulating, a part of the language production (expression) process. The commonality, they said, is derived from the following: (1) formulating and parsing are both lexically driven—they operate from a base of syntactic information stored with individual words of the lexicon; (2) both processes construct a syntactic tree from the information with the words as terminal elements; and (3) both have facilities for expanding, from left to right, the syntactic trees. In addition to formulation, the other parts of the human sentence production system described by Kempen and Hoenkamp are conceptualizing or planning and articulating. The inference is that these latter two processes of production differ from processes involved in perception or comprehension. There are therefore common knowledge areas and performance differences between comprehension and production.

The knowledge of the meanings of language, the representations of the world, the ideas, the objects, and their interrelationship, are common to both comprehension and expression, although comprehension may require a greater breadth of knowledge insofar as the listener needs to understand whatever a speaker chooses to say, whereas the speaker usually chooses to express those ideas that are within the framework of what he or she knows.

The correspondence between production and comprehension appears evident also in the similar results obtained by both processes (comprehension and expression) in dealing with open and closed class vocabularies (see Chapter 7). When both comprehension and expression tests have been given to children, there is a high correlation between these two types of tests, indicating that they both tap a common factor (Carrow-Woolfolk, 1985).

Bloom and Lahey (1978) propose that understanding and speaking represent mutually dependent but different underlying processes and that the developmental gap that often exists during language acquisition varies from child to child and within the child at different times. They suggest that "knowing a word and knowing a grammar, and understanding structural speech and using structured speech, apparently represent different mental capacities" (pp. 243–244). (This will be discussed at length in Chapter 9.)

The argument that Bloom and Lahey provide for considering understanding and speaking as different processes is that children do not have to process the syntax form completely in order to comprehend the

> *Quote 6–8*
> *If, for example, one were to discover that the architecture of comprehension and production is the same, the interpretation may be that the organization of processing systems for language is more heavily determined by informational structure (e.g., that indicated by the rule system of grammar) than by modality-specific aspects of the physical representation of language.*
> (GARRETT, 1982, p. 210).

reference to semantic-syntactic relations when information is available in the situation context, but the children do need to know something about syntax of the language and semantic constraints in order to talk about such relations.

The most *significant* difference between production and comprehension behavior may be in the demands, peripheral to linguistic processing, that the task makes on the user of language. Basically, comprehension calls on recognition memory, whereas production depends on the retrieval of information in the absence of cues from the environment. When a child learns the meaning of a word—associates the phonemic sequence and the meaning it has for him or her—that child must have had experience with the meaning (real, vicarious, or verbal), must commit to memory the phonemic sequence that makes up the word, and must remember how the two, the word and meaning, are associated. If the memory for the phonemic sequence is not sufficiently strong, if the concepts associated with the word are not fully developed, or if the association between the word and its meaning has not been firmly established whereby one elicits the other, an individual will have difficulty with comprehension and expression. Comprehension will be, however, a less difficult task because the verbal stimulus of the speaker will give the listener a model or a cue to use in searching. And perhaps also, as Bloom and Lahey (1878) state, specific knowledge of semantic and syntactic relations is not as crucial to comprehending a message accurately as it is to generating one. In comprehension only half of the association—the meaning—needs to be recalled; the other half is available. Such a model or cue is not available in production. In speaking, an individual has a meaning to express, has to search for appropriate words and syntax without a cue to the phonemic characterization of the words, and has to produce words and word sequences with accuracy and efficiency. One would hypothesize that the former task is less complex in execution than the latter. However, the difference is in performance rather than in competence (although Bloom and Lahey might say there is also a difference in competence requirements for effective understanding and speaking behavior).

Support for the distinction between comprehension and expression is also provided by studies of errors (called speech errors) that occur in language formulation in the face of adequate comprehension for the specific structures that are in error. The literature that was previously referred to, which compares comprehension and production performance on language tests, also indicates that, although there is a significant correlation between the two processes, the relationship is sufficiently different to indicate some difference in the two processes (Carrow-Woolfolk, 1985). In a study by Kamhi, Catts, Koenig, and Lewis (1984) symbolic representational deficits were correlated with receptive language measures but not with expressive ones. They concluded that different factors might underlie receptive and expressive language deficits.

An indication of the importance of the comprehension processing system to the development of expressive language is found in the autistic child. Language experts believe that immediate echolalia in autistic children signals a lack of comprehension combined with some intent to communicate (Prizant, 1983). Even delayed echolalia appears to have communicative intent and utterances are often used in grossly appropriate situations. The autistic children seem to have segmentation processing difficulties with the language input and therefore inadequate storage for the individual elements of meaning. Intervention directed toward developing comprehension appears to improve their oral expression. Their oral language reflects their comprehension difficulties. In this sense, the poor performance in comprehension affects linguistic knowledge and therefore linguistic expression.

KNOWLEDGE/ PERFORMANCE AND LANGUAGE DEVELOPMENT

How do we describe the language acquisition process in the system that must deal with knowledge *and* performance?

In order to develop the *knowledge*, the child must *acquire* rule behavior. This acquisition involves the child's construction of behavior rather than the acquisition of responses. It is a process of *discovery* of complex relations between meaning and linguistic forms and discovery of organizational principles and sets of rules. The role of the adult is to "incline and incite" this discovery (Chomsky, 1980). The environment partially shapes, triggers, and facilitates the internally directed process; thus, the role of the environment is minimal.

To develop *performance ability*, the child must acquire skill behavior. He or she develops strategies for performing language with efficiency and ease. The child learns strategies of access to the data base, retrieval, and coding. Lastly, the child *automatizes* the production of language; he or she perfects the skill. Bruner (1974) states that if the attention that is necessary to regulate an act is reduced, the act is then incorporated into an act of a higher order and a longer-sequence act without disrupting the regulation of the higher-order act. Sternberg and Wagner (1982) suggest that many specific learning disabilities are related to failure to automatize learning skills. Children with these problems continue to perform in a controlled way—with conscious attention—tasks that should be automatic. When the attention is needed for controlled execution, it is not available for other uses. Controlled processing is considered by Sternberg and Wagner to be centrally executed. Since the central processing is needed for adaptations to new tasks, it needs to be replaced eventually by automatic or local processing. Local processing is primarily parallel—any number of local subsystems can operate at once. Ackerman and Dykman (1982) state that some mental operations are innately automatic, while others become automatic through extensive practice. There is some evidence, according to Ackerman and Dykman, that incomplete semantic automatization (naming speed) is in part responsible for the effortful semantic processing that is required in memory and reading comprehension. Repeated behavior is thus necessary for developing the skills. In the development of performance skills, adequate social relations are required if the child is to sustain, replicate, and repeat the intention-directed behavior of communication. The role of the environment in developing performance ability is significant.

KNOWLEDGE/PERFORMANCE AND LANGUAGE DISORDER

How do we describe language disorders, assessment, and intervention if we integrate knowledge and performance in our description of language? The task of assessment in this interpretation of language will be to differentiate between problems of language knowledge and problems in language performance. The study of language knowledge will include a study of the consistency with which specific rules are either not used or misused and a study of the rule relation between surface structure and meaning, meaning to include not only referential meaning but also such meaning as in inference and metaphors both in comprehension and expression. The study of performance, on the other hand, is separate from the determination that the knowledge of the rules is adequate or inadequate. The problem of performance is one of difficulty with using the code efficiently and correctly although the child may recognize the inadequacy. The assessment process needs to identify factors that exacerbate the performance problem, such as the length of the utterances, the complexity of the idea, or the particular situation in which the child is trying to communicate. At what point is there a breakdown in surface structure and under what conditions? In other words, is the communication breakdown and the message inadequacy a function of lack of knowledge of the rules governing the syntactic, semantic, and pragmatic behaviors of the child, or is it a function of lack of ability to perform the rules he or she knows because of poor retrieval, execution efficiency, poor automaticity, or other similar factors?

If we consider language as *knowledge of rules only*, then all language disorders are rule-based problems and all intervention is directed toward developing the rules. Since rule-behavior develops by means of the child's own construction and revision, the role of the clinician is to "incite and incline," to modify the input, and to facilitate.

If we consider language as knowledge of rules *and* performance capacity, we recognize that some language-disordered children, instead of or in addition to having rule-based problems, have problems in searching, in access or retrieval, or in automaticity. The development of skilled behavior in these areas becomes the focus of intervention. Practice is the key to improvement of performance problems. The role of the specialist is to set up meaningful experiences for this practice and to be more directive in intervention.

I believe that if we would visit intervention programs throughout the world, we would find language specialists attempting to facilitate children's acquisition of language rules. I believe we would also find language specialists teaching children to perform language with greater accuracy, ease, and automaticity. I believe, further, that language interventionists have clearly recognized the knowledge and performance distinction in disorders and have adopted intervention procedures accordingly. What has been lacking is a theory that addresses both aspects of language. I am sure it confuses the specialists to read about techniques that are exclusively dedicated to facilitation of rule acquisition if these specialists have within their case load children who do not appear to have a rule-based problem. In some respects, we may arrive at a valid theory of language by backing into it from study of its disorders.

INTEGRATING THEORIES: THE ISSUE OF LANGUAGE MODULARITY

NONMODULAR THEORY

MODULAR THOERY
   Evidence for Separating the Syntactic and
      Semantic Components
   Independence of Pragmatic Component

THE COGNITIVE MODULE AND LANGUAGE
   Relation between Form and Meaning
   Concepts as Schemata

INTERRELATIONSHIPS IN MODULAR THEORY

MODULAR THEORY AND LANGUAGE DISORDERS

   A second issue in language theory that has important implications to disorders, assessment, and intervention is that of the structure and the relationship among the components of language knowledge. The general position of linguistic theory is that language is a code that has syntactic (grammatic), semantic, and pragmatic aspects. Cognition is considered an integral part of language but nonlinguistic in nature. The role of cognition, according to the linguistic position, is primarily one of providing the prelinguistic foundations and the meaning for the linguistic code. This position clearly affects the choice of content in assessment and intervention, that of the linguistic code itself or even more specifically, the linguistic expression (production) of the language-disordered individual. Since cognition plays a secondary role in the theory of language, it also plays a secondary role in assessment and intervention.

THEORY, ASSESSMENT AND INTERVENTION
IN LANGUAGE DISORDERS: © 1988 by Grune & Stratton
AN INTEGRATIVE APPROACH

ISBN   0-8089-1918-0

> *Quote 7–1*
> . . . *we are assuming from the outset that there is something in-identifiable as* **language**, *which is conceptually and empirically separable from something else called* **cognition** *or* **thought**, *which is in turn distinct from another thing called* **social development** *or* **social interaction***.*
> (BATES, BENIGNI, BRETHERTON, CAMAIONI, & VOLTERRA, 1977, p. 257).

If we look at language from the viewpoint of pragmatic theory, we are concerned primarily with the speech act—the speaker intentions and listener effects. The language components are viewed in relation to their role in discourse and other forms of verbal interaction. The primary emphasis is on the pragmatic and semantic aspects of the language system. Although the cognitive system is considered important, the relation between the linguistic components and cognition is not explicitly defined.

If language specialists are to function with validity in the intervention context, the relations among the components of language should be clarified. To do this, we need to answer questions about the linguistic code itself as well as the relation of each aspect of the code to cognition. What are the intrinsic structural characteristics of each of the linguistic components—syntax, semantics, and pragmatics? Do these components follow a uniform system of emergence or do they differ, each having unique characteristics and lines of development? How does each of the linguistic components relate to cognition? Is cognition, in fact, extrinsic to the language? How can we characterize the relationship between the linguistic components and cognition? What type of organization can be hypothesized to describe the manner in which these components interact among themselves and with cognition? How does the theoretical position about the structure and relationship among components affect the way language disorders are described and the manner in which assessment and intervention are conducted?

These questions cannot be ignored. Obviously there would be fewer theoretical problems if we could. If the cognitive psychologists disagree, how can we hope to understand and explain cognition as it relates to language? Studies continue to demonstrate, however, that language-impaired children perform poorly on nonlinguistic tasks. Nelson, Kamhi, and Apel (1987) summarized findings showing poor performance by the language-impaired on anticipatory imagery tasks and symbolic play, and in solving visually presented discrimination learning tasks. In another study, Kamhi, Catts, Koenig, and Lewis (1984) found the language-impaired to be poorer than a control group similar to them in mental age on a haptic recognition task and a portion of a discrimination (nonlinguistic) learning task. Kirchner and Klatzky (1985) found the language impaired to have a broad deficit in processes related to short-term memory. Nelson, Kamhi, and Apel (1987) concluded that language-impaired children's linguistic and cognitive difficulties are caused by less capacity and efficiency in processing verbal *as well as* nonverbal information.

Two theories have been used as a basis for explaining the organizational structure of the cognition/language relationship: the nonmodular and the modular theories. Perhaps both have validity in explaining a portion of the relationship. These theories of cognitive organization are not presented as factual, empirically grounded positions but rather as plausible claims that may contribute to an understanding of language and to the development of new areas of research in language. Of the two, the modular theory has been more completely applied to language and hence will receive broader treatment here.

NONMODULAR THEORY

The application of nonmodular theory to the explication of language is not new. In many ways, Piaget's (1955) theory of language and the cognitive organization theory presented in this book can be said to be of the nonmodular type. According to this theory, the development of cognitive tasks is said to be uniform and undifferentiated at the starting point and across domains. Language is considered one of many cognitive tasks that pass through characteristic and similar operations in the process of learning. The cognitive faculties that are functionally distinguishable are viewed as horizontal (Fodor, 1983) insofar as they provide characteristic and similar patterns of transformations in the development and execution of the cognitive tasks. According to this position, examples of such mechanisms would be those of memory, judgment, and perception. A horizontal faculty such as memory, for example, would operate in a similar fashion across domains of a similar type, that is, either uniformly good or uniformly poor or unequal only because of the interaction of the faculties.

Piaget's *mental structures* could be viewed as falling into a nonmodular system. Mental structures are abstract organizational patterns that form an organizational principle operating across patterns of behavior. These structures are said to underlie and be common to the mental organization of all children and to evolve in a sequence of stages.

By using the nonmodular approach to explain cognitive learning tasks, we might identify some common processes of these tasks (Kirk, 1983):

1. Strategies for problem-solving,
2. Progressive reorganization of component parts, *à la* assimilation and accommodation, and
3. Attainment of two kinds of knowledge—complex relations and strategies for learning and doing.

The same processes are applied to whatever task is being learned, including language.

MODULAR THEORY

Since modular theory has adherents in linguistics and child language, it may be a useful theory for understanding language disorders. Of particular value is the manner in which the theory integrates the components of language.

According to modular theory, the cognitive system is comprised of distinct though interacting modules, each of which is organized according to special principles and properties. These modules are special-purpose structures that are innately specific and autonomous and that develop along internally directed courses. They are described as vertical rather than horizontal (Fodor, 1983).

Chomsky (1980) viewed the language faculty as a module that has its own unique structure—it operates according to principles that are distinct and differentiated from those of other cognitive systems, such as the general perceptual and motor systems. Chomsky (1980) described the "*knowing* the language" module as made of at least two components:

1. The "computational" aspect of language—the rules that form the syntactic constructions of phonological or semantic patterns, and
2. The system of "object-reference" as well as relations (thematic relations) such as agent, instrument, and the semantic component.

Fodor (1983) included an input system in the linguistic module that provides the distal auditory information to the organism and interprets the transduced information. He indicated that this takes place by means of an auditory perceptual system specialized for language. In other words, both the knowledge and performance aspects of the computational aspect of language are language-specific and independent from other cognitive functions.

Hamburger and Crain (1987) included the following in the syntactic module: word order, word category, inflectional affixes, special morphemes (like "by" and "to" in the English passive and infinitive), and so on. Hamburger and Crain asserted that each syntactic structure is, or at least includes, a "labeled, rooted, ordered tree, called a 'phrase-worker'" (p. 108). They believe the evidence is strong for families of phrase types associated with major word categories.

Chomsky (1980) also suggested that the second component, the semantic one, may not be part of the language faculty itself, as is the syntactic component, but part of a cognitive/conceptual module that is

> *Quote 7–2*
> *It is clear that what Chomsky talks about is grammar but what he wishes to generalize about is **language**.*
>
> (SALZINGER, 1975, p. 191).

distinct from the linguistic module. This conceptual module may include the real-world knowledge that results from the assimilation of the sum total of an individual's experiences of every kind, verbal and non-verbal, and from every input source. These modules, the linguistic and conceptual, interact when expressions from the linguistic system are linked to elements of the conceptual system. The semantic component includes the relationships that result from this interaction and could therefore fall in either module.

It is important to remember that *semantics* and *concepts/meanings* are not synonomous terms. *Semantics* refers to meanings in language (see Rice, 1983). Schlesinger (1981) separates the cognitive, semantic, and surface level more specifically as follows:

1. Cognitive level is made up of the concepts and relations in terms of which we perceive the world. (A knife is an instrument.)
2. Semantic level is the funnel that receives the relations of the cognitive level. (The knife can function as an agent.)
3. Surface level is the realization of the structures at the semantic level. This realization can take numerous forms.

According to Schlesinger's definition of the semantic level, the semantics categories are language-specific. This definition would lead us to consider semantics together with syntax within the modular system.

Or we may need to think of semantics as related in different ways to the conceptual and syntactic levels. The meanings that syntactic structures reflect can be thought of in their relations to the world knowledge of the individual that permits him or her to construct meanings from heard utterances that are therefore related to the cognitive level. The classification of the events or objects into role-specific categories and the relations of these roles may also be cognitive. The roles that words of specific meanings can take in relation to other words/meanings in the surface structure may be the aspect of the semantic level that relates to syntax. The child learns the mapping of words and meanings and of roles and permissable syntactic ways of expressing them in a specific language. The language respects the roles and the roles respect the world's "texture" (Schlesinger, 1981).

It appears that semantics can legitimately be placed in either the linguistic or cognitive module depending on which aspect of semantics is being considered. Take, for example, a view of linguistic/meaning mapping from the point of view of internal cognitive processes.

Dinsmore (1987) describes a theory on how the mapping between the context of internal mental spaces and propositions asserted to be true in the real world can take place. Dinsmore's thesis is that the concept of mental spaces (domains used for consolidating certain kinds of information [Fauconnier, 1985]) are functionally motivated and support a general reasoning technique that Dinsmore calls *simulative reasoning*. In simulated reasoning, knowledge is partitioned into distinct spaces or knowledge bases and the contents of each space effectively simulate a possible reality. The meaning of a space is called its *context*, which is regarded as the space's propositional function. In applying his model to discourse, Dinsmore says that people can put together a coherent discourse by describing the objects and relations of any space as if the objects and relations belonged to the real world. Dinsmore is theorizing on what is happening internally at the cognitive level as we express propositions in language discourse. The cognitive aspect of semantics is obviously much broader than meanings encoded in words. Semantics is a complex concept, and this complexity needs to be considered in working with the language-disordered.

The phonological and grammatical (computational) components of language do appear to belong to a single linguistic-specific module. (As previously noted, there is some question regarding the classification of the semantic level.) Rapin and Allen (1983) found a specific syndrome within the general syndrome they call *developmental language disability* that they have labeled the *phonologic-syntactic syndrome*. The main disabilities in this syndrome are in the phonological and morphology-syntax systems. The articulatory and grammatical errors are not the typical developmental errors found in childhood. Children in the phonologic-syntactic syndrome usually have the semantic categories intact and their gestures are clearly ahead of expressive abilities. The findings of Chiat and Hirson (1987) that phonological errors in words and syntactic errors in sentences were related in the language of a dysphasic child led them to hypothesize that phonology and syntax disorders are connected, particularly that phonological constraints can be said to account for certain syntactic problems. These findings lend support to the Chomsky argument that the speech perceptual system and the phonological and syntactic computational aspects of language form a module separate and distinct from the semantic and general cognitive systems.

The independence of the grammatical system can also be argued from the fact that some linguistic knowledge is not directly tied to meaning. McCawley (1971) provides an example in the English speech of constraints that are purely of a formal, grammatical nature and beyond the meanings expressed. For example, a similar meaning is expressed by "Put the hat on," "Put on the hat," or "Put it on," but not "Put on it." Rice (1983) suggests that these arbitrary constraints of the lin-

> *Quote 7–3*
> . . . *Cognition and language can be thought of as a complex of in-terconnecting systems and subsystems. Syntax may represent one system and semantic rules another.*
>   (NELSON & NELSON, 1978, p. 225).

guistic system, the portion of language not accounted for by cognition, may be the area that causes difficulty for some language-impaired children. (A discussion of the independence of the auditory perceptual memory system in processing language is found in Chapter 8.)

Evidence for Separating the Syntactic and Semantic Components

If there is such a structure as a linguistic module, is there evidence to support an assumption that the syntactic and semantic components of language are both members of this module or that they belong to separate modules? Bellugi, Poizner, and Zurif (1982) raised the question of separateness between these components. The implications from theories already presented in this chapter are that the cognitive system is involved with semantics, at least at the functional or operational level. Are there any empirical data that support either position?

Neuropsychological data are helpful in providing information on this question. According to Zurif (1982), there appear to be separate routes for lexical access to open (unrestricted) versus closed (restricted, e.g., grammatical morphemes) class vocabulary. He reported that a number of posteriorly brain-damaged patients presented primarily a word-finding difficulty in the context of grammatically well-formed utterances. Studying Broca's aphasics, Bradley, Garrett, and Zurif (1980) found that these aphasics did not show the capacity to distinguish the closed-class items from the open class. They suggested that agrammatic aphasics are unable to access the systems for grammatically based function words. Zurif (1982) concluded that the semantic facts associated with closed-class items are available in principle to Broca's aphasics;

> *Quote 7–4*
> . . . *the syntactic and semantic structures and processes that are theoretically part of the normal system have been shown to be useful in characterizing various performances that define particular aphasic syndromes. This demonstration not only lends support to the hypothesis that aphasia reflects disruption of abstract linguistic components as they function in different tasks and in all modalities, but it also supports the psychological reality of the theoretical components as they have been described.*
>   (BERNDT, CARAMAZZA, & ZURIF, 1981, pp. 23–24).

the patients, however, no longer have the specific closed-class retrieval mechanism, which Zurif hypothesizes serves as input to a purser, and the aphasics cannot make on-line use of such information. If we consider the open-class vocabulary problems to be problems of semantics and the closed-class problems to be problems of grammar or syntax, the studies by Bradley et al. and Zurif indicate a structural separation between semantics and grammar.

Three occurrences support the distinction between the operational knowledge of open- versus closed-class items, although there is no clear evidence whether the distinction occurs in the data base or in the access to the data. The first support for the knowledge difference between open and closed classes is that of the differential development of these classes in young children. Early language is characterized by open-class lexicon occurring in both isolation and semantic relation to each other. Later, the grammatical morphemes emerge as modulators for the open classes. The evidence from disorders has already been presented; there is a differential loss of closed- and open-class items in agrammatic and fluent aphasics, respectively; the latter preserve what is lost by the former, and vice versa (Saffran, Schwartz, & Marin, 1980; Garrett, 1982). Lastly, there is evidence from the typical errors made by speakers in spontaneous speech situations. Garrett (1982) concluded that, because errors in which two elements exchange position are confined to open-class vocabulary and errors in which a *single* element shifts its position are characteristic of the closed-class items, there are processing differences between these two types of grammatical structures.

In discussing the results of three lexical decision experiments, Katz, Boyce, Goldstein, and Lukatela (1987) found support for the conclusion that inflectional processing (syntactic) functions independently in auditory word recognition. According to these researchers, the inflectional processor "(a) is unaffected by semantic information, (b) operates postlexically" (p. 261). This indicates that there is separability in syntactic and semantic processing.

In addition to the data and reasons just provided, there is another argument for considering these aspects (semantics and syntax) of linguistic knowledge as separate. Some brain-damaged subjects produce grammatically intact automatic speech in the face of lack of meaningful language. Whitaker (1976) reported a case of isolation of the language function in the brain in which there was essentially no spontaneous speech. There was echolalia, however, in which the subject maintained the stress and intonation patterns of the verbal stimuli. The echolalic mechanism was coupled with a "grammatic filter"—the echoed responses occurred when the stimuli were grammatically acceptable English utterances. When presented with sentences that had phonologic or syntactic errors, the subject corrected them half of the time. Semantically erroneous stimuli were never corrected.

This leads us back to the studies of language acquisition that have attempted to distinguish between activities related to automatic speech processes and those related to meaningful language. The question is, do these two aspects of language involve different kinds of knowledge—one of information, the semantic one, and one of automatic skilled behavior, the syntactic one? In an early study, Fraser, Bellugi, and Brown (1963) concluded, after finding imitation to be less difficult than comprehension of the same grammatical forms, that imitation is a perceptual-motor skill not dependent on comprehension.

Semantic information needs to be thought of as including a variety of types of associations in addition to that of the usual dictionary meaning of the lexicon. Semantics links perceptual representations of words to concepts. The associations are between grammatical forms and specific meanings, other stored perceptual representations, visual imagery, and episodic or schematic information. In other words, semantic information is a collection of concepts (Samuels & Eisenberg, 1981). According to Schlesinger (1977), cognitive categories or concepts are formed primarily by the classification provided by linguistic input. The manner in which cognitive data are grouped is partially a function of the way in which language classifies them.

If grammar and semantics are separate in terms of cognitive structure, we would expect to find separate kinds of language disorders in children. Testing would be directed to identifying problems involving the accuracy and automaticity of rules that form syntactic constructions and the facility and accuracy with which grammatical structures are generated to express meaning, as opposed to problems involving the associations between the surface structure and meaning, the access, retrieval, and production of meaningful words, idioms, and other structures, and the understanding of inferred meaning, metaphors, and so on. If semantics belong to the conceptual module instead of the linguistic one, then there would be a need to evaluate the contribution of the cognitive system to a semantic disorder with corresponding attention to this in intervention.

Quote 7–5
The temporary priority given to lexical access over inflectional processing may also be reflected in the developmental pattern of language acquisition: children produce violations of syntax even when they make no semantic violations. . . . [There is] evidence from the first two experiments that the inflectional processor (a) is unaffected by semantic information, (b) functions obligatorily in natural, rapid speech and (c) operates postlexically.
(KATZ, BOYCE, GOLDSTEIN, & LUKATELA, 1987, pp. 260, 261).

Independence of Pragmatic Component

Thus far in the modular theory we have a linguistic module and a conceptual module that interact. The linguistic module is made up of the rules governing phonological and syntactic constructions and the input system that receives language. The semantic aspect may be part of the linguistic module or part of the conceptual module or the result of interaction between the two. Where does pragmatics fit in?

Chomsky (1980) suggested that pragmatic competence may be a cognitive system distinct from the linguistic one, which operates on principles that differ from those of the grammatical module. Foster (1984a) describes pragmatics as the application of general cognitive principles to linguistic material. She claims that the difference between syntax (grammar) and pragmatics is based on differences in the types of rules, and she provides arguments to support her claim. She states:

1. Syntax rules are discrete while pragmatic rules operate according to degree.
2. Syntactic rules are defined within phrasal and clausal boundaries; pragmatic rules operate over messages.
3. Pragmatic rules, unlike syntactic rules, are not special to language.
4. Syntax and pragmatics have separate knowledge bases that come together the instant those knowledge bases are hooked up to the production and comprehension mechanism.

Implied in this position of both Chomsky and Foster is that syntax or grammar and pragmatic rules develop independently of each other, and consequently one does not need to be a prerequisite of the other. Studies comparing language-disordered children with those not having such disorders in pragmatic functions have shown that the two groups are similar, indicating that not all language-disordered children have pragmatic deficits (Fey, Leonard, & Wilcox, 1981; Rowan, Leonard, Chapman, & Weiss, 1983). These findings appear to support a distinction between the linguistic and pragmatic modules. It may be that what are considered linguistic functions, such as turn-taking and topic maintenance, may in fact be cognitive or social functions. Whether or not the cognitive and social components in pragmatics call for a distinct module is not clear. It may be that there is a module of social perceptual behavior distinct from a general cognitive module. Or perhaps they are united in the child during early developmental periods and only later become separated. We may need to study how social theory differs from referential theory in terms of the basic underlying cognitive structures. For example, are the notions of intention and affect even farther removed from linguistic functions than those of turn-taking?

> *Quote 7–6*
> *The theory of speech acts is not an adjunct to our theory of language, something to be consigned to the realm of "pragmatics" or performance; rather the theory of speech acts will necessarily occupy a central role in our grammar, since it will include all of what used to be called semantics as well as pragmatics.*
>
> (SEARLE, 1975, p. 38).

We may find it helpful to establish a distinction between general pragmatics, which deals with the use and purpose of social acts, and linguistic-pragmatics, which deals with the relationship between the linguistic code and its use. This former aspect describes the internal motivation and intention of the speaker to engage in communication, and the latter describes the appropriate linguistic routines and rules associated with specific communicative activities; in this sense, semantics becomes part of pragmatics.

This is not to say that only the linguistic module is language and the conceptual and pragmatic domains are not. All three are essential to the communication of messages. It is unclear why the form of a message is considered language, whereas "concepts" or meanings (organized knowledge of real-world relationships), the other half of language, are not thought of as language; they are often said to be nonlinguistic. Perhaps concepts are *nonlinguistic* if we use the term *linguistic* to refer to the grammatical aspects of language, but concepts and meaning are not *nonlanguage*.

THE COGNITIVE MODULE AND LANGUAGE

Relation between Form and Meaning

The way we state the relationship among the various components of language produces what I consider to be a problem in understanding the nature of language. We usually describe the form of language as having meaning. It would be more accurate to say that we bring meaning to the form. The particular meaning we bring to a form is related to our understanding of relationships among concepts, to the meanings

> *Quote 7–7*
> *. . . **all** of semantics is **essentially** pragmatic in nature. Children do not learn a set of isomorphic sign-referent relations. Rather, they learn how to do things with sounds, continually redefining the appropriate contexts for various language "games."*
>
> (BATES, 1976b, p. 426).

garnered from verbal input, and to the meaning abstracted from external factors such as our experiences and the contexts in which forms are used. Again, form does not have content; we bring the content we have to the form. We attempt to set boundaries for the relationship between form and content so as to have the same meanings that others have and thus to communicate effectively. For the most part we are successful, particularly with respect to referential meaning. The difficulties we do have in comprehending what we hear or read reflect the differences in the content we bring to the form. On the other hand, once we associate forms with the meanings we have, the forms have a way of crystalizing and refining these meanings, particularly when dealing with abstract notions.

This interpretation of the content/form relationship places content and form on an equal basis and not on the basis that content is evaluated through form or the expression of form. This interpretation assists in clarifying the relationship between cognition and language and the variability inherent in the interpretation of form in sentential and situational contexts. It certainly makes it easier to describe the notion of figurative language if we believe that individuals bring their own unique and idiosyncratic meanings and meaning relations to a form. It may also help to refine the distinction of concept development and semantic development, concept development referring to the broad world knowledge we acquire and semantic development referring to the application of this knowledge to the form of language. We should recognize that all our knowledge can be potentially mapped into language, not only that which is in the meanings of words and sentences. This is why words have different meanings to different individuals as their knowledge and experience is brought to bear in understanding and using words.

With respect to the idea that we bring meaning to our comprehension rather than getting meaning from it, I remember telling students who said they did not get anything out of a conference or speaker that they did not have enough knowledge to take to it. Those who took more knowledge to the lectures would bring more back. I have noticed in my own experience that I can listen to a lecturer on the most elementary subject and hear something that excites me, something that I seem to be hearing for the first time although I know I have heard it many times before. My internal schema about language is constantly growing and changing and as it does, old information becomes new.

It may further clarify the issue to use the term *linguistic* to refer to the "computational" aspects of language described by Chomsky (1980) and to reserve the term *language* to a broad interpretation that includes the grammatical *as well as* the cognitive/pragmatic domains and their interrelationship and the internal processing and external contextual variables that accompany and modify the acts of speaking and listening.

In this sense, content and use are nonlinguistic but are not "non-language"; they are an integral part of language. The debate regarding the relationship between language and cognition becomes moot. Cognition is a part of language.

If we include cognition as an integral part of language and view the content associated with linguistic representation as meaning that we bring to the language comprehension and production processes, the consequences will be a better understanding of concepts, their development and their role in language. Intervention with language-disordered children will benefit.

Concepts as Schemata

Concepts may be thought of as organized into schemata (similar to event structure [Nelson, 1986b]) or scripts. Rumelhart and Ortony (1977) define *schemata* as generalized concepts that underlie situations, objects, events and actions, and sequence of actions and events (see also Schank & Abelson, 1977). For example, an action-oriented schema or script may involve all persons, objects, and actions associated with going to the grocery store or going to the movies. Schema can accept other variable information, can even be embedded in one another, and may include procedural information. Schemata are specific to each person—based on her or his own experience, and what goes into the organization and access of schemata depends on the frequency and variability of the experiences of the individual. Samuels and Eisenberg (1981) state that, ". . . the more a person performs an activity, the more specific will be the details stored in the schema and the easier it will be to gain access to the schema from memory" (p. 46). In developing schemata in specific areas, the individual uses knowledge available to him or her in similar already schematized areas (see also the discussion of events and scripts in Chapter 10).

Samuels and Eisenberg (1981) give two functions of schemata that they consider to play important roles in reading. The same can be applied to oral language, particularly to oral language comprehension. The first function is that of providing structure to the information that is received (in reading or listening) by making available previously stored information and by organizing the information into a form that is easily retrieved. A second function is that of providing information not available in the input text. Use of this stored schemata allows the listener to make inferences and also, for example, to understand figurative language. How can a youngster understand her mother saying her best friend is just like cream if she has no real or vicarious experience or schema involving the process of milking and of watching cream rise to the top? To provide intervention on inference or figurative language by focusing on the text or surface structure and not taking into account the expansion of the associated conceptual schemata would be fruitless. At least equal weight needs to be given to the conceptual aspect of figurative language as to the linguistic. Whereas difficulty in comprehending metaphors may be due to poor strategies for interpreting metaphoric language, this difficulty may also be related to inadequate knowledge of the concepts underlying specific metaphors. This is why we cannot think of language as the linguistic form or of semantics as the narrow meaning of the form. We must give an equal and parallel role to conceptualization.

If we apply these ideas to comprehension, we can think of comprehension as a process of generating meaning for language (Wittrock, 1981). As readers read and listeners listen, they *construct* meaning by relating their general knowledge of the world and of linguistic rules as well as their memories of experience and creative imagery. Construction of meaning is dependent on what is already in the memory. Comprehension is a generative task. (This process will be discussed more completely in Chapter 9.)

It appears that the development of the cognitive system is an integral part of the development of language and should go hand-in-hand with the development of the linguistic system. This is particularly true in language-delayed children whose input to conceptualization may be limited due to the failure to develop linguistic skills—one avenue through which concepts develop. The language disorder-related processing difficulties produce a further disorder by limiting the development of world knowledge and corresponding concepts and their classification. The disorder contributes to a delay, and that delay together with disordered language itself contributes to a deprivation of general cognitive development. The intervention implications are clear. A total program of language intervention must include a systematic plan for expanding concepts and world knowledge in addition to the facilitation of rules and the teaching directed to improved performance of the process of language.

Quote 7–8

Language, however, contains many terms that have no "portrayable correlates". . . . It is this line of reasoning that has led me to feel that one cannot easily dismiss the idea that language may make a major contribution to thought, even to the thought of a young child. If it is to be meaningful, however, any search for the contribution of language to thinking should be carried out not in the realm where other modalities do an equal, or even better, job, but in the realm where language may have unique properties for organizing our experiences.

(BLANK, 1975a, p. 45).

In this view of language as composed of parallel and interacting systems of linguistics and cognition, it is not appropriate to speak of cognitive prerequisites to language because cognition is part of language and could not properly serve as a prerequisite to itself. It would be more accurate to refer to other cognitive prerequisites to symbol use, to the comprehension of linguistic symbols, or to speech—the production of linguistic symbols. You could also talk about linguistic prerequisites to speech, meaning that the development of some linguistic rules that underlie language knowledge and even the comprehension of some of these rules may predate their use in language production.

It may be useful to consider all aspects of the language system as nonmodular except that of the linguistic computational (grammar) aspect. Thus, such cognitive strategies as problem-solving and rule induction would be important to language learning but not completely responsible for the acquisition of grammar.

INTERRELATIONSHIPS IN MODULAR THEORY

If we accept the theory of modular components in language, there needs to be an accompanying explanation of just how these modules interact both in terms of the development of the various functions as well as with respect to the processing of information through and between the modules. Cognitive psychologists (e.g., Hamburger & Crain, 1987) describe attempts to disentangle the effects of syntax, semantics and response plans, or algorithms in responding to a sentence in specific circumstances since these are viewed as independent targets of empirical investigation. They believe that there is a path in verifying the claims of modularity (at least cognitive/linguistic) and the specific structures within each of these modules. Some work, already cited (Katz, Boyce, Goldstein, & Lukatela, 1987), has demonstrated separability of syntactic and semantic processing. Hamburger and Crain (1987) caution that the postulation of an independent existence of various modules does not imply that they act in serial fashion. In experimental research, descriptions in which each module completes its work and passes its results to the next module may provide clarity to the study. However, it is probably more accurate to envision the passing of partial results, parallel processing, or bidirectionality.

The interrelationship among modulars as well as modularity structure may be responsible for difficulties children have in language processing. The dissimilarities among structures may demand complex processing even if the modules themselves are simple (Hamburger & Crain, 1987). Rice (1983) reviews studies that indicate cognition/language mismatches and concludes that linguistic acquisition is somewhat distinct from general understanding and cognitive processes.

MODULAR THEORY AND LANGUAGE DISORDERS

Where does modular theory (the theory that views the computational aspects of language—syntactic and phonological—as different from other cognitive tasks, the former task possessing special properties and guided by special principles developmentally) lead us in terms of language disorders? What effect on language disorders does the classification of linguistic (grammar), pragmatic, and conceptual domains into separate but interacting modules have on the interaction with language-disordered children? Modular theory might generate disorder descriptions similar to those generated by clinical experience. Chomsky (1980) and Foster (1984a, b) have also provided a few possibilities, which are discussed in the following sections.

Possibility 1. The first possibility is that the conceptual system can be immature or disordered while the linguistic system is fully matured or intact. Kamhi, Catts, Koenig, and Lewis (1984) refine this hypothesis by stating that a language-impaired child might have a relatively severe symbolic deficit without an associated *expressive* (not receptive) language impairment.

Possibility 2. A second possibility is that the linguistic system can be immature or disordered while the conceptual system is intact. According to Kamhi et al. (1984), a language-impaired child might have intact symbolic skills but still suffer from an expressive language deficit.

Possibility 3. Another possibility is that a child can have full grammatical competence and not pragmatic competence—reduced ability to use a language appropriately although syntax and semantics are intact. (This problem is evident in inappropriate behavioral posturing in social situations.)

Possibility 4. A fourth possibility is that there may be a problem with the interconnection between modules. Children may develop grammar semantic and pragmatic skills but be unable to employ them

---

Quote 7–9
Deviant use of language surely does not logically entail an impairment of linguistic capacity per se. Just as the components of linguistic models interact with each other, so too must linguistic capacity interact with other components of human cognitive capacity. In attempting to develop precise functional analyses of cognitive deficits that arise concomitantly with brain damage, it is essential that there not be pretheoretical conflation across domains.

(KEAN, 1982, p. 180).

in interactive-automatic routines. Hamburger and Crain (1987) refer to this as mismatch between modules. In a study of a child with developmental dysphasia, Chiat and Hirson (1987) found that although the child could express complex conceptual intentions, they were not mapped into conventional language structures—a mismatch between syntax and cognition. Problems in the interface of syntax and semantics in language-impaired children have not yet been thoroughly investigated (Rice, 1983). Rice believes that such studies may clarify some of the linguistic processes involved in language acquisition in language-disordered children.

Possibility 5. Last is the possibility that problems in pragmatics may be related to problems in general cognitive functions such as attention and abstraction.

If we examine the implications of such a framework for language disorders to assessment and intervention, we can compare this modular theory with others that classify language components:

1. Nonlinguistic cognitive behaviors would need to be studied throughout the language life of the child, not only at the beginning stages of language. The emphasis on the role of cognition would be of particular value in the adolescent years when skills in the use of inference, analogies, metaphors, humor, sarcasm, and so on are so essential to language understanding and use.
2. The position that cognition, pragmatics, semantics, and syntax are distinct but interrelated systems will require that all be examined independently as well as in the manner in which they interact. We would not only look at words and their referents or utterances and their content, speech acts and their use, messages and their intention, but we would look at all of these. For example, behaviors that relate to social interaction would need to be observed outside as well as inside the framework of language. The relative emphasis of the various components in intervention would depend on the level of language of the child.
3. Patterns of language disorders would be more clearly defined if language is viewed more broadly than through linguistic eyes only. For example, even when evaluating linguistic functions, there would be attention given to the distinction between open- and closed-class structures. Rice (1983) suggests that each child's perceptual, cognitive, and linguistic constraints must be known if remediation is to be effective.
4. If we consider conceptual (real world knowledge) and linguistic (form) to be equal partners in semantics instead of defining semantics as the meanings of words, then semantic structure development will take on the dimension of enriching concept

> *Quote 7–10*
> *The paradigm that comes out of this perspective is one in which one views language behavior as the result of internally interacting mental structures. One such mental structure we might call "syntax," another "the system of illocutionary acts," another "the system of cognizing certain aspects of the world." Different kinds of facts are explained by each structure.*
>
> (Beaver, in Glucksberg, 1975, p. 40).

development by including the relationships among the functional, spatial, and temporal specification of objects as well as the manner they act or can be acted on instead of simply developing the meaning of a word by indicating the object it refers to.

5. Grouping children for intervention purposes would take into account the distinctions based on modular factors. Children with purely computational problems, the rules that form the syntactic construction (closed classes), would be grouped separate from those having cognition-related problems of semantic or pragmatics. In other words, there is some validity to grouping phonological and syntactic problems together and separate from semantic and cognitive disorders.

6. Lastly, and most importantly, the divergent points of view regarding the role of the environment described by the linguistic theory and the communication theory would be integrated by a modular theory. It could be hypothesized that the acquisition of the computational aspects of language, governed by the linguistic module, would depend primarily on the child's own organizing system to construct rules of syntax and semantics, whereas the acquisition of concepts and social interactions governed by a cognitive module would depend on the interactions with the environment for the child to develop the appropriate behavior repertoire that serves as a basis for language.

Whether or not these interpretations of language are accepted depends on how they fit with our data and observations. For ultimately, the path of paradigm development should be that of bringing data and theory together. We should not try to force all our data into a neatly organized unidimensional theory because the theory sounds good, but we need to generate a series of interrelated theories that can account for the multidimensional characteristics of language disorders.

8

INTEGRATING THEORIES: AUDITORY PERCEPTION, MEMORY, AND LANGUAGE

In Chapter 6, I argued that it was important, from the standpoint of disordered language, to distinguish between knowing language and performing it. Chapter 7 presented a position about the relationship among the components of language knowledge—cognitive, linguistic, and pragmatic. This chapter discusses the performance of oral language, the relation among the various performance tasks in language, and the relation of these tasks to the acquisition of language knowledge. What role do auditory perception and auditory memory play in language comprehension and what relationship does access and retrieval of language

THEORY, ASSESSMENT AND INTERVENTION
IN LANGUAGE DISORDERS: © 1988 by Grune & Stratton
AN INTEGRATIVE APPROACH

ISBN   0-8089-1918-0

have with memory? Why is it important to attempt to understand this relationship in general and with reference to the assessment and intervention of language-disordered children? To omit discussing the role of performance strategies in a book about language would be to omit a significant aspect of language in humans. Bever (1970) concurs when he says, "While the grammatical rules make possible the extrapolation of new sentences from old ones, the system of behavioral strategies make more efficient the perception [comprehension] and *production* of sentences." However, this aspect of language is ordinarily left out of general discussions of language, its development, and disorders. In fact only two theories of the six presented in this book provide explicit descriptions of perception and memory and specify the role that these processes play in language, the neuropsychological and information process theories.

Nelson (1986b) suggests that immediate perception and subsequent representation need to be distinguished, and this distinction is important in understanding the cognitive functioning of young children, particularly since the cognitive processes such as categorization, pattern analysis, and inference operate not on the real world phenomena but on the mental representation of them. She states that the acquisition of new knowledge is influenced by the initial perceptual representation in the same way that prior knowledge influences perception.

McNeil and Kimelman (1986) describe *listeners* as active, creative gatherers of information. Operations that are active and cognitive, performed on information, and independent of the speech code are referred to as *processing operations*, and it is in this sense that I am using the term to describe auditory perception and memory.

The emphasis in this chapter is on the role of auditory memory and auditory perception in language development and language performance. This is not to say that only the auditory perceptual system influences language. There are equally strong positions explaining the role of the entire perceptual system on the development of the cognitive system, particularly on the quality of internal representation of reality that forms the conceptual framework for the meaning side of language.

In this chapter I will focus on the relation between auditory processes and language. It is my position that no theory of language that accounts for disorders of language is complete without an attempt to

---

Quote 8–1
The question of how one defines the relevant relationship between stimulus parameters and perceptual response is perhaps insoluble in any plausible way if one is restrained from characterizing the stimulus by reference to the structural system which the perceiver brings to the analysis process.
(GARRETT & FODOR, 1968, p. 461).

> *Quote 8–2*
> *It is important to realize that the effects between components are never perfectly proportional and not completely predictable. The dependence, cumulative, and interactive effects exist between components that may in turn relate to other components in different or similar ways. . . . This indicates that the components cannot be considered as independent aspects of language, nor can any one of them, alone, be viewed as encompassing the totality of language.*
> (CARROW-WOOLFOLK & LYNCH, 1982, p. 207).

integrate the auditory perceptual and memory processes with oral language. At some point in the history of language disorders it became bad form to talk about the relation between auditory perception, auditory memory, and language. As soon as the subject was brought up, someone in a professional gathering would be sure to exclaim, with raised eyebrows, "Not again!" So for many years the literature has kept relatively silent about perception and memory—I guess hoping that the whole idea of such a relationship would go away.

There are probably many reasons for the reluctance to talk about how auditory perception and memory relate to language. One major reason is that research findings regarding the correlation between perceptual-memory factors and language are inconclusive—at least early research findings with the language-disordered have been. Rees (1973) reviewed numerous studies concerning auditory deficits and found discrepancies among the findings. She concluded that even if a primary perceptual difficulty was isolated in language-disordered children, there would still be little evidence to suggest that such a deficit was systematically related to language. The major fallacy with much of the type of research with language-disordered children that Rees reviewed is that it assumes that children with language disorders comprise a homogeneous group and therefore the characteristics studied should be present in all children or that the correlation between the variable and language disorders should be high in order to indicate a relationship between the variable and language disorders. The fact is that language disorders are not all alike. Children with these disorders exhibit various patterns, only some of which show a relation between auditory perception, memory, and language. Whether or not a correlation between the above variables in a group of language-disordered children is significant is not relevant. Whether or not some language-disordered children with specific kinds of comprehension and/or expression problems may also have auditory perceptual and/or memory problems is relevant. It is the presence of such co-occurring deficits that makes the theoretical integration of these variables important. We need to try to understand how auditory memory, perception, and language are related, not to infer a causal relation, not to try to "remediate" at the perceptual memory level so as to improve language, but to help us understand the kinds of language disorders children have, how all related cognitive systems contribute to their difficulties with using language, and what we can do in intervention to make it easier for them to learn.

Recent research by Tallal (1980), Tallal and Stark (1983), and Kamhi, Lee, and Nelson (1985) has shown that some children with language disorders do demonstrate auditory processing problems. Similar studies of children with reading and writing disorders indicate that some children with these disorders also exhibit auditory processing and memory disorders (Vellutino, 1979; Tallal, 1980).

In a comparison of language-impaired children with normal-language children on tests of speech perception and language ability, Bernstein and Stark (1985) found that although the two groups at early ages differed significantly in discrimination, sequencing, and rote processing of and serial memory for synthesized /ba/ and /da/ stimuli, the performance of both groups was at or near ceiling in follow-up. Bernstein and Stark concluded that from a developmental perspective, they could not reject the hypothesis that perceptual deficits are causal in language impairments. They suggested that disabilities may persist as a result of inadequate processing of sensory information during early childhood even after the original processing deficit may no longer exist. This may be another reason, according to Carrow-Woolfolk and Lynch (1982), that studies of the presence of auditory processing problems in children are in disagreement. The finding of such a problem may depend on the age at which language-impaired children are tested.

It is not my purpose here to review the literature on auditory perception nor to attempt to defend the existence of such problems in children with language disorders. My own clinical experience has convinced me that certain types of language disorders do co-occur with certain types of auditory processing and memory problems and I would go so far as to say that they are related to one another. I also believe that it is important to know when a child has such problems.

It would be impossible within a small section of this book to develop a complete theory that integrates auditory processing, auditory memory, and language. However, some thoughts as to how perception, memory, and language fit together might be helpful. What makes this integration particularly important is the theory that the auditory processing skills that are used in language are considered part of the linguistic module (see Chapter 7) and as such are independent from those cognitive-perceptual functions that do not process language (Fodor, 1983). If it is true that these processes are unique and serve language specifically, then we cannot dismiss their role in language acquisition and language disorders. Kean (1982) believes that a theory of linguistic capacity "is responsible for accounting for the mapping between the sound realization of a string and its semantic interpretation" (p. 181).

In this discussion of auditory perception, memory, and language, there is no attempt to present these in any type of model or level of processing. Duchan (1983) has been persuasive in her arguments that any type of description of these processes that implies a discrete identity for each of them (as in box models) fails to consider the integration among them and their reciprocal interaction during processing. She states that concentration on the bottom-up (superficial to deep) and serial organization denies the importance of parallel and top-down processing (Fig. 8–1). Ultimately, the processing of the acoustic-phonetic input must be studied within the context of the syntactic and lexical processing systems (Frauenfelder & Tyler, 1987; Pisoni & Luce, 1987). There is and needs to be a two-pronged attack at the understanding of the processing system, one of formally representing the phonetic and phonological information in speech recognition and developing algorithms for using this information in acoustic signal analysis and one represented by the psycholinguistic approach of making mental structures and processes explicit in lexical processing (Frauenfelder & Tyler,

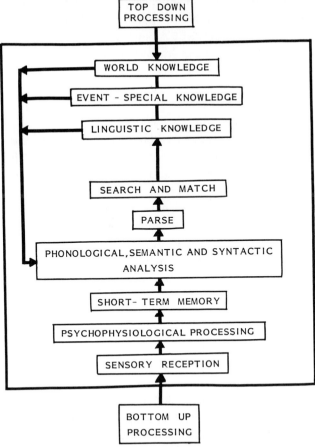

FIGURE 8–1. An illustration of bottom-up and top-down processing in auditory comprehension.

1987). I am limiting the information in this chapter to a simple description of the auditory perceptual system and its role in language. Some of the other issues will be or have been discussed in other chapters, particularly in Chapter 9. I also need to point out, as I have done previously (Carrow-Woolfolk & Lynch, 1982), that the effects of disordered processing vary with the relationship between the language processing components and other cognitive and linguistic components in each child, with the stage of language development at which a processing problem may interact with language and with the efforts a child makes to handle learning within the system's constraints.

RELATION BETWEEN AUDITORY PERCEPTION AND LANGUAGE

My purpose in this section is to argue that there is a performance link between the process of receiving and perceiving speech through the auditory system and the process of developing and using oral language. This argument will be theoretically and logically based, although empirical findings will be used to strengthen theoretical positions wherever possible.

Speech Perception as a Language-Specific System

A first step in the argument is that the neurological bases for both, auditory perception for speech and language, are in the left hemisphere. The literature that locates language in the left hemisphere is abundant. There is also evidence that there is a right-ear (left hemisphere) advantage for the perception of verbal materials, an advantage that cannot be accounted for in terms of memory, attention, and other faculties (Satz, 1968). A corollary to this is the finding that speech perception is a process that is unique and different from the perception of nonspeech sounds (Liberman, Cooper, Shankweiler, & Studdert-Kennedy, 1967). So language and speech perception are considered different from corresponding nonlinguistic tasks in each of their related areas.

Aspects of the language task, especially the computational aspects, are thought by Chomsky (1980) to function as a module separate and independent from other cognitive modules (see Chapter 7). Fodor (1983) appears to include the speech perception input system *as part of* the language module; it works in domains that have language properties. Fodor says also that the input mechanisms are similar to reflexes in that some of the same conditions are present. Both are triggered automatically by the stimuli that they apply to. Studdert-Kennedy and Shankweiler (1970) support the position that the sounds of speech are integral to the hierarchical structure of language and consider it reasonable to expect that among the language processes that are lateralized in the dominant hemisphere are mechanisms for the speech perception. Liberman et al. (1967) state that the perception of the complex speech code is *basic* to language. There appears to be support for an integral relationship between speech perception and language both from a neurological and functional viewpoint. Both speech perception and language are found in the dominant hemisphere; they both are unique and distinct from processes that are nonlinguistic, and both are considered, at a theoretical level, to be part of the same system.

The speech recognition system appears to be particularly responsive to the universal properties of language (Fodor, 1983). The special perceptual mechanism serves as decoder for a very special kind of code, one that requires efficient and parallel processing of successive phonemes (Liberman et al., 1967) instead of serial processing (phonemes processed one at a time). Parallel transmission may increase the difficulty of the task of perception but allows the speaker to transmit phonemes at a rate of 15 per second.

Another characteristic of speech perception that is not shared with other kinds of perception and that makes it particularly suited to the perception of spoken language is categorical perception. In categorical perception, a listener is unable to discriminate among acoustic stimuli he or she identifies as belonging to a single category but can discriminate well among stimuli belonging to different categories. In the perception of speech sounds, the listener does just that: most speech sounds are perceived categorically (even though the acoustic cues for individual phonemes overlap in continuous speech) but most nonspeech sounds are not (Liberman et al., 1967).

An even stronger connection between speech perception and linguistics is the postulated relation between the motor production of speech and perception. The claim of the theory is that the distinctive parameters for acoustic stimuli at the phoneme level are based on articulatory patterns; speech is perceived by reference to production. Liberman and colleagues (1967) suggest that the interdependence of the perceptual and productive processes may be similar to that at higher levels of grammar. Perceiving by grammatical rules of the language would engage the encoding process at higher levels.

The Breadth of the Perceptual Process

The perception of speech may therefore not be limited to discrimination of the distinctive cues of the input signal that are presented at a specific rate; perception may also describe a deeper level of processing. At this deeper level there is perceptual segmentation that translates

> *Quote 8–3*
> . . . *typical language processing models have deficiencies be-
> cause they incorrectly assume that listeners begin by hearing the
> signal and then, in a step-like manner, continue through and
> passively process until an interpretation is made. Instead, per-
> haps even before the signal is introduced, there is an active
> higher order processing going on which selects the relevant sig-
> nals and processes their contents in parallel fashion.*
> (DUCHAN, 1983, p. 89).

external structures to internal ones. Gibson (1971) believes that in reading, four classes of features—phonlogical, semantic, graphological, and
syntactic—are processed independently and sequentially in a type of
hierarchy. If this is true for processing spoken language as well, the
need for an adequate perceptual mechanism is emphasized.

At all the levels of perception there is interaction among all aspects
of processing. The individual's knowledge of syntax and semantics or
even his or her experience with what "sounds" correct will influence
how and what the individual perceives and will consequently influence
comprehension. Misperceptions can be due to problems in distinguishing auditory cues as well as problems in segmentation related to deficits
in the grammatical aspects of language.

Numerous theorists have attempted to describe the sequence of
events in the processing of word recognition internal to the process of
feature and phoneme perception. New descriptions have evolved from
an interface between acoustic-phonetic processes and the process of
word recognition (Pisoni & Luce, 1987). Frauenfelder and Tyler (1987)
say that the process of recognizing a spoken word begins when a
representation from the sensory input makes contact with the lexicon—
the internally stored form-based representations (the representations of
words) associated with each lexical entry. After the activation of a subset of the lexicon, sensory input continues to accumulate until, through
processes of activation and inhibition, the appropriate entry is selected.
This selection phase has been labeled as a *process of differentiation* by
McClelland and Rumelhart (1986), as *reduction* by Marslen-Wilson
(1984), and as *search* by Forster (1976). The goal of lexical processing
(Frauenfelder & Tyler, 1987) is that of making the stored knowledge
available with a word, available for interpreting the spoken utterance.
The stored knowledge has phonological, syntactic, semantic, and pragmatic properties. The decision as to whether this process consists of a
serial flow of input through autonomous systems (bottom-up) or an interactive process in which information at different levels interacts with
one another (top-down) has not been made. There are equally convincing arguments for both points of view (see Cutler, Mehler, Norris, &
Segui, 1987; Grossberg, 1987; Pisoni & Luce, 1987). Cutler, Mehler,
Norris, and Segui (1987) suggest that both positions probably have

validity and the selection of processing depends on attentional factors and is independently motivated.

The Auditory-Vocal Link

I have argued that there is an aspect of auditory perception that is particularly suited to the perception of the speech sounds that comprise language and that both may belong to a language-specific system that has specific neurological origins.

Another tie between perception and language may be the low-level almost reflexive connection between the auditory and vocal systems. The first evidence we have of an automatic vocal response to a stimulus to the auditory system is in the infant who first responds by general vocalization to a caretaker's verbal caresses and mimics or parrots aspects of what he or she hears. Later, the child imitates what is heard. Obviously the input has been perceived adequately for it to be repeated vocally. This, of course, is accomplished in the absence of comprehension of the stimulus. This same phenomenon occurs in autistic children who echo what they hear even though they may not understand. The echo of autistic children usually preserves the phonemic and syntactic structure of an utterance. A third instance of the auditory-vocal linkage in the absence of comprehension is of patients with brain injury. Patients who are said to have an injury that "isolates the speech area" are able to echo speech with excellent articulation with no evidence of comprehension of language (Geschwind, Quadfasel, & Segarra, 1968) and in some cases to "correct" grammatical structures in their echoed speech that were provided incorrectly in input (Whitaker, 1976). What is rendered in the isolation of speech areas from the rest of the cerebral cortex according to Marin (1982) is a speech machine that has attributes for correct decoding and encoding of speech but without access to meaning or use of the language for referential purposes. These examples seem to indicate that the auditory perceptual, phonological, computational, and productive aspects of language are related. I believe that this linkage permits the automatic syntactic productive behavior previously described— with the vocal production linked to external auditory stimulation. This automatic production of speech is not always available when syntax or surface structure is linked to meaning. The integration of automatic production and meaning may be difficult for some children. An illustrative case is a child I once had for intervention whose language was error-free in articulation and syntax in echolalia but who, as soon as he learned to generate meaningful language, demonstrated the typical developmental errors of other children.

Contributions of Perception to Comprehension

The auditory perceptual mechanism for speech contributes to the task of understanding language and so impairment of the mechanism may impair comprehension. To begin with, what the listener receives is not perfect speech. The wave form of speech is variable. In the wave form, phonemes are rarely realized as a "linearly-ordered sequence of discrete acoustic events" (Pisoni & Luce, 1987, p. 23). In addition, speakers coarticulate phonemes that are adjacent. The variance and nonlinearity contribute to problems in utterance segmentation. Furthermore, spoken language does not occur in a soundproof environment. It is the job of the perceptual system to convert this imperfect data to meaningful units. The system restores or replaces sounds that have been masked out by surrounding noise. It constructs meaningful phonological units from partial data. It stores incomplete information until there is sufficient data provided in the subsequent content to interpret the missing part. If these abilities are impaired, subsequent comprehension abilities may likewise be impaired.

Tallal and Stark (1983) found abnormal development of the ability to respond correctly to selected spectral and temporal cues at the rate these cues occur within speech in language-impaired children. Furthermore, they found that this deficiency in ability to process rapidly changing sensory information is related to the level of delay of receptive language, that is, the greater the delay, the greater the perceptual deficiency. Although Tallal and Stark do not claim a causal relationship between these two deficiencies, it can be hypothesized that such a deficiency in processing temporal cues may in fact impair discrimination of the incoming speech signal and thereby cause problems in comprehension. Highnam and Morris (1987) found that language-disabled children handled auditory input—segmental or suprasegmented—less efficiently than nondisabled children. Furthermore, the language-impaired found a linguistic stress task (judgment of appropriateness of linguistic stress for prerecorded pairs of question-answer triads) to be more difficult than a semantic interpretation task. Most language specialists know of language-disordered children who have difficulty in processing speech, have to request constantly that utterances be repeated, and who even verbalize their difficulty in comprehending what others say, particularly in noisy situations. So at least at a theoretical level and possibly at an empirical one, we can claim a relationship between the ability to discriminate adequately and the ability to comprehend.

The Influence of Perception on Language

I have attempted to show how the perception of speech is intertwined with language, at least at a theoretical level. There is evidence to support this relationship. Remaining at a theoretical level, I would like

> *Quote 8–4*
> *. . . complex perceptual mechanisms specialized to regulate speech are innate in man and function at some level in infancy even though the young infant cannot understand the precise information about reality that speech is intended to convey.*
> (TREVARTHEN, 1983, p. 64).

to describe the effects a perceptual deficit may have on language development and language use.

Perceptual learning is accomplished by an active mechanism, one that searches the language input for clues relative to the best approach to decoding. Since so much processing segmentation and parsing of language occurs at the perceptual level, it is imperative that the signal that is received be an accurate reproduction of what is presented so that the processing of the signal is valid. Otherwise problems in comprehension could arise. Since the vocal system appears to be tied to the auditory system at the grammatical level, one could theoretically propose that problems in perception could cause problems in phonological and grammatical usage at the production level.

The effect of a perceptual problem at the developmental level could be one of *delay* in comprehension and production of language. Articulation and grammatical errors would persist until sufficient exemplars would be available for appropriate abstraction of the invariant aspects of phonological and grammatical forms. Frequency would compensate for degraded quality of the input. Redundancy of input in a variety of contexts would ultimately provide sufficient correct data from which to induce rules in the face of a perceptual deficit. Some residual of the problem might remain for some children. They may continue to misarticulate or have grammatical errors and thus need intervention. (Perhaps one reason we do not find more children with articulation problems having auditory perceptual deficits is because the perceptual difficulty is "outgrown" but its effects on articulation are not.)

The long-term effect of a continuing perceptual problem, particularly if it includes a memory disorder, would be on "on-line" comprehension. Even after the rules of language have been mastered and are used adequately in production, there may be problems in comprehending the ongoing stream of language. Individuals with this type of decoding disorder get messages wrong, misunderstand instructions, ask for directions to be repeated, and misarticulate new words and the names of new friends. Their knowledge of language rules permits adequate comprehension if a message is simple or if it is repeated or if background noise is eliminated. These individuals have a language disorder even though a sample of their language may not reveal it and problems in the production of language forms or a test of their knowledge of language rules would probably indicate average or above average performance.

Intervention for Children with Auditory Processing Disorders

Lubert (1981) speculated that language-impaired children, who are unable to perceive some speech sounds normally, cannot do so because their "feature-detecting" is too slow or inefficient to allow them to perform higher level tasks. If this is an accurate assumption, Lubert suggests, these children will have extreme difficulty in abstracting language rules from the degraded, fragmented, and often ungrammatical language signal that they receive.

My point in this brief discussion of auditory processing is to show that this aspect of performance may have significant effects on language. In instances where input is consistently misperceived, it may affect the manner and type of storage of language thereby affecting the rule system and production. The overall effect of a serious problem of this nature on a child's ability to receive accurate messages cannot be underestimated. Does this mean that we should include auditory processing techniques in intervention? Unfortunately, training does not improve perception substantially. But recognition of a problem of this type can help us help the child with such a problem.

If a child has difficulty abstracting language rules from degraded, fragmented data, and if a child has difficulty, as a consequence, in decoding the input language, he or she will need a greater *amount* of input and a variation in the coding of messages for learning to take place. The degree of language stimulation, including the language of instruction, must be far greater than that provided for the normal child.

The child's own awareness of the difficulty may make him or her more attentive in situations such as a classroom. The use of note-taking and audio recording devices will allow reexamination of parts of instruction that are misunderstood. The use by teachers of visual aids such as figures and graphs and of written instructions on the chalkboard will help all children who are visual learners. I believe that our obligation to a child with such a perceptual problem includes helping him or her to cope with it in real life situations as much as it is to teach him or her to use grammatical and pragmatic rules.

RELATION BETWEEN MEMORY AND LANGUAGE

As is the case with auditory perception, the studies of the relationship between auditory memory and language disorders are not consistent. My clinical experience has indicated that in some instances, poor memory and disordered language co-occur at least. It is because of this and because I believe a discussion of language would be incomplete without a discussion of memory that I have included this section. It is by no means a complete thesis on the subject. It is meant to stimulate thought on the importance of memory to language and to move us away from the idea that auditory memory has to do with recalling digits.

The study and understanding of the memory process in the human being is difficult at best. An attempt to understand the relationship between memory and language is even more complex, particularly if one includes within the framework of memory the retrieval of linguistic information. As with perception, the understanding of memory is a theoretical one and the knowledge that is arrived at is obtained through inference from behavior and through metamemory activities of the theorist. The significant role memory plays in language makes it imperative that specialists in language disorders continue the quest for insight into this relationship.

Views of Memory

There are numerous approaches to the study of memory as well as numerous theoretical models for its function and organization. A brief review of some of these approaches may provide insight into the role that memory plays in language and the manner in which this understanding can assist in the intervention of children with language disorders.

Early models of memory focused on distinguishing between short-term and long-term memories or primary and secondary memories, and this focus led to the concept of a series of storage capacities. The multi-store model included a sensory register, a temporary working memory (short-term), and a permanent storehouse of information (long-term). Theorists believe that once words are processed into sentences, the output of the process is accommodated in a secondary storage system. In fact, Gough (1972) stated that items pass into secondary memory only when they are related. If the initial words of sentences exceed the capacity of the primary memory before their grammatical relations can be discovered, they will not be understood. According to Gough, this is true of sentences that are embedded to a degree of two or more.

In a discussion that addresses short- and long-term memory, it is important to distinguish between two aspects of cognitive processing. First, there are the structural features of the system that are resistant to modification and function outside of conscious control (e.g., the capacity of short-term memory, the durability of memory traces, and the speed with which the system's processes operate). The other aspect of cognitive processing includes the information and skills that are learned through experience—the long-term memory content with its corresponding knowledge of the world, the habitual ways of thinking, and the rules and strategies that guide performance in tasks. The latter features can be changed by instruction (see Torgesen & Greenstein, 1982). It is these that merit our attention.

A way of distinguishing between types of long-term memory has been suggested by Tulving (1972). He distinguished semantic memory and episodic memory, not as a proposal for a new theory of memory, but as a useful delineation of memory types. Tulving described *semantic* memory as a "mental thesaurus, the organized knowledge a person possesses about *words* and other *verbal symbols*, their *meaning* and referents, about relations among them, and about rules, formulas, and algorithms for the manipulation of these symbols, concepts and relations" (p. 386). This memory is independent from specific events. *Episodic* memory stores information about temporally dated events or episodes and temporal-spatial relations among these events. These data are stored in terms of their autobiographical reference as opposed to the cognitive referents of the input signals in semantic memory. Episodic memory is more susceptible to memory loss than is semantic memory.

Some theorists draw a distinction between episodic and event representation (Nelson, 1986b). The episode is seen as a member of the class, event. For example, a child might experience an episode of an event. The internal representation of each of these differs even though both are derived from initial experiential data. The episodic memory is represented in a more concrete fashion than the event, the latter being incorporated into a schema. The general event representation (GER) derives from specific experiences or sets of experiences and thus interacts with episodic memory. Nelson (1986b) believes, however, that these are two distinct types of representation. Since both events and episodes include the verbal scripts that accompany the actions, participants, and other components of the event or episode as an integral part of it, the concept of this type of representation has considerable implications for language—in both the semantic and linguistic components.

A memory distinction made by Schank (1975), similar to that of Tulving, produces a different way of separating general and specific aspects of language. Schank describes a *lexical* memory that stores information about words, idioms, common expressions, and other language items. The lexical items are linked to a *conceptual* memory comprised of *language-free* associations and relations between concepts that are a result of personal experience and therefore episodic in nature. According to this view of memory, there is no special memory that embodies all of semantic knowledge per se. There is a general knowledge base that is derived from episodes and remains close to them, and this is tied to the lexical memory.

Schank's lexical memory appears to be a more probable construct than the semantic memory of Tulving. Schank does not limit the lexical memory to dictionary-type entries but allows for the idiosyncratic meanings provided by the individual's own episodes and experiences to enrich the definition and to bring a unique interpretation to the meaning

> *Quote 8–5*
> *. . . it is obvious that the lexical system reflects the language system of the child's community, while the conceptual system is derived, at least in part, from subjective experience represented at a less general, episodic level . . . . the considerations brought out here have indicated that understanding the child's semantic development requires understanding the development of his knowledge system, that is, of the structure of relations within and between concepts.*
>
> (NELSON, 1978, pp. 75–76).

of the words. Tyler (1981) states that there are strong arguments in favor of the claim that the meaning of a linguistic expression involves extralinguistic sources of knowledge. This idea of lexical memory is also consistent with what is seen in bilingualism. When we learn a second language, we do not develop a whole constellation of new meanings to attach to the words in the second language. We usually just add a new word to the already existing meaning. In cases where translation is difficult, it is because a dictionary entry for a specific meaning is not available in the first language. The particular slice of reality is not labeled in the first language and so we need to add a new entry with its meaning.

Whichever way of organizing memory that we choose, we must recognize, according to Nelson and Brown (1978), that long-term memory knowledge emerges from episodes and is stored in a form that reflects them directly. All other organizational forms—cognitive maps, scripts, semantic and categorical relations, and others—are derived drom this knowledge. Nelson and Brown further suggested that the organized language-based semantic system is freed (but not completely independent) from experiences that are originally multimodal (verbal, imagic).

It seems logical to also theorize a syntactic memory as well as a semantic one. A syntactic memory stores the rules for the computational aspects of language, a memory that ordinarily permits easy access during the parsing and phonological segmentation phases of comprehension and easy retrieval for the rapid grammatical utterances of speech. The memory connects the auditory input and expressive systems in such a way that it allows imitation and also correction of utterances

> *Quote 8–6*
> *From a developmental point of view, then, the conflation of semantic (i.e., lexical) memory and real-world knowledge is unfortunate; for an understanding of semantic development, the two must be considered separately and the contents of each examined.*
>
> (NELSON, 1978, p. 42).

with syntactic errors (see discussion of the auditory/vocal relationship in previous section of this chapter). The frequency and temporal contiguity of occurrence of specific morphemes make possible the automatic functions of speech and bring closure without direct attention to meaning. It permits the system to use the linguistic code effectively without having to access the semantic memory for every single morpheme used.

Some theorists propose a phonological memory that contains units that are related to acoustic *and* articulatory inputs. (Articulatory units are included in phonological memory because of the theory that the kinds of articulatory-motor responses made in performing speech may also be involved in the perception of that sound.) According to Samuels and Eisenberg (1981), the units in phonological memory include distinctive features, phonemes, syllables, and morphemes. This memory may be the same as the syntactic memory just described.

There should also be a memory category in which to place non-meaningful associations. By nonmeaningful I mean new associations between perceptual events that do not have frequency of occurrence. If words have to be understood before they enter secondary memory (Gough, 1972), what happens to nonmeaningful words? If what is remembered from a sentence is the gist or meaning, what happens when we have to remember exact words without cognitive meaning, for example, when we want to remember the name of a new friend? How many times are you introduced to someone and then turn around to introduce the same person to someone else and fail to come up with the name? How many times do you have to be exposed to names and places in *Trivial Pursuit* before you can remember them? We must have auditory storage for sequences of sounds that are not dictionary entries. If we do not store them well, we have difficulty retrieving them. The storage of these nonmeaningful data requires a deliberate effort to remember—to allocate the item(s) to secondary memory—whereas the storage of meaningful information can be entered into existing episodic frameworks easily. Content is stored more easily than form.

These descriptions of memory indicate that theorists presently believe that there is a network of memories between which information can be exchanged and which have concepts that relate to one another. Components from various memories are joined into schemata.

Cognitive Processes and Memory

There appears to be a reciprocal relationship between cognitive processes in general and memory: (1) the memory allows for the integration of incoming with existing information; (2) cognitive processes operate on *representations* of external events; and (3) a child's cognitive organizing skills assist in ordering material to be remembered.

Memory is thought to be directly involved in a number of cognitive processing stages: there are storage, encoding, and retrieval phases of memory (Lange, 1978). There is memory involvement in the interaction between the perceptual processes in decoding and encoding processes. If the cues for item retrieval are to be effective, the encoding of that item must associate the cue with the item. In order for the encoding to occur in that manner, the relationship between the cue and the item must be identified during the perceptual process. Lange (1978) states the "organizational processing at the perceptual and encoding phases is a necessary precondition for the organization we see at retrieval output" (p. 104). The recall of items appears to vary with the extent and stability of their organization in memory.

Memory permits us to represent the events and scripts of the external world. The cognitive processes of pattern analysis, sequencing, rule induction, and so on act on the representation of the world, not on the world itself. Inadequate representations because of inadequate perception or memory can produce inadequate thinking and talking.

It follows that the memorizer's organizational abilities and experience with the input items influence the accessibility of the item. Salient cues and an effective structure will result in operative retrieval. If there are organizational failures, they may be due to a failure to establish a "clearly definable and stable organization of the stimuli" (Lange, 1978, p. 111) that is termed an *input failure* or a failure to make use of the organization to access the items *(integration failure)*.

Cognition and memory are also related at the level of comprehension. One way in which memory aids comprehension is by permitting recycling of information. By recycling, new information is added and is integrated with what is already in memory and the input is understood more clearly. Memory also assists in constructive comprehension skills, such as those involved in drawing inferences from sentences (Paris, Lindauer, & Cox, 1977). Inferring requires relating what is heard or read with what is already in the memory system. Drawing inferences in turn enriches and deepens understanding by increasing the number of relationships discovered about an event (Paris, 1978). Although inferences are usually thought of as operating on verbal information, they utilize nonlinguistic material as well.

Early memory improvement is probably due to an increase in the knowledge of the child. As the child develops, memory improvement is probably related to growth of control processes (techniques for moving information among the memory stores) that in turn improves memory. Past 5 years of age, the use of deliberate rehearsal, organization, or retrieval strategies may be the source of improved recall (Myers & Perlmutter, 1978).

Recall improvement for syntactic structure input seems to be related to the child's general growth in linguistic ability. Tyler (1981) reported studies of memory experiments with children who were instructed to repeat verbatim the last sentence they heard when a story to which they were listening was stopped. The 5-year-olds differed from the older children and adults in their lack of clausal structuring of recall. The younger children tended to use a global interpretive reproduction rather than a syntactic one. Tyler suggested a plausible interpretation of her findings to be that the age differences in recall reflect differences in 5-year-old children's versus the older children's dependence on syntactic as opposed to interpretive factors during the original processing of the material.

It would appear that the organization type and strength of memory stores would affect the ease with which retrieval of information takes place. One could hypothesize that individuals who have difficulty in the immediate recall of what they have heard would also have difficulty in retrieving linguistic structures when there is no auditory stimulus serving as an input. Leonard, Nippold, Kail, and Hale (1983) found that language-impaired children had longer response latencies than their age controls in a naming task and that frequency of the name of the depicted object significantly related to the language-impaired children's naming time. In one explanation of the phenomenon of retrieval, Leonard et al. suggested "that in the network of associations that constitute semantic memory . . . , associations involving frequently used words, are stronger—and hence retrieved more rapidly—than associations involving less frequently used names" (p. 613). Their second explanation related to storage limitations of the language-impaired realized in the form of words with few representations in memory having less associative strength.

It would appear to be obvious that auditory memory is basic to auditory perception and vice versa. The perceptual function provides the data that the memory stores. The act of recognition of a perception, even a basic phonological one, implies prior experience with like perceptual events and the memory of the events. In other words, the memory imposes a particular structure on the incoming stimulus.

Memory and Language Disorder

So much of language is dependent on memory that it is difficult to imagine how language can be described without it. The relationship is not only to the storage and encoding of language information, as just described, but also to the manner of retrieving the information once it is stored. As in perception, the effect of an auditory memory deficit may not impair the acquisition of linguistic rules as much as it may interfere with the facility of *understanding and producing an ongoing stream of language* (for example, language use in Alzheimers disease). If it is valid to hypothesize that there are different kinds of memories, there may be different kinds of memory problems that may interfere with processing different kinds of information. We do not yet know exactly how the constraints of memory affect language. We do know, however, that memory and language interact with one another at every level of knowledge and processing. We cannot stop looking for the manner in which they interact. As we increase our understanding we will do a better job of helping children with language disorders.

Implications for Intervention

Perhaps the greatest value of information on memory is that of recognizing its role in many of the skills we assist children in acquiring. If memory is viewed from a constructive approach, as an active system, we can recognize the need for children to be able to provide organization for the sensory input from the child's abstractions and concepts in order for memory to function well. Perhaps we can assist them in developing strategies that will help them to remember facts they need to learn in school, strategies that will help develop a network or schema of episodic memories so that ideas and events can be related and common elements and differences explored, and that in turn will assist in comprehension. Take, for example, a closet that has pegs, shelves, hooks, and rods—organized so that everything that is entered has a place. The time taken to place or replace objects in this closet is clearly reduced compared with a closet in which everything is disordered. Furthermore, access to specific needed objects is easy and quick. Some individuals need help in organizing, and they profit from it when it is provided.

This framework of memory representations, which permits us to classify, identify patterns, conduct abstractions and inferences, and in general perform other cognitive functions, is labeled by Nelson (1986a) and others as *event knowledge*. Our cognitive operations are influenced to some extent at least by what is represented in our mind and in what form it is represented. Event knowledge is not only a knowledge of objects and relations, but also knowledge of them within a dynamic, holistic structure that has internal changes over time. Nelson (1986b)

Quote 8–7

*According to the former hypothesis [one-store notion], information is stored in memory through an abstract format connected with, but separate from, both languages of a bilingual. For instance, the encoding and retention of the words **shame** and **verguenza** would both depend centrally on some single representational format that contains some deep abstraction of their meaning.*

(CROWDER, 1978, p. 349).

> Quote 8–8
> *The most obvious behavioral constraint on language acquisition is the development of memory in the young child. The child's immediate and long-term memory must constrain his language ability in vocabulary size, utterance length, and amount of material in the external structure of sentences deleted from their internal structure.*
>
> (BEVER, 1970, p. 350).

suggests that the initial content of mental representations are changes of state that in turn are the basis of the derivation of stable mental elements. The event knowledge is derived form exposure to everyday experiences and events. The implications are considerable. The need for repeated experiences or events that combine verbal and situational input cannot be underestimated.

If I understand anything about language at all, it is because early in my studies I developed a framework for classifying the components of language and their interrelationship. The basic framework that I wrote about in 1968 and again in 1975 has not changed in essence (Carrow, 1968; Carrow-Woolfolk, 1975). I have modified and expanded it, but new knowledge has not made me discard what I have and start over again. The internal organization has been flexible and reflective of the reality I have attempted to know. Instead of viewing apparently conflicting ideas as incompatible, I have always tried to see how they fit into the schema. Where this has not been possible, I have put the aberrant one on hold until I can find a place for it. I rarely discard an idea completely. Most ideas can be found to solve at least one part of a puzzle.

As was mentioned in the discussion of perception, we may need to help children compensate for a memory problem. For example, teachers may need to provide instruction in written form to preserve the input for study, or the child may need to learn to write everything down that he or she needs to remember. I am not saying that we need to work with drills for improving short-term memory capacity. These have no useful purpose. But we can teach children techniques for helping them remember the facts they need to know in order to function well in communicating with others.

Rice (1983) also believes that understanding and evaluating internal processing factors is useful clinically. In fact, she states that effectiveness of remediation is related to the knowledge of each child's perceptual, cognitive, and linguistic constraints. She states that the "recent recognition of cognitive factors has balanced the earlier enthusiasm for behaviorism in that it has returned the clinical focus to the internal capacities of children as well as to environmental events" (p. 354). She further suggests that we should be open-minded about language-specific processes so that the understanding of language-impaired children may be based on a recognition of individual differences and not on the "simple observation that children vary in their linguistic aptitude" (p. 354).

9

INTEGRATING THEORIES: LANGUAGE COMPREHENSION

WHAT DOES "COMPREHENSION" MEAN

MODELS OF LANGUAGE COMPREHENSION

FACTORS THAT INFLUENCE COMPREHENSION
  External Factors
  Internal Factors
    Phonemic Categorization
    Procedural Knowledge
    Knowledge of the Rules

Role of Short-Term Memory
Long-Term Storage
Propositional Knowledge

COMPREHENSION DEVELOPMENT

COMPREHENSION AND EXPRESSION

DISORDERS OF COMPREHENSION

COMPREHENSION INTERVENTION

In the early sections of this book, I reviewed the six theories of language that I believe have been and are the basis of assessment and intervention procedures with language disorders. As indicated in these reviews, the neuropsychology and cognitive process theories are the only two that describe the role of comprehension in language in an explicit manner. The behavior theory ignores all internal processes, while the cognitive organization theory describes the internal processes in terms of the strategies such as problem-solving, symbolization, and rule-development that are common to all cognitive systems; special attention to comprehension is not provided. The linguistic and pragmatic theories are concerned primarily with analysis and description of production and with the speech act, respectively. Although linguistic theory (Bloom & Lahey, 1978) does describe the developmental relationship between understanding and speaking, it suggests that to include comprehension in

THEORY, ASSESSMENT AND INTERVENTION
IN LANGUAGE DISORDERS: © 1988 by Grune & Stratton
AN INTEGRATIVE APPROACH

ISBN   0-8089-1918-0

intervention, a child should be exposed to contexts that combine content/form/use at the level of the child's productive development. Its emphasis is, however, on facilitating the production of language. Pragmatic theory is concerned with listening and comprehending because it contributes to the accuracy of messages in any type of language interaction. The contribution of pragmatic theory is in terms of understanding the role of context and the variation introduced by the intentions of the speaker in comprehension. This contribution, then, is significant.

In Chapter 6 I described briefly the relation of comprehension and expression in reference to the knowledge/performance distinctions in language. I suggested that the factors common to knowledge and performance are primarily in the area of linguistic and conceptual knowledge (although there is probably some difference even here, particularly during the period of language acquisition) and the differences between comprehension and expression in the area of performance. More will be said about the relationship of comprehension and expression in this chapter.

The main focus of the chapter is comprehension itself. Because comprehension is an internal process and not conducive to behavioral observation and analysis, there has been a tendency in the field of language disorders to treat the whole process of comprehension in a superficial manner. It is much less difficult to describe changes in production as a result of intervention than it is to decribe changes in comprehension, so the tendency is to direct intervention toward expressive language, particularly since specialists such as Bloom and Lahey (1978) have stated that comprehension is not necessarily a prerequisite to expression and that there actually may be an opposite order of emergence of these systems developmentally. I believe, however, that if we make a distinction between the comprehension of linguistic forms specifically and the comprehension of language in general, our understanding of the comprehension process will broaden and we may be in a better position to provide the kinds of language intervention that will assist the language-disordered not only in the areas of teaching productive skills when they are young but in those areas of language that are needed throughout their school career. In other words, I see intervention with comprehension not as a means of improving expression but as a means of improving language.

As I hope it is clear from discussions in previous chapters, I interpret language as a union among systems, particularly the conceptual (to include social) and linguistic. Language is more than the use of correct grammatical rules in production and the use of correct interactive rules in pragmatic speech. The use of language is also a means of obtaining and relating concepts and ideas, verbal as well as nonverbal. The conceptual component of language is as important a focus for development as is the linguistic component. It is through comprehension (of both oral and written language) that we can develop the kind of language and general understanding of the world that will be a basis for success in learning school subjects. It is for this reason that I will attempt a brief description of the comprehension process. I will attempt to describe comprehension as a cognitive process as well as a part of the pragmatic system of communication.

_____

WHAT DOES "COMPREHENSION" MEAN

When we speak about comprehension, we usually mean the behavior by which we attach meaning to coded symbols and signs. The code may be received aurally in response to spoken language or visually in response to the code as written or signed. In order to comprehend, *an individual must know the rules of the code*, the particular combinations of phonemes, morphemes, and syntax and the meanings they have when used in specific ways in a particular language. I cannnot understand German even though I can discriminate all the phonemes when it is spoken and may be able to repeat or echo what is said. I must have general and specific conceptual knowledge (depending on what is being communicated) and attach this knowledge to the form of the language in order to comprehend. Even if I have an extensive knowledge of a language, for example, the English language rules, I still may be unable to understand what is happening at a baseball field by listening to a ballgame over the radio. Only a baseball aficionado would understand the following: "He got pure heat right up among the letters," or "He put that split finger right through the trap door," or "Ashley, in the on deck circle, will squeeze it." I can understand the language, but not comprehend the meaning.

A second aspect of comprehension involves the *clarity and accuracy of transmission of language through the auditory system.* An individual may know the rules of language and have an adequate conceptual knowledge for bringing meaning to the code, but have difficulty understanding because the auditory perceptual processing system lacks precision in the discrimination or categorization of phonemes or in the parsing or segmentation of units of language input (also see Chapter 8). There may be a problem in the speaker's articulation or the level of background noise that causes a disturbance in the message transmission. Redundancy in the linguistic or situational context and the familiarity of

---

Quote 9–1
Speech has developed into a fairly independent acousticovocal system, with peculiarities that set it apart in perception, production, and cognitive organization.

(MARIN, 1982, p. 51).

the listeners with the context will often compensate to a great extent for the lack of clarity, but that may not be enough for a person with processing impediments.

A third aspect of comprehension has to do with utilization of messages. Bridges, Sinha, and Walkerdine (1981) say that in constructing an interpretation, a listener also identifies the intentions of the speaker for the utilization of the message. The listener formulates together with the literal interpretation of the utterance a "sense" of what the speaker desires in terms of a response—linguistic or nonlinguistic. It appears that these are simultaneous processes and integral parts of comprehension.

Listeners may have difficulty understanding and comprehending if they do not decode accurately and may have difficulty comprehending if they do not understand the code, but they can decode (as in another language) without understanding and they can understand (as in the baseball analogy) without comprehending. For this reason we should make a distinction between decoding, understanding, and comprehending and should clearly state this distinction when discussing comprehension. This distinction is particularly necessary when discussing disorders of comprehension in which the nature and the effects of problems related to different aspects of comprehension differ.

Much of what is called *comprehension development* is the development of representation of two kinds, representation of the nonlinguistic aspects of language, the meaning acquired by the internalization of the world, and the representation of the linguistic aspects of language—the grammar, and the association between these two kinds of representation. When we test for comprehension or even engage in what is called *comprehension intervention*, we are actually probing to see if this association has taken place. Much of what passes for comprehension intervention—pointing to pictures or acting out in response to a linguistic stimulus—is simply a way of verifying this internal association.

We also need to recognize differences between terminology that refers to the process of actually carrying out the comprehension process as opposed to learning to carry it out. Learning to comprehend involves developing a complex matrix of interacting systems to include, among others, (1) linguistic and nonlinguistic representation, (2) related semantic notions, (3) relations among notions and between notions and their linguistic counterpart, and (4) interpretation and storage of the contexts in which actions and events take place to use in expanding and refining meaning. Adults who "carry out" the comprehension process have, at least it is assumed they have, the internal stores of meaning and the linguistic data base. Their task is to decode a message that may be awkwardly phrased by a speaker, that may contain terminology that they do not know, or that may enter their processing system in a degraded fashion because of insufficient loudness or background noise. Their system needs to accurately transmit the message for comprehension. Children must accomplish the task of the adult as well as their own. They are in the process of building, and using while they build. This makes it difficult for us to identify their deficiencies when they cannot comprehend. The greatest mistake we can make, I believe, is to treat comprehension as a simple process.

MODELS OF LANGUAGE COMPREHENSION

Models of language comprehension are developed for different purposes and, consequently, the components they include and their basic designs differ. I will describe four models of comprehension so that the various aspects of the comprehension process can be more fully appreciated.

Woods (1982) designed a model to use for developing a computerized speech understanding system. The components of Woods' model are seen in Figure 9–1. In this model the component *feature extraction* takes over or extracts the basic features (acoustic) from a continuous stream of words. *Lexical retrieval* searches for words that match the phonological or acoustic features. Once certain words are hypothesized, the component of *matching* checks the low-level acoustic data to determine to what degree the evidence supports the hypothesis. When the string of words has been hypothesized, *syntax* checks whether it is well formed. The *semantics* component checks whether it is meaningful and *pragmatics* whether it is relevant to the context in which it was spoken. *Control* distributes attention among the various components and decides when to switch hypothesis if the first one does not fit the evidence. *Bookkeeping* keeps track of all the hypotheses that have been considered. The way that Woods tested his components was to allow humans to carry out all the tasks except that of lexical retrieval, which was handled by a machine. The data he gathered from his experiments provided information for developing the computerized program.

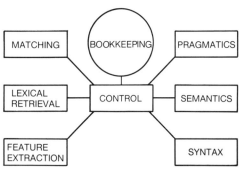

FIGURE 9–1. Components of a speech understanding system. (Reproduced with permission from Woods, W. A. [1982]. HWIM: A speech understanding system on a computer. In M. A. Arbib, D. Caplan, & J. Marshall (Eds.), *Neural models of language processes* (p. 97). New York: Academic Press.

Although Woods did not intend the model to be used as a basis for describing the entire comprehension process, the identification and separation of components in the model illuminate the complexity of speech perception and the kinds of processes involved in comprehension. It is for this reason that I have included it here.

Marcus (1982) schematized the process of understanding past the point of word recognition (see Fig. 9–2). Marcus assumed that the incoming word stream is the input to a parser called *Syntax*, which analyzes the syntactic structure of the input. The syntactic structure that is the output of Syntax may be in the form of a tree structure (S → NP + VP, etc.). The syntactic representation serves as input to the *Semantic* processor. The Syntax component may be bypassed if either the Syntax produces only fragmentary information or as an interim procedure for associated analysis by Semantics while waiting for the syntactic analysis. The Semantic component produces some meaningful representation that is logically compatible with the input structure. The meaning obtained from Semantics goes into the *World Knowledge* of the individual. Marcus makes the point that semantic processing is sufficiently robust for determining meaning with a fragmentary input from syntactic analysis.

Bloom and Lahey (1978) used a different approach to schematizing comprehension. In describing comprehension in the absence of an external event that may assist in understanding what is being said, they identify four components. *A* is a linguistic signal that is processed at *LP*, the linguistic processor. Information from the *LP* is compared with what the child already knows by using *INFO* in cognitive memory. Input from *INFO* is received in *C*, consciousness, where a mental representation of the content of the message is obtained. The message is then understood (Fig. 9–3).

When comprehension takes place within the context of an external event, the process is described differently. The additional component is termed *discourse context* and is included in a comprehension model called an "on-line interactive model" by Tyler (1981). This model evolved from experiments with on-line (immediate) processing tasks with adults (Marslen-Wilson & Tyler, 1980). Tyler's position claims that the processing involved in comprehending is conducted with immediate

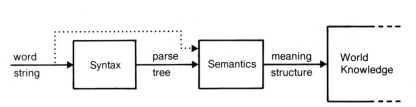

FIGURE 9–2. Postulated information flow of the undersdtanding process. (Reproduced with permission from Marcus, M. P. [1982]. Consequences of functional deficits in a parsing model: Implications for Broca's aphasia. In M. A. Arbib, D. Caplan, & J. Marshall (Eds.), *Neural models of language processes* (p. 117). New York: Academic Press.

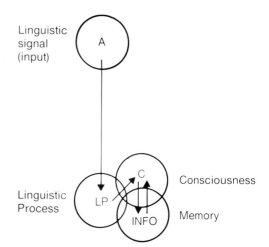

Linguistic signal (input)

A

C

Consciousness

Linguistic Process

LP

INFO

Memory

FIGURE 9–3. A description of the comprehension process in the absence of an external event that may assist in undersdtanding what is said. (Reproduced with permission from Bloom, L., & Lahey, M. [1978]. *Language development and language disorders* (p. 258). NewYork: John Wiley and Sons).

reference to the discourse context in which the comprehension takes place. The interpretive representation that a listener constructs is the result of the interaction between nonlinguistic (specific discourse context and general knowledge of the world) and linguistic properties of the utterance. This view differs somewhat from that of Marcus in that Tyler states that "the syntactic and semantic properties of utterances, as linguistically defined, do not correspond during processing to computationally distinct syntactic and semantic 'levels of analysis'" (p. 150). She states that syntactic knowledge functions during processing as a guide in assigning structural relations within the interpretive representation. Furthermore, she suggests that semantic properties of words are analyzed together with their interpretation in some "context of use" and not as an independent stage of processing. (The issue of processing stages will be discussed in a subsequent section of this chapter.)

These brief sketches of four comprehension models provide an insight into the comprehension process and the internal activity that must take place for comprehension to occur. Woods' (1982) model emphasizes the various comprehension components and the way in which a control component shifts back and forth from the various analysis nodes and proposes various hypotheses before arriving at a match between the evidence and the meaning. Marcus' (1982) parser illustrates the need for correct segmentation in order for correct meaning to be elicited; he also stresses that this meaning can be obtained even if there is degradation of the input. Bloom and Lahey (1978) point out that utterance meaning must be obtained from what is already stored in the memory if it is not present in the context in which the child is the listener. Tyler (1981) includes the discourse context as an integral part of the component and suggests simultaneous processing as opposed to that of stages. The components that Woods describes I will refer to as the *decoding* aspect of comprehension. If adequate parsing takes place as in Marcus' model to include the situational context as part of the processing as suggested by Tyler, a meaningful structure is presented to what Bloom and Lahey call *consciousness* and I call *understanding*. But not until the information *INFO* from past events and those of the discourse context are associated with the linguistically analyzed structure can comprehension really take place.

FACTORS THAT INFLUENCE COMPREHENSION

If we are to provide adequate assessment and intervention for comprehension disorders and to have insight into what may be possibly contributing to the disorders, we need to identify factors that influence the quality of comprehension. I would like to group the factors into external, those that occur outside of the individual's processing system, and internal factors, those that have to do with the adequacy and efficiency of the input processing system.

External Factors

One of the main external factors that influences comprehension is the context in which an input is received. Most adult conversation would be totally incomprehensible if taken out of the situational context within which it occurs. The objects, events, and actions that surround us when we are speaking often become the silent subjects or verbs or prepositions in our utterances. It is particularly apparent in language development that children rely to a great extent on visual cues for their comprehension of the language of a parent or caretaker. Language specialists often recognize that many children whom they examine do not, in fact, comprehend as well as their parents believe they do. So much information is transmitted by their environment in requesting certain behaviors that it is often unnecessary for a child to understand every single word. This is particularly true if specific objects are the focus of concern and therefore are more noticeable to the child.

The particular individual from whom we receive input also influences our comprehension. If we know this individual well and we know his or her past experiences and knowledge and his or her intentions, it is likely that he or she will make implicit references to people and events that comprise a shared knowledge, and therefore his or her utterances will be completely comprehensible to us even though they may not be understandable to others. Recognition of the linguistic style of another person also aids comprehension. Some persons customarily use indirect statements for the purpose of requesting something. It is important to recognize these for what they are. Children particularly need to learn to recognize covert and implicit messages in contrast to overt and explicit ones.

Bridges, Sinha, and Walkerdine (1981) suggest that the listener not only represents the context to which an utterance refers but must understand how the speaker intends for the listener to modify his or her representation of the context: to act on it, to assert something about it, and so on. This process of bringing meaning to an utterance, relating it to the speaker's intentions, and accommodating the new information into the original representation, Bridges, Sinha, and Walkerdine refer to as *construction* and *deconstruction*. Within this framework, comprehension is a product of the relationships between message, intention, and context. Therefore, according to Bridges et al., context is an intersubjectively constructed frame of reference. Its relationship to the utterance itself is specified by the intentions of the conversational partners.

Linguistic structure and linguistic context also play roles in comprehension, particularly in the decoding aspect of comprehension (Fischler & Bloom, 1979). With regard to linguistic structure, it is universally recognized that grammatical forms differ with respect to the cognitive requirements underlying their understanding, that is, the meanings of some forms are more complex than others in their level of abstraction, in the number of notions expressed, and so on. There is also a difference in comprehension related to the type of encoding used to express an idea, such as free versus bound morpheme, simple versus embedded sentences, sentence length and cohesion, or density of propositions. Bloom, Merkin, and Wooten (1982) suggested that the syntactic function of forms and their contingency relations in discourse influence sequence of acquisition and therefore comprehensibility. Some forms always occur in a specific linguistic environment that differs from the environment of other forms and therefore influences the difficulty and comprehensibility. An individual's ability to understand is influenced by the particular forms chosen by the speaker for encoding his or her ideas.

The framing used by a speaker is a linguistic means of aiding comprehension. A frame is a standard or routine linguistic package that precedes, follows, or envelopes the message. Usually, in children, the parts of the routines or frames may not be understood as isolated units, but because they are heard repeatedly together, they provide a verbal context to the message, a prediction of its meaning, and therefore a trigger to its comprehension. Special frames are specific types of text material such as narratives. The degree to which a story or narrative follows the typical path and uses the elements or frames that follow the rules of a story grammar influences the degree to which the story or narrative can be understood.

The linguistic topic provides the same type of aid to comprehension as does a situational object or event. If a listener is aware of the subject matter that is being discussed, she or he can more easily tune in to the discussion and bring to the comprehension task his or her own knowledge of the subject. We sometimes experience this when listening to a conversation in a foreign language in which we have some ability. A totally incomprehensible exchange can be converted to an understandable one if someone tells us the topic being discussed.

There are purely physical characteristics of the input that also influence the decoding aspect of comprehension. The clarity, loudness, and articulatory precision of an input is important to the accurate reception of the code. The signal to noise ratio must be within the limits that a typical ear can accept and still decode the message. In the previous chapter I pointed out that even under the best of circumstances, something of the physical characteristics of an input is lost in the transmission to the ear. But the nature of our perceptual mechanism permits a certain portion of the degradation of the message without loss of meaning by restoring what is missing.

Internal Factors

I have summarized briefly some of the factors external to the listener that influence the accuracy with which a listener comprehends messages. There are internal factors that influence comprehension and that can be accounted for by the processing strategies and knowledge of the listener. Aspects of the listener's processing system interact with the input at various levels of decoding and the storehouse of information carried by the listener's memories interact at every stage of the comprehension process. This storehouse of information, in addition to world knowledge organized into various memories, contains the procedural knowledge necessary for decoding at the processing level and applying the propositional knowledge, which is knowledge about things, events, and so on, to the decoding process.

Phonemic Categorization

At the lowest level of processing the perceptual system must categorize the incoming speech sounds in their correct phonemic classes. If the phonemes are not identified correctly, the input that is presented for further analysis will contain wrong words and therefore will be misunderstood. This categorization, although it appears to be an easy task, may not be so for some individuals. The dialects used by native speakers can cause variations in phoneme production that for other listeners cross phoneme boundaries. If the listener has difficulty in making accurate overall judgments of meaning, taking into account also the syntactic and semantic information, she or he will not arrive at a correct interpretation of the message.

Procedural Knowledge

Procedural knowledge is what is used to decipher information that is not explicitly available in the input. At the lowest level of analysis, we use procedural knowledge to segment a continuous stream of language into words and words into syntactic and semantic units that are acceptable within the structural grammar of a particular language. No information is provided in the input as to how it should be decoded; the decisions for segmentation and parsing belong to the listener. Obviously, there are rarely if ever sentences stored that are exact replicas of the ones we hear. What is required, therefore, is the evaluation of segments on the basis of stored lexical, syntactic, and pragmatic information (see Woods' model in Fig. 9–1).

Knowledge of the Rules

In order to segment and interpret grammatical structure accurately, an individual must have an adequate knowledge of the basic structural rules of the language. Experience with many grammatical frames is needed for judging and classifying a specific input. One problem in comprehending school-level materials presented by a teacher is the typical child's lack of exposure to grammatical structures other than those basic ones used in the home and social activities. The teacher's oral text quickly increases in complexity as she or he explains complex subject matter, and the children are expected to understand even though they have not been exposed or taught to decode lengthy and complex textual material.

Role of the Short-Term Memory

If input sentences are long or the input is in the form of many sentences, the short-term memory plays an important role, particularly with individuals who have difficulty with the input analysis. Woods (1982) suggested that we set up hypotheses about what sentences mean and then go about verifying these hypotheses by syntactic, semantic, and pragmatic analysis. Although for most individuals the time taken for this procedure is minimal, for individuals with decoding problems, the hypothesis testing may not be simple and the extra time needed is made possible by holding a part of the input in short-term memory while analyzing another part. For some, the auditory-vocal tie described in the previous chapter reinforces the short-term memory store by an internal

---

Quote 9–2

. . . the function of linguistic input is to deal with the categorization problem: after he has constructed a map of the world through his extralinguistic experience, the child utilizes linguistic input to draw in the borders between adjoining categories. Now we suggest that linguistic input may also be responsible for constructing certain parts of the map itself.

(SCHLESINGER, 1977, p. 161).

repetition or rehearsal of what is being held-in memory and thus helps to prevent decay. Individuals with processing problems may not be able to decode with sufficient rapidity to keep up with the speaker. They are either delayed in their responses to short inputs or they ask for input repetition to give them another chance at decoding.

Long-Term Storage

Long-term storage capacities for syntactic rules and lexical units are also integral to this process. To decode, an individual must first have memory banks equipped with information about syntax, semantics, and pragmatics. Whether these data are stored together or separately has been the subject of previous chapters. But regardless of how or where they are stored, data about language are essential to the decoding and comprehension of input. It is against this stored information that new information is compared. These data provide information that may be missing from the text input. Rules allow predictability in comprehending. There is nothing in the text itself that describes how it is to be decoded.

Propositional Knowledge

At a higher level of processing, the listener relies, for sentence analysis, on his or her propositional knowledge. According to Samuels and Eisenberg (1981), propositional knowledge is knowledge of the things in our mind and in our world. This knowledge is of perceptual concepts such as size, shape, and loudness or of abstract concepts of events and is received through all the sensory input systems and analyzed and categorized partially through language. The knowledge

---

Quote 9–3

. . . an adequate model of parsing and lexical look-up simply does not constitute an adequate model of auditory sentence comprehension . . . . The model needs also to take into account the processing of the prosodic structure of an utterance, which takes at least in part the form of an active search for the location of the main sentence stress . . . . the comprehension of spoken sentences involves the construction and testing of hypotheses about the content of the input and that the location of a sentence's semantically most central portion is actively sought in order to facilitate the construction of the correct hypothesis.

(CUTLER, 1976, p. 147).

Further, it has been noted that the proper understanding of certain sentences must be based on a semantic representation which is not identical with the literal meaning of the sentence, and that some sentences bear presuppositions which are demonstrably available to the listener once the sentence has been comprehended.

(CUTLER, 1976, p. 141)

may be of episodes; it may be in the form of a schema or network of information. Propositional knowledge tells us about things and what they do, about ideas and what they mean, about relationships and how they are bound together. This knowledge ultimately is what helps us to comprehend. If we do not have a sufficient breadth of knowledge or we do not know schemas about specific events, we cannot bring this knowledge to our understanding of what is being said. As pointed out in an earlier chapter, comprehension is not getting meaning from what is said but bringing meaning to it. We must have the basic knowledge to begin with. If the knowledge is not available in some form within our memory systems, we cannot understand what we receive. This is not to say that children cannot understand something they do not yet know. Certainly they can. But in order to do so, they must at least develop primitive knowledge of the basic vocabulary and concepts referred to. Inference comes from filling in the missing parts from one's own background.

It appears to be useful to think of comprehension as a process of generating meanings for language by relating what is heard to knowledge and memories of experience. Wittrock (1981), in his description of reading comprehension, suggests that we construct or reconstruct meaning from the input. On the one hand is the speaker's intended meaning; on the other are the extensions, inferences, and embellishments brought by the listener, together with alternative interpretations not intended by the speaker. In some instances, comprehension of the verbal input adds new knowledge by tying together parts of old knowledge and filling in the gaps. Table 9–1 lists the factors that influence the construction of meaning in comprehension.

TABLE 9–1. FACTORS THAT INFLUENCE THE CONSTRUCTION OF MEANING IN COMPREHENSION

External
    The actual words spoken.
    The context in which the words are spoken.
    The intentions of the speaker.
    The accuracy with which the speaker encodes the intentions.

Internal
    The listener's representation of world knowledge.
    The listener's propositional knowledge.
    The listener's knowledge and recall of the specific event or context.
    The listener's knowledge of word and grammar meanings.
    The accuracy with which the listener's processing system analyzes, delivers, and parses the message.
    The listener's ability to decode the literal meanings of the speaker.
    The listener's ability to decode the implicit or covert meaning of the speaker.
    The listener's ability to extend and embellish to new interpretations.

COMPREHENSION DEVELOPMENT

As we reflect on the complexity of the comprehension process, we must recognize the importance of the development of comprehension and particularly that of syntactic and lexical knowledge. The way in which concepts are acquired will be reflected in the form and context of the lexical entries to a child's system. Gaps in this system will be reflected in the child's performance.

Johnson-Laird (1987) lists two obvious processes by which meanings of words can be acquired: a child can be told what a word means or the child can infer what it means by encountering it in use. Establishing the set of referents or features for a word is not simply an association between a word and the action or event or object it denotes, and therefore the pairing of word and meaning cannot simply be a function of conditioning. Johnson-Laird (1987) reminds us that many words have no perceptible referent or are parts of speech for which the notion is irrelevant.

If comprehension is a constructive process, children cannot be passive receivers of object-word associations. Bowerman (1978) suggests that children entertain their own hypotheses about the meanings of words, and Clark (1982) describes how children coin their own words if they do not have an appropriate term to use. Children must learn words through hearing them used by others—within linguistic and nonlinguistic contexts, probably embedded in structures containing words they already understand (Johnson-Laird, 1987).

Some words, according to Johnson-Laird, have a complete semantics—no conceivable advance in human knowledge would add to their meaning (for example, herd). Other words are not complete; their boundary lines are not clearly specified. Children may have incomplete semantics for many words. They may grasp the sense of the word without really knowing it. They may act as if they comprehend but may in fact not do so. It is important to provide the raw data from which children can build their knowledge of the world and of language. These raw data cannot be in the form of single words or even single sentences. Constructive comprehension is learned through ongoing verbal interaction in which the listener processes connected utterances within a context that supplies portions of meaning. If the data are thematic, they will generate stability of reference (Karmiloff-Smith, 1981). In this manner, a child learns not only what utterances mean, but what speakers mean when they use specified utterances.

There are times when all of us have difficulty in comprehending a particular sentence or series of utterances. This is particularly true of children who have not yet developed the knowledge base they must have in order to comprehend. In these cases they tend to use strategies based on what they do know to decipher the meaning of the unknown structure (Chapman, 1978). Van der Lely and Dewart (1986) define a comprehension strategy as a shortcut for arriving at the meaning of a sentence without utilizing all the information in the sentence. One method is that of "probable event" in which an utterance is interpreted according to what appears to be most probable or reasonable regardless of what is stated. Van der Lely and Dewart (1986) found that the language-impaired children they studied relied more heavily on semantic cues (as opposed to syntactic information) and consistently applied a probable event strategy in comprehending. Word order is also used to determine meaning even if the agent is not the first noun in the sentence. And because we usually speak of events that are probable or because the agent is usually first in an utterance, the strategy works.

It is important for us, as language specialists, to discover if and when a child comprehends. If in fact a child is not comprehending, it may tell us that his or her internal processing systems are not functioning adequately or that his or her knowledge base is not sufficiently developed, or that he or she is using strategies that interfere with comprehending.

We must be clear in what we mean by *comprehension development.* The process of acquiring the rules of language and their storage and the process of internalizing the world is another way of talking about the process of learning to comprehend. Once we have acquired the rules and have an adequate data base, the process by which we compare incoming signals with the data base and arrive at meaning is also comprehending. This is why I said in Chapter 5 that the naturalistic method of intervention, which facilitates the child's own induction system to acquire language rules, is similar to the method espoused by Winitz (1973) in which he teaches comprehension rather than expression.

COMPREHENSION AND EXPRESSION

One of the main reasons for including a chapter on comprehension in this book is to point out the complexity of the process of comprehension and to illustrate the performance difference between comprehension and expression. As pointed out in Chapter 6, comprehension

---

Quote 9–4
. . . the child will learn the grammar for those sentences which he can understand (at least partially). Conversely, the child will have difficulty in learning the putative grammatical structure underlying sentences that he has difficulty in understanding. Thus, the child's system of speech perceptions constrains what he can understand and consequently restricts the kinds of grammar he can learn.

(BEVER, 1970, p. 312).

and expression seem to use the same data base and even may use some of the same access mechanisms to the data base. Studies that I reviewed previously (Carrow-Woolfolk, 1985) demonstrate a high correlation between performance on tests of comprehension and tests of expression. I concluded then that the tests measure a common linguistic factor, the knowledge of the relationship between the linguistic code and its meaning. The knowledge is utilized in decoding a received message and encoding one for production. The fact, however, that many studies demonstrate a difference in test results between comprehension and expression in language-disordered children may indicate that in some children there is a performance difference between these two processes and the problems language-disordered children show in one over the other are problems of performance, not knowledge.

Bloom and Lahey (1978) speak to this performance difference. They state that in comparing understanding and speaking in the absence of an external event, speaking may very well be easier than understanding. In speaking, the content of the child's message originates with an idea from memory (he or she ordinarily speaks about what is known.) In understanding, they say, the content of a heard message depends on the complicated task of extracting information from the input signal (which may contain many unknown words and ideas) and relating that information to what a child already knows.

It may be that at the higher level of performance, the conceptual one, expression is easier than comprehension for the reasons just given by Bloom and Lahey. Perhaps at the lower performance level of decoding and encoding using the computational knowledge of syntax and the semantic storage system, comprehension may be easier than production, since there are linguistic cues available for searching and matching in comprehension but the retrieval of linguistic information for the expression of an idea must be retrieved without such cues, but quickly and in sequence for production.

Bloom and Lahey (1978) themselves stated that the *production* of grammatical forms and lexical items requires that a more refined distinction be made among the specific features involved in the grammatical

---

Quote 9–5
The reason for listing goals for production instead of or along with goals for comprehension is simply because more is known about the development of children's production of content/form/use interactions than is known about the development of children's comprehension of these interactions. . . . In intervention, all content/form interactions are presented in a context that represents the meaning being coded. Input is stressed throughout. Thus comprehension is being facilitated at the same time as production.

(BLOOM & LAHEY, 1978, p. 377).

> *Quote 9–6*
> *A modicum of cognitive development must precede any learning of language, because language remains meaningless unless referring to some already interpreted aspect of the environment. However, once some structuring of the environment has occurred and some primitive utterances can be understood in accordance with this structure, there is room for an influence of the form of these utterances on the child's cognitive development.*
> (SCHLESINGER, 1977, p. 166).

forms and lexicon, and that greater knowledge of word order is necessitated in the expression of sequences and other linguistic forms than in their comprehension. Production of an utterance requires knowledge of specific properties of every unit of the utterance as well as the sequence in which the units must be presented. Comprehension of the same utterance does not pose the same requirements. Comprehension could occur by understanding only segments of the utterance, the main information carrying words. Bloom and Lahey use this argument for focusing on production rather than comprehension in intervention. The demands for making linguistic distinctions are greater in production, and therefore by using production in intervention, more specific linguistic learning takes place, which in turn assists in comprehending these same units. Information can be missing and comprehension can still take place; expression requires that the details of syntax and morphology be present.

Although I agree in essence with the arguments of Bloom and Lahey, I would like to add two cautions. The conclusions that readers may reach regarding the comprehension/expression relationship is that children can use forms they do not comprehend or have never heard. Because it is through auditory input that linguistic information is originally received and stored, it is impossible for children to generate language they have never heard. It is possible for children to use grammatical morphemes correctly even though they do not understand them because of the frequency with which specific ones occur together in speech; the occurrence of one predicts, so to speak, a subsequent one with which it is frequently associated in temporal contiguity. It is also possible for children to use and practice new structures in new contexts and to use them with greater precision in production than is needed in comprehension. In production the need to choose among a number of possible forms, the exact one for a specific meaning, helps to reinforce the correct choice once it has been made. It is this interpretation that I believe Bloom and Lahey describe. The second caution follows from the first, and that is the misinterpretation that there is no need to intervene in comprehension. If we do not provide additional linguistic and conceptual data to a child through his or her comprehension system, he or she may refine the knowledge already possessed but will not add to it.

> *Quote 9–7*
> *If our interpretation of the strong correlation between performance on the PPVT and the haptic recognition tasks is correct, then it follows that a symbolic representational deficit would explain better the receptive language deficit that the expressive one. This hypothesis implies that a language-impaired child might have a relatively severe symbolic deficit without an associated expressive language impairment or, conversely, have intact symbolic skills but still suffer from an expressive language deficit.*
> (KAMHI, CATTS, KOENIG, & LEWIS, 1984, p. 175).

From the point of view of intervention for *accuracy* of production only, the exclusively expressive approach to intervention is probably valid. Siegel and Vogt (1984) taught two of four retarded children the plural rule by means of what they termed *comprehension* (pointing to single and multiple arrays of objects) and then in production (labeling the same arrays). The other two children were taught in the reverse order. The sequence in which comprehension and production were taught did not affect the facilitation.

DISORDERS OF COMPREHENSION

From the description of the three levels of comprehension outlined in this chapter, it is possible to project three types of comprehension disorders. Comprehension disorders may be related to a problem in the perceptual/memory processing system that interferes with the clarity and accuracy of the message as it is transmitted through the system. This type of problem continues throughout life even after the rules of language have been acquired. A second kind of problem has to do with inability to segment or parse correctly because of deficiencies in the knowledge of the phonological, syntactic, or semantic rules. A third kind of problem relates to the inadequacy of the conceptual system to bring meaning to the linguistic input that is received, thereby causing semantic problems. (Wolfus, Moskovitch, and Kinsbourne [1980] found that children with comprehension deficits also exhibited significant semantic impairments). All of these types of comprehension problems interfere with message reception and thereby can make it difficult to add new information to the linguistic or conceptual systems. The comprehension problems may only slow the acquisition process down by requiring more exemplars than are normally necessary to master specific linguistic rules. According to Fey and Leonard (1983), children with marked comprehension problems may also exhibit deficits in conversational skills. They suggest that children with comprehension problems probably have difficulty in understanding the message of their partners.

> *Quote 9–8*
> *I should therefore like to propose that the development of these conceptual skills flows not from encounters with the physical world but rather from encounters with certain forms of complex dialogue. If children have not had the opportunity or need to engage in such dialogue (i.e., the dialogue necessary for the mastery of **why** and for the mastery of many other words referring to intangible phenomena), then it follows that a wide range of their problem-solving skills will be adversely affected.*
> (BLANK, 1975a, p. 56).

Fey and Leonard did not find such a pattern with children who had expressive delays only. They concluded that the possibility that deficits in the participation in conversation vary with impairments in comprehension of language structure and content, and therefore an explicit description of the comprehension abilities of children with specific language impairment is essential.

COMPREHENSION INTERVENTION

A major theme of this book is that of giving equal time to the conceptual aspects of language as is given to the linguistic and pragmatic aspects. This should be particularly true in comprehension intervention. What is usually recommended for comprehension is what I call "lip-service" intervention, that of "pairing" events, objects, or pictures with a linguistic structure in hopes that a child will infer what the structure "means."

Although the identification, refinement, and learning of distinctive features of linguistic forms is probably best accomplished by focus on production, the exposure to these forms under numerous and various conditions is the manner in which the variant and invariant aspects of each unit can be identified and stored. Some knowledge, even if undefined, must be available within the memory system in order for specific distinctions to be made expressively. Linguistic input to the child is essential as a foundation on which to build.

If comprehension is necessary for receiving knowledge and storing it, expression is necessary for the ultimate "cementing" of the knowledge. Until one's own words are used to express an idea, the structure or the word is not ours. It is in the actual moment of expressing *in a generative manner* that final learning takes place. Imitation and repetition drill do not yield the same results. I used to tell my students that the level of their knowledge was indicated to me if they could formulate in their own words the ideas I was attempting to teach and even better if they could relate ideas to each other. If they could recognize ideas as being true only by indicating true or false or selecting a right

> *Quote 9–9*
> *. . . It appears that some children with language problems can learn to produce as well as comprehend new words without intervention focusing directly on production skills.*
> (LEONARD, SCHWARTZ, CHAPMAN, ROWAN, PRELOCK, TERRELL, WEISS, & MESSICK, 1982, p. 562).

answer from among some alternatives or filling in or completing statements to make them right, their knowledge was incomplete. Anyone who understands a foreign language well but has difficulty expressing himself or herself in it recognizes the need for practice in real-life oral expressive situations even in the face of good understanding. Both are needed.

Language, however, is not, in my opinion, only a learning of linguistic rules (which is what expressive intervention does best). Language is also the ability to decode what is being said so that communication can take place. Decoding, as we have seen, does not only involve knowledge of linguistic rules. It involves procedural knowledge for phonological analysis, segmentation, and parsing. It involves an ability to discover the propositions in the input and to search for specific lexical meanings and general syntactic meanings. It involves the individual's construction of meaning using the listener's entire system of world knowledge, episodic knowledge, semantic knowledge, and the network tying all of these together. Comprehension is an active and constructive process, and we should engage in helping children become active in comprehension.

At the lowest level of decoding, children can be taught to understand sentence frames. It may be that only a few types of constructions have been available in their environment. Teaching them to understand frames both of small units such as sentences and later even of larger units such as narrative and expository material will help them focus on the information rather than the structure. Response to structure should be automatic.

From a cognitive framework, the child can learn to look for essential elements in the input, the propositions—the noun phrase, the verb phrase. Gradually, the input can be increased in complexity so that the search for propositions is accomplished in a context that replicates the classroom instruction. Attention can be directed to the essential elements by asking the questions needed to make the discovery: Who . . .?, What . . .?, and so on. The child will learn to search for these elements in trying to understand verbal input.

As children get older, they can learn to translate what they hear into visual pictures that may take the form of diagrams, outlines, or any other type of drawing that illustrates meaning. This helps to retain information visually as well as auditorially. Older children also need to

> *Quote 9–10*
> *. . . experiments show that intensive exposure to a construction in an experimental situation facilitates productive use and improves comprehension of that construction in similar situations. But the limits of these training procedures with respect to generalization to new situations, different lexical items, and different semantic relations are still being mapped out. . . .*
> (DE VILLIERS & DE VILLIERS, 1982, p. 147).

know how and when to analyze what they hear in terms of the general purpose of instruction—to analyze for meaning or to analyze for remembering detail. Different kinds of material and different purposes influence the approach to comprehension. Teachers should indicate to students what outcome is expected from a listening task.

One difficulty in dealing with language-impaired children is that they do not or cannot communicate to others their own problems in comprehending. Brinton and Fujiki (1982) reported that normally developing 5-year-old subjects produced three times as many requests for clarification as language-impaired children. Children who have problems in comprehension should be aware of these problems and taught to deal with them. Dollaghan and Kaston (1986) suggest an intervention program for improving children's ability to monitor their understanding of what they hear. Comprehension monitoring would provide language-impaired children with a survival skill that may facilitate many of their academic and interpersonal interrelations. Teaching the children how to request clarification could also become part of this survival skill. The following sequence of teaching is suggested by Dollaghan and Kaston (1986): children are taught (1) to react to signal inadequacies—insufficient loudness, excessive rate, or presence of a competing noise; (2) to react to inadequate information content—inexplicit, ambiguous, or physically impossible commands; and (3) to react to unfamiliar lexical items—excessive length or excessive syntactic complexity.

I have pointed out that the listener's own experiences and ideas are the single most important aspect of comprehension. A child who does not have breadth of experience and has not been a participant in a vast array of episodes will have little to bring to the comprehension task. If we begin early to develop real, verbal, and vicarious experiences together with their corresponding vocabulary, if we begin early to fill their memory store with all sorts of information, and if we constantly require the child to use his or her information for solving problems, making inferences, and so on, we will have fewer language problems in adolescence. I believe language grows by seeing, doing, listening, and speaking. If we can eliminate language deprivation, we will do a better job of working with language disorders.

Relating the idea of the need for comprehension and expression to the six types of instructional strategies provided in Chapter 5, I would like to suggest the following integrated model for using both comprehension and expression in intervention with young children:

1. Begin intervention by using types I and II informal approaches, which focus on the input (1) to provide a purposeful and salient linguistic environment for the child's induction of the syntactic, semantic rules of the code, and (2) to provide exciting episodes around themes, for enriching the child's "world" memory stores for events, objects, and people and related vocabulary.

2. Use types III and IV for children who do not use target forms within a realistic period of using the purely "facilitative" approach or for children who have difficulty performing the forms appropriately even when they try and appear to know the rules. Type IV can be combined with type V for children who need and can profit from the extra structure.

3. Use type VI interactive approach as a follow-up to all intervention to provide for the child the opportunity to express and therefore to truly learn language and to perform it accurately, efficiently, and appropriately.

The ratio of comprehension to expression will vary with the needs of each child, but both are important to effective communication.

10

INTEGRATING THEORIES: LANGUAGE DEVELOPMENT

Although the topic of language development/acquisition has been briefly presented in a number of chapters of this book—for example, a brief discussion of the theoretical positions on the issues of innate versus environmental contributions to language provided in Chapter 2—I decided to attempt to tie together many comments on development that are sprinkled throughout the book because theory of language development has had and still has such a strong influence on intervention preocedures. This is particularly necessary because there appears to be some misuse of developmental terminology in its application to intervention. In the current literature on intervention one finds terms such as *naturalistic*, *facilitator*, *interactive*, *self-driven*, *constructionistic*, and *inductive* all used within the context of a single intervention procedure.

THEORY, ASSESSMENT AND INTERVENTION
IN LANGUAGE DISORDERS: © 1988 by Grune & Stratton
AN INTEGRATIVE APPROACH

ISBN   0-8089-1918-0

183

If these terms and the notions they represent are traced back to their theoretical origins, however, many of them reflect not only different but contrasting viewpoints about development. This is not to say that contrasting viewpoints cannot be integrated, but there should be a logical process by which this is done. Current terminology should not be used for the sole purpose of providing credibility to intervention techniques. A rationale based on theory and/or empirical findings should be the basis of any intervention approach and the *raison d'etat* for using it.

The theme of this book is the relation between theory and practice. The implication is that intervention and assessment should be based on theory—theory of language, theory of language development, and theory of language disorders. This position is defensible, however, only if the theory has validity, that is, if it represents reality insofar as it is possible to understand language, its development, and disorders. It is important, particularly wherever theory is used as a basis for action, that there be an attempt to reconcile the data about language behavior and language disorders with that theory. A theory can never be accepted as if it is fact. Therefore, intervention procedures that are generated from a theory that has not been tested adequately cannot be thought of as the best or only approach to changing the language of children, no matter how adaptable that theory is to practice.

DISTINGUISHING ISSUES AMONG THEORIES

Theories about language development are plentiful. No one complete theory has been generally adopted by specialists in language development. The basic issues on which theories vary are the issues of relationship among language, cognitive and social roles in development, and that of the location of control in shaping the direction that development takes in a child. These two issues, which are the focal points of theoretical differences, will be discussed in this chapter. Subsequent to the discussion, I will present two theories of language development that I believe are prototypes of current theories on which intervention procedures are based, the interactive theory and the constructionist theory. I will also include the positions of those theorists who have attempted to integrate the cognitive and social factors in development.

Because the two theories, interactive and constructionist, are used as bases for intervention with language-disordered children, each will be treated in terms of the manner in which they handle the two issues, the relationship among components and the control for shaping the language in learning. The application of these theories to intervention will be discussed. Finally, I will comment on the possible integration of theories of language development.

> *Quote 10–1*
> *Although children can shape their behavior to coincide with the empirical events that they see and hear, learning a linguistic code waits on the conceptual capacity for a linguistic induction, and such an induction is schematized by the interaction and overlap among content/form and use . . .*
>
> *The development of language results from the interaction between the child and the context—specifically, the interaction among the child's changing needs and changing capacities, and the different situations in the environment.*
> (BLOOM & LAHEY, 1987, pp. 71, 72).

The Issue of Component Relationship

Although the theories that have evolved from the innatist point of view consider the development of language structure to be independent from other cognitive tasks and the language structure itself to form a module separate from other cognitive modules (see Chapter 6), most other theoretical descriptions of language postulate an interdependency among cognition, socialization, and language. What separates these latter descriptions from one another, however, are the explanations about exactly how this interaction takes place. Bates, Benigni, Bretherton, Camaioni, and Volterra (1977) have, based on earlier work by Jenkins (1969), identified six major positions that relate language and cognition and have shown how these same positions could apply to cognition and social development and to social development and language. If theorists were to choose one position for describing cognition and language, another for describing cognition and social development, and still another for describing social development and language, there would be a possibility of generating 216 possible positions (Bates et al., 1977). If added to this, the positions would describe a degree of dependency with "partial dependence, partial independence, and isomorphism based on the nature of systems rather than a shared source" (Bates et al., 1977, p. 285); about 30,000 models could be generated for describing the interrelationship of the three systems. This illustrates the difficulty of arriving at a single theory with which all theorists can agree.

The basic relationship among the components (social, cognitive, and language) can be described according to five models or positions (see Bates et al., 1977):

1. Language and thought are the same, language is thought and thought is language.

2. Language, cognition, and social development are derivative. Thought derives from or is dependent on language or on social development, language derives from or is dependent on thought or social development, and so on. If all of these are considered valid, it would lead to an interaction position in which the three components develop in interaction with each other; these are bidirectional or tridirectional processes. A more specific description of the dependent point of view is one defined by a system of "priors" in which, for example, development of very specific cognitive tasks must be mastered prior to the emergence of very specific linguistic structures, and so on. Shatz (1981) says that for such a direct relationship to be valid, only certain kinds of prior systems will work: those that provide directly and clearly the structural information needed for the acquisition of new linguistic knowledge. Any indirect relation assumes that the internal properties of the child mediates the acquisition.

3. The three components interact but are independent. A form of this position is taken by the nativists who consider language structure to emerge (at least partially, for some theorists) independently from cognition and social development. Bates and colleagues (1977) suggest that there are various forms of this position and some theorists change direction with changes in the developmental stage of language.

4. Language, thought, and social development derive from a third system, that is, they have a common origin. This type of relationship is called a *homologue*; the common origin produces components that are similar in structure and therefore function in a similar manner. Bates et al. (1977) suggest that Lenneberg's (1967) idea that categorization and extraction of properties play a role in human cognition and language development is an example of a homologue in which both these systems derive from perceptual processing. These same researchers, Bates et al., used this interpretation in their own research—that both linguistic tasks and cognitive ones are dependent on underlying operative schemes shared by the two domains.

5. Language, cognition, and social development are parallel (not similar) in structure and sequence because of their adaptation to similar problems; they have a common historical origin (Bates et al., 1977). This type of relationship is called an *analogue*. For example, translating turn-taking in social activities at a prelinguistic level (mother claps, child claps, mother claps) into turn-taking at the communicative level may be termed an analogy.

> *Quote 10–2*
> *. . . some—if not many—developments in children's language*
> *cannot be explained by reference to the addressee's interaction*
> *with the child. Rather I shall submit that processing demands*
> *from the child's own point of view must also be invoked in any*
> *explanatory model of language acquisition.*
> (KARMILOFF-SMITH, 1981, p. 121).

It is obvious from this description of the various positions explaining the role of the components in language development that any research or intervention resulting from theory must be specific with respect to the position taken regarding component relationship. It is not enough to state that one component is a prerequisite to another or that one is dependent on another. The nature of the relationship should be specified clearly and in detail, and the logic of the application of the theory to practice should also be delineated. Some theories may hold to one position to explain one stage of development and another for another stage of development. This too needs to be made clear.

Part of the confusion in discussions of language development may be related to the use of the word *language*. Some language development theorists use *language* to mean the entire spectrum of behaviors, internal and external, knowledge and performance, code, meaning, and use. Other theorists restrict the use of the term to the linguistic structure aspect. This difference alone may account for a large portion of the apparent conflict between theoretical accounts of language development. Whereas some descriptions of language development may in fact be describing the development of the semantic or pragmatic aspects of language, others may be limited to the emergence of language structure. This needs to be noted in any discussion of language development.

After reviewing the literature on contemporary accounts of the cognition-language relationship, Rice (1983) concluded that the different explanations focused on different aspects and levels of linguistic competence, and therefore the relationship between cognition and language vary as a function of age, linguistic abilities, and the type of cognition involved. She labeled attempts to characterize the relationship in global terms as misdirected.

The Issue of Control or Shaping

Implied in each of the positions just described regarding the relationships among components is the specification of the central control for guiding and directing the course of acquisition. The theories that describe a strong role for the caretakers in the environment place the

> *Quote 10–3*
> *Recently, a rather different model has been proposed for the relation between language and context. In this model, context does not just **cause** language, but is an integral part of the **structure** of language. Meanings are conveyed through a creative combination of utterances and social settings.*
>
> (BATES, 1976b, p. 412).

responsibility for shaping language development on the environment. The theories that hold that the child's own system chooses from the possible language inputs, incorporates new linguistic information with that already organized and stored, and constructs the rules by which he or she generates language, are based on the assumption that the language-learning system is innate and separate in structure from other cognitive systems and the acquisition of language is a function of the child's own construction abilities. These two points of view are very different even though the clinical literature often treats the concepts that relate to the constructionist and interactive theories as if they were the same.

Issue two, the shaping issue, *appears* similar to issue one, the relationship among components issue, but they are in fact different. It is possible for aspects of a component such as social development to occur prior to linguistic development without being the cause and the shaper of the linguistic development. The degree to which one component (social, cognitive, linguistic) is responsible for the other with respect to general developmental schedules as well as with respect to specific one-to-one structural correspondence between these components and the degree to which the source, environment or child, controls the direction of learning, reflect the degree to which theories differ.

AN INTERACTIVE THEORY OF LANGUAGE DEVELOPMENT

The "Unified" Model

To serve as an example of an interactive theory of language development, I have chosen the "unified model" of Lewis and Cherry (1977). This model is defined by the assumption that, because all are aspects of the same individual, the social, cognitive, and language knowledges are interdependent and interrelated. The three components are considered to have a social origin insofar as they develop in the course of the interaction of an individual with others. Because each component is one aspect of interaction, it cannot form a discrete domain.

In one version of this model (a), the interrelationship of linguistic, social, and cognitive knowledge is defined as a dynamic flow that is in a

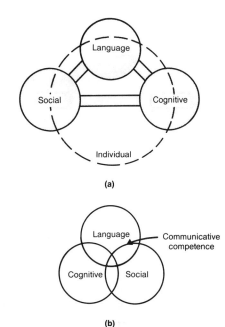

FIGURE 10–1. The unified model of language development showing two versions of the model: (a) in which the interrelationship of linguistic, social, and cognitive knowledge is represented as a dynamic flow existing within and without the individual; and (b) in which the relationship exists as an interaction of the three domains. (Reproduced with permission from Lewis, M., & Cherry, L. [1977]. Social behavior and language acquisition. In M. Lewis, & L. A. Rosenblum [Eds.], *Interaction, conversation, and the development of language* [p. 231]. New York: John Wiley and Sons.)

state of constant change that exists internal and external to the individual. In a second version of this model (b), there is a core knowledge developed from social, cognitive, and linguistic knowledges that exists as a product of the interaction of the three domains; i.e., the interaction among the three components forms a core of related knowledge and this in turn results from social interaction with others. See Figure 10–1 for both versions of the unified model.

The developmental process in the unified model involves changing from a unified and highly integrated system of knowledge to one that is highly specialized by means of gradual differentiation among components. The resulting end products of the three domains are functionally independent of one another. An example of this differentiation, provided by Lewis and Cherry (1977), is that of context embeddedness of the child's early comprehension, and the gradual independence of linguistic comprehension acts from context as the child develops. The model implies that causal chains among linguistic, social, or cognitive behaviors pass through an individual before resurfacing as new behavior in one or the other domain.

A specific theory that falls within the unified model is one that Lewis and Freedle developed in 1973 (reported in Lewis & Cherry, 1977). This theory specifies a communication network between an infant child and the mother that develops as a language analogue superimposed on the social-cognitive system. The sociocognitive behaviors, thought to underlie language behavior, are referred to as *interactional competence*. The analogues are illustrated by the parallels between "social grammar" of early mother-child interaction and later patterns in verbal interaction. For example, "the approach of the mother, the presence of the mother, and finally her departure could be used as the prototype of tense" (Lewis & Cherry, 1977, p. 241). Another prelanguage prototype of linguistic rules involves the chains of behavior between infant and mother that are governed by rules of chain occurrence, chain length and duration, chain initiator and terminator, and so on. Lewis and Cherry liken the chains to sentences with the individual words making up the sets or to words with the letters making up the sets. Thus the source and pattern for the interaction among social, cognitive, and linguistic components is the pattern of early caretaker-child interaction. Lewis and Cherry (1977) believe that "the child's acquisition of knowledge (both meaning and grammatical constructions) are dependent on his early transactions with the social world" (p. 242).

One would deduce from the explanation of this theory that social interaction is a *sine qua non* of language development (as well as other development), and that within the context of social interaction, language is also dependent on the simultaneous emergence of cognitive and social behaviors with which it interacts. This analogue-type of relation between language and social interaction (position 5 provided earlier in this chapter) implies parallel structure between social interaction and language, but, according to the theorists, also implies a system of priors in that in early development very specific social interactions are the precursors to specific forms in linguistic grammar. Later, interaction between social, linguistic, and cognitive components appear to be tridirectional and interdependent. The theory thus is representative of two or three of the possible relations among components listed earlier.

Interactive Theory and Language Disorders

The interpretation of language disorders within the framework of this theory is directed to the adequacy of social prerequisites to language. If the three components, cognitive, linguistic, and pragmatic, have a social origin, developing as they do from the interaction of an individual with others, then an inadequate social interaction will not provide the needed stimulus to linguistic development. The first level of the structural analogue on which linguistic behavior builds will be missing. If the further development of the three components is a function of gradual differentiation of behaviors from a unified and holistic response that takes place as a result of interaction, the absence of interaction will affect this differentiation. Language, according to the unified theory, is originally linked to cognitive and social behaviors, therefore it is passive and dependent. The disorder in language is therefore primarily external to language behavior itself. The transition from dependency to relative autonomy as a result of interaction implies a functional separation from the other behaviors (Deutsch, 1981). Here, too, failure of interaction inhibits the separation.

Interactive Theory and Intervention

Application of this theory and all theories of this type to intervention practice carries with it the notion that there are certain social interaction patterns that are precursors to the gradual differentiation of the child's behavior. Using this theory as a base, intervention procedures would need to incorporate interaction protocols between the language-disordered child and the individuals in his or her environment. Such protocols would simulate those found in the normal home setting during the early period of child development. The linguistic development would need to wait for appropriate social interactive patterns to be established. Control for the shaping and direction of linguistic patterns is in the environment, and in this sense the child plays a passive role in the selection and shaping of improvement in language intervention according to this theory. Also according to this theory, working on language without ensuring appropriate social interactive prelanguage experience would be fruitless, particularly if analogue patterns are considered to occur on a one-to-one basis between social interaction and language—the extent to which linguistic form is derived from and subsequent to social interaction. No amount of language stimulation in naturalistic situations or increase in saliency of linguistic input would assist in the development of forms that have not yet been patterned in social interaction or patterns that a child has not yet internalized.

The second aspect of the unified theory that has application for intervention with language-disordered children is that of the gradual differentiation among components as a result of the interaction of these components as the child interacts with the environment. This aspect of the theory describes a process by which tasks that require behavior in all three components—social, cognitive, and linguistic—facilitate the emergence of each of these components by virtue of the presence of the other two. The focus is not only on the relationship of the components to each other, but on the effects on each of the components of an individual child's interaction with the environment in a task that utilizes all of the components. This aspect of the theory does not address the issue of priors or relationship. It does specify that a child's original response to the world is in a holistic, integrated manner, with each component gradually separating from bondage to the others. Neither does this aspect of the theory imply how this interaction affects the acquisition of linguistic rules; it does not specify if, in fact, linguistic rules can develop without the interaction. It would be unreasonable to suppose that the acquisition of each linguistic rule would need to be a product of an interaction among three components. The usefulness of this aspect of unified theory to intervention would be the notion of the strengthening and gradual independence of language production as a function of interaction. The initial performance unity of cognitive, linguistic, and social behaviors establishes the associations between the form, meaning, and use of the language. This unity is an integrative one, not simply a sum of separate components. The separation of these behaviors (decontextualization) at a later period permits the use of one of the behaviors, such as the linguistic one, to represent the others.

The thrust of intervention in both stages of development described by the unified theory is on interaction. Social interactions should precede language and be the pivot around which the linguistic system develops. The settings for intervention should be naturalistic because it is in this type of setting that normal interaction takes place. Naturalistic settings for children are those involving play and caregiving. Verbal exchanges should be child-directed and centered on everyday topics. The kinds of cueing, responding, instructing, and intervening usually and naturally provided by the caregiver should be what is given in intervention. Because social interaction is the source of development, it shapes and directs language. In simulating this interaction in intervention, care must be taken to encompass the totality of interactive exchanges usually available to the child in a home.

Comments on the Interactive Theory

A process somewhat different to that presented by Lewis and Cherry is described by Bloom and Lahey (1978). Instead of the initial aspects of development beginning with a gestalt behavior in which cognitive, social, and linguistic behaviors are unified and only subsequently differentiated, Bloom and Lahey indicated that content, form, and use represent separate threads of development in early infancy and come together only when children begin to use language, around the second year. Instead of a social prerequisite to language, Bloom and Lahey propose a seriation between cognition and linguistic development, ". . . learning a linguistic code waits on the conceptual capacity for a linguistic induction" (p. 72). The induction is gradual, according to Bloom and Lahey, and is influenced by as well as influences the continuous acquisition of the "precursory capacities for linguistic behaviors" (p.72). Although Bloom and Lahey state that language develops as a result of interaction between the child and the context, they apparently consider the internalization of the context to be represented by separate social, cognitive, and linguistic threads.

> *Quote 10–4*
> *The first crucial point about the mother's role is that she drastically tailors output at the start to the nature of the task and to the child's apparent competence. . . . If a child responds, the mother responds to him, and if he initiates a cycle by pointing or vocalizing, she responds even more often. Her "fine tuning" is fine indeed.*
>
> (BRUNER, 1981, pp. 166–167).

Shatz (1981) and others provided arguments that may temper the wholehearted and exclusive acceptance of the unified (interactive) theory. I would like to summarize these along with presenting one or two of my own.

1. The translation from interaction to linguistic structure, as for example from actions such as giving and taking to word order, is not necessarily direct or transparent (Slobin, in press). Shatz (1981) states that the data regarding conversational strategies and syntax acquisition indicate that these "strategies may have little effect on the progress of syntax acquisition, and that the two tasks being accomplished by the child may go on relatively independently of one another" (p. 29).
2. Children's interactive responses may be based on primitive social strategies (Shatz, 1981), therefore the assumption that interactive responses are based on social knowledge may not be accurate.
3. The child may acquire grammar in a way different from the mappings provided him or her in social interactions. Although social interactions differ from child to child, the stages of emergence of linguistic forms do not.
4. The facts of interaction do not support the position that mothers are sufficiently tuned to their children's development to provide them with the ordered and regularly changing data that will account for the order of acquisition (Shatz, 1981; Gleitman, Newport, & Gleitman, 1984).
5. The order of acquisition of grammatical forms is relatively the same in second language acquisition as it is in the primary language, although the second language is often acquired after the basic social and cognitive behaviors are relatively developed.
6. Children follow unique and creative paths to language, over-generalizing some forms and using forms not present in the adult language (Cazden, 1968; Karmiloff-Smith, 1979).

A major difficulty with some interpretations of the interactionist position is that it does not account for the role of the child in language development. Shatz (1981) goes so far as to say that this type of theory is incompatible with relating social interaction and syntax acquisition because it discounts the internal activities of the child.

**A CONSTRUCTIONIST
THEORY OF
LANGUAGE
DEVELOPMENT**

The "Bootstrapping" Construct

The basic tenet in the constructionist theory of language development is that the child is an active participant in the creation of his or her language. One particular model that describes the method by which the child, by means of his or her own operations, achieves a conventional communicative system is provided by Shatz (in press). Shatz calls the approach she uses to explain language acquisition, the *bootstrapping construct*. This theory specifies the following regarding language development (Shatz, in press):

1. The executive control of language learning is housed internally in the learner.
2. Because the learner is a limited capacity processor and cannot learn anything and everything at any moment in time, the learner selects and houses language data for later analysis. By doing so, the learning functions even within an environment that may not be sensitive to his or her needs.
3. The process that children utilize in the construction of an adequate language knowledge base is that of using what they know to learn more; they bootstrap.

Shatz (in press) describes three bootstrapping operations: elicitation, entry, and expansion. Each of these operations helps the child to use partial knowledge to acquire additional knowledge. The logical order for the occurrence of these operations is from elicitation to entry to expansion, and they take place in cycles or waves of data entry, analysis, and reorganization. These operations are used reciprocally between syntax, semantics, and pragmatics—whichever aspect is known is a means of discovering the unknown.

The child as center of control in shaping the direction of learning is clearly illustrated in the elicitation operations. By means of these operations, the child identifies those aspects of reality about which general or verbal knowledge is needed. The child may elicit this information via gestures. Gestures encourage the members of a dyad to attend jointly on the same events or objects, and to do so particularly during the period where speech is not sufficiently developed for accomplishing this purpose.

Shatz provides other examples of elicitation behaviors that she classifies as children's response behaviors: (1) pulling familiar labels from adult utterances and acting on the objects mentioned; (2) using phrases they observe being used as responses and adapting them (often inappropriately) to their own needs to respond; (3) responding to com-

> *Quote 10–5*
> *Correspondingly, the belief that various systems of mind are or-*
> *ganized along quite different principles leads to the natural con-*
> *clusion that these systems are intrinsically determined, not*
> *simply the result of common mechanisms of learning or*
> *growth. . . . Those who tend toward the assumption of modularity*
> *tend also to assume rich innate structure, while those who as-*
> *sume limited innate structure tend to deny modularity.*
> (CHOMSKY, 1980, pp. 40–41).

mon (yes/no) questions sometimes indiscriminately, recognizing the
need to respond with one or the other words but not sure which one; (4)
using discourse-cohesive but semantically inaccurate responses; and
(5) using imitation to keep the conversation going. All these responses
use the partial knowledge of the child for signaling the child's interest
in continued participation and for keeping the parents involved in the
process. The kinds of parental responses to a child's response and child
elicitations, which assist the child in acquiring new data on which to
operate, provide additional speech input to the child. Shatz believes
that without elicitation behaviors few parents would have the fortitude
to pursue the unrewarding task of "talking to an unresponsive listener"
(p. 23).

Shatz calls the second kind of bootstrapping in child language,
entry operations. Through entry operations, information is entered into
the language learning system in a format that assists the child's analysis
of it at a rate and time that is within the child's ability. The entry units
represent an input that is longer than the word and consists of new
words within the context of known words or utterance frames, rote
phrases, familiar exemplars, and so on. Storing new and old information
together (*tall* tree) may help to cue the meaning of the new word (tall).

The last bootstrapping technique Shatz calls *expansion operations.*
By means of language practice and play as well as spontaneous repairs,
the child combines and substitutes words and manipulates previously
stored unanalyzed strings. Words begin to be classified into grammatical
categories, inferences are made regarding the functions of specific
categories, and rules are induced. The external signs of these operations
are the idiosyncratic forms that children create from overgeneralizing
and misunderstanding rules. Shatz says that children build up and break
down word sequences in operations that explore common constraints
among words and patterns.

Although Shatz' focus is on the acquisition of structure and the examples she gives are structure-based, she states that the bootstrapping
approach applies to semantics and pragmatics as well and the direction
of facilitation (using old knowledge for new) among grammatical structures, semantics, and pragmatics is reciprocal.

Language Disorders and Constructionist Theory

The patterns of language disorders in this theory would follow inter-ruptions in the bootstrapping operations. If the child does not assume the role of initiator or elicitator, it is likely that the adult provisions of new material for learning will be limited. Shatz implies that if children do not accept unanalyzed sentences into their own system, they will be unable to develop broad productive expression. Holding unanalyzed strings for future attention requires an adequate storage system. If this is not available, there will be little internal data for the child to work on. The behaviors of language play and practice require some metalinguistic ability on the part of the child. Not all children have the capacity to engage in language manipulation and therefore to expand and improve their language knowledge. These then would be language-disordered children.

Constructionist Theory and Intervention

There are intervention principles that flow naturally from the con-structionist theory of language development. The position that the initiator for learning language is the child requires that the role of the caretaker or language specialist with young children become one of facilitator. The main function of the facilitator is to respond to the child's response to the environment. The facilitator does not manipulate the environment to produce specific responses; instead, the facilitator allows the child to direct the linguistic flow by his or her questions, comments, and other elicitation techniques. There needs to be a rich source of data from which the child selects portions for taking into his or her system, and there needs to be time provided for the analysis, reanalysis, and organization to take place. Immediate change and use of new information will not occur. The specialist may need to encourage and structure opportunities for language play and practice if these metalinguistic behaviors are difficult for the child. The setting for intervention is not naturalistic in the same way as intervention for the interactive theory. Although the role of the specialist in the constructionist theory is that of facilitator, the specialist assumes the responsibility of providing appropriate responses to the child. This involves greater awareness of the child's linguistic needs and the best avenues for satisfying those needs. The specialist, however, does not plan or direct the course of acquisition.

Comments on the Constructionist Theory

Elements of Shatz's theory are akin to the nativist's position that each child has a language acquisition device that operates independently from other cognitive systems within the child and from direction from the environment. Although Piaget's (1952, 1955) position differs from that of the nativists in that he considers language to be an integral part of a sensory-motor-symbolic system, the aspect of expansion in bootstrapping resembles Piaget's assimilation and accommodation processes in which a child takes in and organizes new information within the context of the existing knowledge.

Shatz' entry operations in which the child internalizes sequences containing both old and new information for subsequent analysis can be compared to Bruner's (1975) suggestion that prosodic and phonological patterns are place-holders learned through imitation, which function as an envelope or matrix for inserting morphemes, or Chomsky's (1980) suggestion that the child inserts the elements of language into a schema with empty slots with which a child is "pre-armed." This theme has been supported by Clark (1974) who proposed that children's early sentences are unanalyzed and imitated and the first novel sentences are simple modifications of imitations. These positions encourage the necessity of a rich environment for development whether the control is in the child or in the environment.

Shatz's theory presents a logical approach to the acquisition of linguistic structure by children. The self-driven and self-regulated procedure by which structure is acquired could account for the variability of the performance of children in language tasks, each child functioning on the basis of his or her own linguistic needs. The theory implies that neither cognitive factors nor maternal linguistic input can explain the course of language development.

Arguments in addition to those presented by Shatz for the child's possession of a language device that controls the language acquisition process can be found in Chomsky's (1980) writings and those of other nativists. Specialists in language disorders are familiar with the unique communication systems that evolve between twins. Idioglossia is a rule-based system that is ordinarily spoken and understood only by the two siblings, usually twins. Their ability to formulate novel rules, which are not induced from their environment, shows at least how independent the grammatical rule-development aspect of language can be.

However, arguments on the side of the caretaker's influence on language have support also. Studies have shown that semantic complexity (which is external to the child's system) does influence the acquisition of linguistic structure (Brown, 1973; Cromer, 1976). Slobin (1973) suggested that the awkward or idiosyncratic forms used by children indicate knowledge of meaning for which they do not have forms. Freedle and Lewis (1977), whose position was presented earlier in this chapter, state that there is some evidence that formal linguistic behavior has its origins in a general prelinguistic social communication system. Studies show some correlation between maternal input of a

> *Quote 10–6*
> *The evidence is mounting that young children, in whatever culture, are spoken to in special ways, and that there are no cultures in which children learn language by mere exposure to it—by simply observing adults in discourse with one another, for instance.*
>
> (BERKO-GLEASON & WEINTRAUB, 1978, p. 214).

linguistic nature and the subsequent child behaviors; at least, mothers may be facilitators for young language learners (Berko-Gleason & Weintraub, 1978; Gleitman, Newport, & Gleitman, 1984). We also know that there are specific developmental patterns in the acquisition of structure by children. It is unlikely that these patterns would exist if the direction of acquisition were totally dependent on the child's needs for new information. Specialists who work with children who have a delay in language have experienced situations in which, by only modifying the social responses to a child and his or her needs, there is a dramatic improvement in language, indicating that the environment can and does play a significant role in language development.

INTEGRATING THEORIES OF LANGUAGE DEVELOPMENT

It appears from the descriptions of the two theories of language development presented in this chapter that they represent two opposing points of view. If we would select adjectives that are descriptive of each we might have a listing as follows:

Unified Theory	Constructionist Theory
Interdependent	Modular
Naturalistic	Naturalistic
Environmentally driven	Self-driven
Functionalistic	Inductive
Intentional	Facilitative
Interactive	Active
Informative	Syntactic
Socially based	Cognitively based

Although the adjectives differ, we often find modifiers from both groups used within the same theoretical position. Perhaps this is because both positions have validity in describing language development. We need to understand in what manner they can interface in the developmental sequence.

We also need to identify language constructs that neither theory addresses satisfactorily. The idea of the intentions of a child to inform

> *Quote 10–7*
> *In place of considering language uses as something to be learned after the basic elements of language—syntax and lexicon—are mastered, an organismic approach should be taken in which the uses to which language may be put form the basis of language training. In this view, the uses of language become the motivating force for learning language as well as the major determiners of which language forms are to be learned.*
>
> (REES, 1978, p. 261).

and the need for information to be successfully imparted in the messages for the intentions of the child to be realized needs to be a part of a developmental theory. Although the idea of functionalism is compatible with both theories, it is not explicitly and logically stated.

How can a broad theory of language development account for both positions—that of the child's role in constructing and shaping his or her language and that of the environment's role in helping in the shaping process? We know it cannot be a simple or unitary explanation of the process. The degree to which each part of the system—child and environment—plays the major role may vary with the age of the child, the child's stage of language, the quality of the environmental input, and the special learning capabilities of the child.

A way of integrating these developmental accounts may be to use the constructionist-type theory to explain the acquisition of linguistic structure and the interactionist-type theory to describe the manner in which this structure is related to both semantic and pragmatic development. This approach does not necessarily negate the role of bootstrapping in semantics and pragmatics, but perhaps it gives the environment a more important role than does Shatz. There are many skills that need to be acquired in learning language, and probably all the theories have validity in explaining at least some part of this acquisition.

Bloom and Lahey's (1978) explanation of language development, which I have briefly described previously, attempts to integrate the concepts of precursors, induction, and the interaction of cognitive, social, and linguistic behaviors acquired within a social context. Such a theory implies that the relationship of language development to the various processes of acquisition—precursor, induction, interactive—changes with time and with respect to the degree of their involvement in the developmental process. Their attempt to integrate the processes appears to have significant validity.

Another possible direction that this type of integration might take is suggested by Bruner (1981). The child's early communicative acts need props and formats (highly rehearsed routines) to provide a "scaffold" for interaction. These props might take the form of highlighting or focusing attention on communication in general or on specific aspects of form or content that results in joint attention and action on, for example,

> *Quote 10–8*
> *An interactive approach requires us to consider not only the child's communicative intent, but also the child's success at achieving the conduit of interaction as a sequence of meaningful exchanges. We can consider meaning in this context to be construed as "making sense," that is, that meanings are conceived not only with perceivable content or with the ability to construct interpretable messages, but more especially with the resolution of a sequence of social actions between two or more participants, such that the exchange of talk and action* **demonstrates** *some appearance of a satisfactory outcome, a happy resolution.*
>
> (COOK-GUMPERZ, 1977, p. 104).

a cup or a ball. The adult begins to act as a scaffold in order to provide continuity to the child's emerging control. As the child develops, according to Bruner, the child, using his or her own library of scripts, begins imposing his or her own formats on communicative situations. There is a gradual transfer of initiative from the adult to the child. Bruner believes that the adults *are* finely tuned to the child's internal readiness and demonstrate this by "modifying" speech not so that the child will imitate, but rather to exaggerate important features or highlight phrase markers and high-information elements for a system that can recognize grammatical distinctions. In a way, according to Bruner, the mother or caretaker consciously takes on the role of language tutor who serves as a facilitator rather than a director. I have always believed that a good teacher, whether parent, classroom instructor, or clinician, can learn to read children rather than teach them. By reading a child correctly, the child's learning is directed to the child's own interests and concerns and therefore is more successful.

Waryas and Crowe (1982) also attempted to integrate the environmental and organismic factors in development by describing the environmental interactions between the linguistic, cognitive, and social inputs to the child as a series of challenges and responses from the child to the environment (child-controlled acquisition), determined by the child's neurological maturation, and from the environment to the child (the environment's fine tuning), determined by the child's ability to respond to increased stimulations.

Another position that appears to integrate the cognitive and social roles in language development has been described by Nelson and her colleagues (Nelson, 1986a). Although Nelson describes this position as falling within the interactive model because it emphasizes the role of experience and the integrated manner in which this experience enters the knowledge system, she also illustrates how the cognitive system operates on the internal representations of events, thus separating the content of the input from the organism's use of it, which I believe essentially separates the constructionist and interactive theories. Nelson sees change as an inevitable outcome of the organizing system that organizes and utilizes differently the representations resulting from different experiential data structures. Furthermore, Nelson states that the knowledge that the child acquires is not exclusively a function of cognitive operations on representations of experience but also of cognitive operations on abstractions of this representation. However, she points out that the constraints on the available data are experiential. She states, "what children represent of an experience has important implications for their possible abstract cognitive organization based on that experience" (Nelson, 1986b, p. 6).

Nelson's (1986b) theory describes the events that she and her colleagues consider to be the starting point of the child's knowledge. These events involve people in purposeful action with objects and other people engaged in a structured, sequential, hierarchically organized, global-oriented activity. Each event has its own structure (grocery shopping, eating at a restaurant, etc.) and the child's internal representation, which Nelson calls the *general event representation* (GER), follows the structure of the event itself—to the extent that the child internalizes the event's characteristics. However, the child's verbal description (public verbal representation) of the event may incompletely reflect the actual event structure.

Particular emphasis in Nelson's theory is on the script model, which she considers to be a type of general event. A script specifies the roles of actors, the actions, and the props needed to carry out a goal in a particular spatial-temporal context. The script specifies the requirements for filling in "slots"—the essential elements of the event. When a child understands a frequently occurring situation well enough to understand its general structure and to develop a script for it, the child can predict the necessary components in any specific occurrence of the event. A scripted event facilitates the formation of a GER because its strong temporally invariant structure and its frequent occurrence assist the participant in understanding the goals, roles, and props involved. According to Nelson, scripts are learned by means of adult direction—the child is taught to take his or her part. Although the adult role is considered important, Nelson (1986b) states that the "degree to which script structures result from inherent principles of cognitive organization and the degree to which they are dependent on structural guidance from adults are open questions" (p.15).

Slackman, Hudson, and Fivush (1986), like Bruner, liken event structure to a scaffold in that the child, once event relations are fully understood, is free to transform and manipulate the sequences of the event. This is because the child understands cause and effect contingencies. The organization of knowledge that results from event knowledge may be the basis for later abstractions and decontextualization of knowledge.

Thus, we can see a beginning of the integration of the interactive and constructionist view of language development.

Although the adequacy of the child's system for representing reality and acting on these representations is an essential condition of learning, we cannot ignore the need for experiences to serve as the data for these operations. Nelson and her colleagues have not only presented a developmental theory based on event structure but have demonstrated that children's performance of activities, such as talking, are more complex in contexts of structured events than in free play or object-oriented tasks. When a mother and her child share event knowledge for an interactive situation, the child's competence in using language in that situation is enhanced (Lucariello, Kyratzis, & Engel, 1986).

Based on the event structure notion of Bruner and Nelson, Van Kleeck and Richardson (in press) described stages in helping a child acquire new linguistic behaviors. The process emphasizes the change from other-regulation to self-regulation. In stage 1, the adult role is to introduce the event structure and entice a child's participation. A daily routine is chosen in which the adult embeds the targeted language, and this routine is repeated. In the second stage, the child participates more freely in the familiar event. The child is supported for whatever role he or she can play. (The adult provides a scaffold.) The remainder of the task is filled in by the adult. The task is varied and extended in stage 3, and the child is permitted to initiate segments, structure the task, and even reverse roles with the adult. The target behaviors are stabilized and automatic. In the fourth stage, the participants begin to think and talk about the activity instead of just acting it out. The adult models verbally, and the planning of the activity and the target behaviors are produced outside of the context of the activity. The child monitors his or her own production and can generalize his or her behavior to new contexts.

Integrative Theories of Development and Intervention

I would like to suggest that there may be phases of language development, each with a different balance between the child's role and that of the environment. These phases may be simulated in stages of intervention and are discussed below. (Such stages were suggested in Chapter 5.)

1. The prelanguage stage in which the child interacts with the environment and through this interaction begins separating linguistic, social, and cognitive aspects of behavior (unified theory) or bringing them together (Bloom and Lahey's theory). In intervention with very young children, a strong program of social interaction (event

structure development) would be provided. Behavior arising from a child's intentions would be responded to.

2. A beginning linguistic structure stage in which the child begins to assume control for his or her own language growth. The environment serves primarily to respond to the child's initiative—to be the source from which a child can draw needed linguistic information and to provide the listeners whom he can inform. The specialist in intervention becomes a "responder" allowing the direction of learning to be guided by the child (constructionist theory).

3. A teaching stage in which, as the child language system becomes complex, the adult begins to take a more direct role by increasing the saliency of some features over others through exaggeration, repetition, and isolation of the specific features. In this sense, the adult facilitates the child's own constructive abilities by making the induction and organization processes less difficult. With children who have special problems, there may be a need to increase this direct role by the adult. The ultimate goal, however, is to make the child responsible for his or her own learning. In intervention, the specialist's involvement may need to be temporary—to assist children with special performance problems through either direct manipulation or metalinguistic means. This may be particularly true with children whose errors have become "fossilized."

4. The final learning takes place in interaction as the child converges his or her automatic grammatical skills with his or her high-level cognitive processes in an attempt to communicate ideas. The only way in which these two processes can converge is in a real or pragmatic situation in which the child really wants to convey a message or idea. Only then is his or her language really learned. The intervention task is completed only when a child is provided with interaction opportunities for communication and can do so effectively. The demands on the system made by the need to communicate forces the system to respond with the highest level of accuracy, fluency, and refinement of which it is capable.

Language development theory has been and still is a valuable source for principles to guide intervention in language disorders. As helpful as these principles are in developing intervention procedures, we must continue to examine them with reference to language impairment. We cannot forget that language-impaired children may not and often do not learn language in the same manner as the nonimpaired child and the simple reconstruction of events to provide for development may not be sufficient for this learning. A good rule of thumb to use in adapting normal development theory in language intervention is to monitor the process carefully to observe where there may be a learning breakdown and to vary the procedures at every stage until success is achieved. The variation in procedures may be in areas such as the length of time spent on a stage or part of a stage, in the amount of repetition given to events, in the degree of difficulty of the structure of the event, and in the amount of support given by the environment. The exclusive acceptance of any one of the theories presented here may serve to limit the influence of other valid positons on intervention.

11

INTEGRATING THEORIES: ORAL AND WRITTEN LANGUAGE

THEORY, ASSESSMENT AND INTERVENTION
IN LANGUAGE DISORDERS: © 1988 by Grune & Stratton
AN INTEGRATIVE APPROACH

ISBN   0-8089-1918-0

We assume that the relationship between oral and written language is obvious to most people. However, because oral language emerges prior to school and reading is taught as an academic subject in school, these two aspects of language are often thought of and usually treated as separate behaviors. The fact that the study of the nature and function of written language belongs to a different academic discipline than that of oral language contributes to the attitude that these two behaviors are discrete.

The fact is that oral and written language are inextricably intertwined. The elements that they share are essential to the nature of each of these processes. To wit, in western civilization, the written code is actually mapped on the oral code. Furthermore, in many types of language disorders, deficits can be found in both oral and written language, indicating either common structure in their codes or common internal cognitive processes used in performing them, or both—probably both. In a way, the relation between oral and written language starts at birth and changes as the child matures in both tasks, the interaction and dependency varying with the level of proficiency reached in each task.

Some language theories explicitly include reading in their description of language and some do not. By not including reading in our theoretical and practical dealings with language we are depriving ourselves of rich information regarding the language-learning and language-using system in humans. We limit ourselves in understanding disorders of oral language and disorders of reading. This compartmentalization, according to Wallach and Lee (1980), may also cause specialists to devise tasks contrary to the manner in which written and oral language actually develop.

There are many ways of approaching a discussion of the relationship between oral and written language (see Carrow-Woolfolk & Lynch, 1981). In a discussion directed to integrating these behaviors at a theoretical level, it may be fruitful to identify the elements common to both oral and written language or those in which they share similar functions as well as in which they differ. The identification of common and distinguishing factors will assist us in understanding other theoretical issues, for example, the issue of knowledge versus performance as well as in carrying out the language assessment process.

COMMMON AND SHARED ASPECTS OF ORAL AND WRITTEN LANGUAGE

The Code

At their most basic level, oral and written language are comprised of the same linguistic code. The same sounds and combination of sounds make up the words of the code, and the lexicon, word order, morphemes, and other aspects of syntax are the same. The semantics in oral and written language is the same; the words and word combinations mean the same thing whether they are spoken or written. The basic text structure and format are the same. The same basic code is used in reading and aural comprehension and in speaking and writing.

Language Knowledge

A second aspect of commonality between oral and written language is that both require that the rules of the code be internalized in order to form the individual's language knowledge base. Although written language requires the internalization of additional rules (which will be discussed under differences between oral and written language), the data base, which is made up of the abstracted rules of language, forms the foundation for both. This is why instruction in syntax and morphology, sentence construction, and vocabulary will improve both oral and written language behaviors, regardless of which input system is used.

Conceptual System

Another common aspect of oral and written language is the conceptual knowledge system. The child's world view provides the content or meaning that is brought to the interpretation of the same language forms in auditory comprehension and in reading. The greater the development of experiences for learning about the world whether vicariously through language or through direct contact, the greater will be the child's comprehension ability—his or her understanding of both spoken and written language.

Language Processing

Bradley and Forster (1987) argue that models of lexical access developed for the written form are also appropriate for speech if the differences due to physical characteristics are taken into account. While it is obvious that listening and reading differ in that they decode from inputs in separate modalities, they also converge at the same level to reach

> *Quote 11–2*
> *The present study offers evidence of essentially similar lexical decision processing for written and spoken words. Further, and more importantly, it suggests that syntactic (inflectional) information and semantic information are initially processed by different, separable, mechanisms.*
> (KATZ, BOYCE, GOLDSTEIN, & LUKATELA, 1987, p. 259).

their common goal—language comprehension. The question is—where do the two processes converge? Bradley and Forster (1987) suggest that a mechanism by which input tokens are associated with mentally represented types is possibly a common area. They conclude that "the lexical processes for print are as they are, exactly because they have been straightforwardly inherited from the speech domain. Commonality has its basis in borrowing" (p. 133).

Rule Induction

In learning oral language and in learning to read, the child is active in inducing the language rules. The first set of rules, the rules of phonology, morphology, and syntax, that the child induces are received through the auditory-vocal system and these rules—the knowledge base of the language—are used in speaking and listening as well as in reading and writing. In learning to read the child needs to induce an additional set of rules—sound and letter correspondence rules that are different from but built on the basic linguistic rules. The beginning reader will make progress in decoding only when he or she can function on the principle that the written language is founded on the spoken language.

Comprehensibility of Text

Because both use the same language system, the comprehension of oral and written language is influenced by the comprehensibility of the input text. The particular words used in the text, their frequency in the language, the degree of embeddedness of sentences, and the density of propositions may influence how well or how poorly individuals understand what they hear or read. Physical characteristics of the text and environment also influence both, but in different ways. Reading is influenced by the shape, style, or size of the letters and the amount of light, whereas listening comprehension is influenced by the distinctness of speech of the speaker, the loudness of the speech, and the background noise.

Degree of Organization of the Input

The manner in which a writer or speaker organizes what is written or said influences the listener's or reader's ability to understand. The logic and cohesive devices used in the text make it easier to decode what is meant. Many times difficulty in comprehending is related to poorly constructed texts. Examine the differences in these two texts and note the assistance provided in the second example by the use of connecting devices.

Example 1:
It's raining outside.
I'm not going to school.
I am going to the store.
Mother can't leave me alone.
It stops raining.
I will go out to play.

Example 2:
Because it's raining outside, I'm not going to school. But I am going to the store because Mother can't leave me alone. When it stops raining, I will go out and play.

When the input lacks cohesion, the receiver needs to integrate and organize it on the basis of his or her own knowledge. This type of integration is particularly important when reading lengthy passages.

Perceptual and Motor Requirements

In reading and in the comprehension of spoken language, the two input systems need perceptual integrity. Reading needs the ability to discriminate and remember visual information, whereas auditory comprehension requires the ability to discriminate and remember auditory information. On the output side, both require a performance system, the vocal system for speech and the motor system for writing (or finger spelling used by some hearing-impaired individuals).

Closure

There is need for closure in both reading and comprehension of spoken language. Neither process can function with the speed at which the human actually understands the spoken or written word; that is, we understand much faster than it takes our mechanism to actually process the input. This discrepancy occurs because we are able to fill in those parts of the message that we do not actually perceive (either visually or through audition) or that we perceive poorly. We bring closure to the message and comprehend it by this "filling in." Syntactic or semantic information can be missing or distorted and we will still be able to understand what is said.

Syntactic: _____ lady _____ go _____ the party.
Semantic: My _____ makes _____ go to _____ every day.

Our knowledge of the language helps us to fill in the parts that we miss in rapid processing and therefore helps us to understand.

Automaticity

In the use of oral and written language, the behavioral process must become automatic in order to be effective. The individual using oral or written language must be able to become so proficient in the processing of the input and output that he or she can perform without conscious effort. Only in that manner can the necessary attention be given to the content of the messages that are being communicated. If a child has to labor over decoding, he or she will not be able to use language or reading for other purposes, nor will it be pleasurable. Being able to verbalize and talk about rules is not the same as internalizing them and using them with efficiency.

Practice is required for automatization. The child is given much more time for the automatic behavior to take place when learning oral language (3 to 4 years) than when learning to read. We expect fluent reading in 6 months of school. Individual differences and different rates of acquisition are acceptable concepts in oral language development, but not as acceptable in learning written language. We forget that children may vary as much as 1 year in age when they begin school.

Role of Metalinguistics

Oral and written language can both be subjects of metalinguistic attention. Although early language is learned without conscious effort, in later stages of development, a child begins verbal play in which he or she enjoys repeating rhyming words and "silly" phrases. Later as parents and teachers draw attention to a child's phonemic and grammatical inaccuracies, the child increases his or her awareness of the language. Many children begin reading without metalinguistic awareness of the written words. Exposure to written words pronounced by a teacher or parent provide the exemplars from which the child induces the rules by which the written form of the language conforms to the oral form. The child moves quickly to automatic reading skills. For some children, the process of induction functions more slowly than for those described previously. They need a greater number of exemplars and time for rule development. Because this is not often provided in the schools, teachers begin teaching children the rules of letter/sound con-

> *Quote 11–3*
> *. . . the use of phonetic codes is a highly automatized skill for normal readers. We are scarcely aware of the phonetics of what we read as we are reading it. The sounds just seem to pop into mind and are all but ignored in favor of a close inspection of semantic content.*
>
> (STERNBERG & WAGNER, 1982, p. 6).

version (phonics) and give practice in decoding combinations of sounds. Beginning reading becomes a metalinguistic process for these children. In the study of language as an object of knowledge, metalinguistic awareness is important; in the use of language as a means of communication, metalinguistic awareness may interfere with the early development of the automatic performance needed in order to attend to meaning. Both oral language and reading use metalinguistic skills to improve performance in advanced language tasks.

DIFFERENCES BETWEEN ORAL AND WRITTEN LANGUAGE

Visual Versus Auditory Inputs

One of the major differences between oral and written language is that written language uses a visual code to represent the sounds of the oral code. The letters represent the sounds of the oral code that are a representation of reality events, objects, and ideas. The input of the code for reading is through the eyes instead of through the ears. Since the original storage for language is auditory, the initial visual input is probably converted internally to a form of auditory input to the storage system that probably accounts for the subvocalization in some beginning readers. When the reader becomes proficient in reading, there appears to be some type of direct access to meaning without the need to go through the complete auditory system except for words or sentences that are especially complex. I learned Spanish through the auditory system exclusively and have done relatively no reading of Spanish. I still need to read aloud to understand any level of Spanish except the most simple (see Fig. 11–1 for hypothesis regarding the internal route from visual perception of text to meaning).

Unfortunately, the coding system from letters to sounds is complex. In addition to single letters representing single phonemes, the visual code has letters representing more than one sound (a for /æ/ and for /a/), single phonemes represented by more than one letter (/k/ by c and k), combinations of letters representing one sound (ph for /f/), and combinations of sounds represented by one letter (/aɪ/ by i). Perhaps this was done originally for economy, with the thought that one letter-one sound

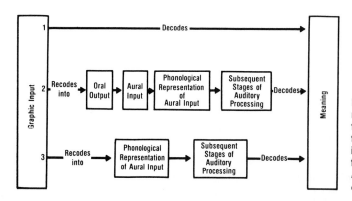

FIGURE 11–1. Three major hypotheses of the relationship between listening and reading: (1) the direct access hypothesis; (2) the subvocalization hypothesis; and (3) the phonological recoding hypothesis. (Reproduced with permission from Carrow-Woolfolk, E., & Lynch, J. [1982]. *An integrative approach to language disorders in children* [p. 315]. New York: Grune & Stratton.)

would result in too many letters for ease of manipulation. The actual result has been to create problems for children learning to read and spell.

Suprasegmental Phoneme Differences

A second aspect of the difference between oral and written language involves the information that is provided in oral language by suprasegmental phonemes such as intonation, stress, and pauses. When using the oral code the speaker can convey meaning by using specific intonational patterns. A rising intonation at the end of the utterance, "You went to church," means surprise at such a happening. The oral code also provides a means to distinguish meaning for words that are spelled alike but pronounced differently and therefore have more than one meaning (read as /rid/ or /rɛd/) when sufficient information for determining meaning is not available in the linguistic context. The pauses between thoughts in oral language are represented by the punctuation marks in written language. Word boundaries, not identifiable in oral language, are provided in written language by spaces between words. One natural boundary in oral language, the syllable, is not made explicit in written language. Since the unit of spoken language is a vocalic with modifying consonants, the syllabic aspects of words are clearly defined. These boundaries are absent in written language, and it is the task of the reader to induce the rules for word segmentation and to perform this task automatically. In fact, one of the most important tasks in decoding for the beginning reader is that of recognizing syllables instead of individual sounds.

Shared Knowledge

Another difference between oral and written language has to do with contextual information that contributes to the meaning of the code itself. In oral language, the communication between two individuals does not occur in a vacuum. The speaker and listener have shared knowledge that at least on the surface is accepted or inferred. There are certain basic facts that an adult assumes another adult possesses without needing to provide background data. When you ask "Where is the Chinese restaurant?" you assume at the least, that the listener knows what a restaurant is and the one you're looking for is in proximity. When two individuals are acquainted with each other, they have additional shared knowledge that comes from having common experiences and friends. This shared knowledge is not ordinarily available in reading. Unless one is reading a letter from a friend, in the typical reading experiences, the reader has no shared knowledge with the author except the expected world knowledge for a specific age group. When there is a discrepancy between the expected shared knowledge of the speaker or writer and the actual knowledge of the listener or reader, there is a problem in comprehension.

Differences in Context

Another variable that influences the interpretation of the code is the context within which the code is used. In using oral language, a speaker and a listener are usually in proximity to one another, except for telephone or television use. The environment within which they communicate offers information that can be referred to in the conversation. This context permits the speaker to economize in the amount of information imparted by the surface structure itself since some of the information is available through other sources. On a recent trip to New Orleans, my husband commented, "It's picking up," as we left Baton Rouge. My daughter who had been asleep during the early part of the trip did not understand what he meant. I did, for I had noticed a change in the amount of traffic we were encountering. Context had provided the necessary information for comprehending. The immediate context is not available in reading. Usually when individuals read, all the information for communication needs to be explicitly stated in the text except for pictures, which do provide contextual support for text. Even in cases where there are charts and figures, the text usually needs to stand alone with the information in the visual aids serving to clarify, but not substitute for, the information in the text. When children begin writing, they need to be taught to include everything, the topic, the purpose, the characters, or whatever is applicable to a complete and explicit written form. My daughter used to argue when writing an essay that she did not need to include information that her teacher already knew. She had not been taught the difference between and oral and written production.

Exchange Formats

The very nature of oral communication involves a type of interaction between speaker and listener that does not occur in reading and writing. The give and take of good conversation, for example, requires the oral language user to be adept at taking turns, maintaining or changing topics, revising surface structure when the meaning is not clear to the listener, and so on. The situation of listening to a lecture does in some ways resemble that of reading, however. The lecture listener, like the reader, must try to understand what someone else is trying to communicate without having the opportunity to respond—at least in the case of a lecture to a large audience. One advantage the reader has is that if a portion of the communication is not understood, he or she can reread and mull over what is read. The listener to an oral language lecture usually has just one chance, unless he or she is blessed by having someone who rephrases and repeats a message (or if the listener uses an audio recording device.)

These factors may be one of the reasons that most children prefer speaking and listening rather than reading and writing. In speaking and listening, the topic can be controlled both with respect to the subject matter and its complexity. Reading material cannot be controlled, particularly in a school situation. It is difficult to maintain the interest and concentration of a child when using materials that have no relation to his or her life situation.

Linguistic Style of the Text

Because the various modalities of communicating differ with respect to purpose, context, and so forth, the linguistic style of the text in these modalities also differs. The written language of a textbook is much more complex in surface structure than the written language of a letter. Both of these differ from the surface structure used in a conversation. One of the reasons a child has to "learn" to read and write, in addition to learning the decoding aspect of reading, is because of these differences. Written language uses linguistic structures and vocabulary that differ from that ordinarily used in oral language, vocabulary, and structure that most children have not been exposed to prior to beginning reading. This is particularly true of children who have not been exposed to a variety of language experiences because of social or cultural deficiencies in their environment.

A further difference in linguistic style is related to the fact that most texts for beginning readers are in a story format. For children whose experience with language is all functional and who have had little opportunity to hear stories, the story format and content is difficult to understand and possibly uninteresting. In a beginning reading program I developed (Carrow-Woolfolk, 1980), the beginning reading tasks are comprised of functions similar to those found in communication: following directions, informing, and exchanging ideas. The changeover from an oral to a written code is made with greater facility when only one aspect is changed at a time.

Sequence of Analysis

Comprehension of oral language, because it is received serially, requires primarily a "bottom-up" analysis of individual sentences and propositions with a gradual construction of an overall structure and meaning (although there is some reciprocal effect of higher level functions on decoding). Comprehension of reading, although it can be in terms of "bottom-up" analysis also, uses a "top-down" procedure based on a prior knowledge of the overall text structure and purpose with gradual elaboration of specific propositions. Headings, titles, and other markers help in the top-down method.

Differences in Production Requirements

In comparing speaking and writing, some of the same kinds of observations can be made as those made in comparing listening and reading. Whereas both speaking and writing require retrieval of linguistic forms to be associated with the ideas ready for expression, the speaker must retrieve these forms quickly and utter them at a pace that corresponds with the formulation of the idea. The writer, on the other hand, has the time to be deliberate in the choice of lexicon and syntax and also can revise to a much greater degree than the speaker can. The reasons many people find it harder to write than to speak is that there is no feedback for encouragement, and it is difficult, if not painful at times, to try to express an idea fully and then have to go back and reread what was said.

Differences in Use of Standard Language

For the average listener and reader, the written word is more standard in the use of the language than the spoken word. The spoken word reflects the great variety of speech and language structure patterns that exist in any heterogeneous groups of speakers within a broad language community. Comprehension requires the ability to recognize the members of distinctive phonemes even when the phonemes used by a speaker deviate to a greater extent from that which is ordinarily accepted in a language community. Dialects and foreign accents can be so different from the mainstream language as to cause difficulty for others to comprehend. The problem may be reversed for the person who has a dialect or accent. Writing uses mainstream phonology and structure. Since early reading passes through the internal auditory processing and storage system, what is read may not match what is already there. This discrepancy may cause a problem in comprehending what is read.

A model of language provided by Carrow-Woolfolk and Lynch (1982) illustrates the common elements in oral and written language: the cognitive units of language content (the meaning), and the units of the linguistic code (the basic rule-based components, the form) (see Fig. 11–2). The only rule-based knowledge that is added is that of graphology, the relation between phonemes and letters. The performance unit differs since reading uses the visual system and listening the auditory. The units in which oral and written language differ to the greatest extent is that of the communicative environment since there is no dialogue with a reader and little context in reading.

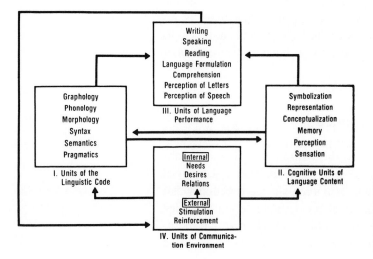

FIGURE 11–2. The role of reading and writing in a four-dimensional model. (Reproduced with permission from Carrow-Woolfolk, E., & Lynch, J. [1982]. *An integrative approach to language disorders in children* [p. 315]. New York: Grune & Stratton.)

**READING DECODING
AND READING
COMPREHENSION**

In the previous chapter I described the difference between decoding an oral language signal and comprehending it. It is important to make this distinction in reading also because, I believe, it is important to distinguish differences in reading problems related to decoding and those related to comprehension.

The first aspect of decoding is at the sound letter association level. To be able to read we must know the sounds the letters make. If we see a character such as

we cannot begin to decode it (unless we know Chinese) because we do not know the character and because it is an abstract symbol rather than a sound-related word. If we see Greek letters, we cannot decode because the letters do not correspond to the letters we use in English. In a language that has letters that correspond to those we use in English, we can translate from a visual to an auditory signal even though we cannot understand the signal because we do not know the language. For example, if we see the Spanish sentence: "Yo no voy a su casa a llamar mi prima," we can probably read it aloud (translate from the visual to the auditory code), but unless we know Spanish lexicon and grammar, we will not be able to understand it. When we decode a written sentence in another language we do not know, we use the phonemic categories of our own language for pronouncing the words; for example, we will probably say the word "llamar" with an [l] in the initial position instead of the correct [j] sound. We also recognize that the Spanish sentence above is not English because some of the letters do not occur in certain positions in English orthography, as the final [u] in *su*.

The next level of decoding is the grammatical level. If we see a nonsense sentence such as the following: "The sholl is freeping on the zoop," we will get some grammatical meaning even though we do not understand the lexical items. We will know among other things that the "sholl" is probably a singular thing or event that can act upon another thing or person, that the action, "freeping," is happening now on the zoop, which is a thing. The grammatical level of decoding is an important one and one that needs particular attention in teaching reading, particularly since some grammatical constructions in reading material frequently do not occur with any regularity in spoken speech. The search for meaning in reading is made even more complex by the degree of embeddedness of long phrases and clauses and the complexity of the lexicon used in written language. The skill of looking for the basic elements of propositions in long complex sentences needs to be taught.

Without the ability to decode grammatically, the young reader will have difficulty understanding what he or she is reading.

As in oral comprehension, the attachment of meaning to a decoded visual signal will also depend on the child's knowledge about events and things in the world, on his episodic memory. The more a child knows about a subject, the better that child will understand what he or she reads. Conversely, because reading is used to teach new information about the world, the better the child reads, the more world knowledge he or she will obtain. If the child cannot decode adequately, phonologically or grammatically, or if the child does not understand the lexical items, he or she will not be able to learn what is being explained. The problem evolves from a problem of poor decoding to one of comprehension (misunderstanding what is read) and then one of learning (failing to understand and learn new things through reading).

Thus we find that reading adds a dimension to both the decoding and comprehension of oral language. In decoding, the reader must learn to analyze complex and lengthy sentences—sentences that are rarely spoken —and also must add vocabulary that ordinarily occurs only in written language to the already existing store of words learned in speaking and listening. Once the decoding skill of reading is mastered, the task in reading shifts; reading becomes a means of knowing instead of an end. The store of world knowledge, episodic knowledge, and semantic knowledge expands through reading (see Chapters 8 and 9 for a discussion of the role of memory in comprehension). As this knowledge expands, there is more for the child to bring to the reading comprehension process. We do not teach children reading comprehension. We teach them to decode the grammar, the style, and the format of what they read, and we help them develop knowledge that they can bring to the printed word and so understand it. Comprehension is a constructive process; we generate meaning from our own knowledge of language and the world and the ideas and concepts we have developed. Therefore, the better the knowledge of language and of the world, the better will we be able to comprehend what we read. In that manner is comprehension improved.

What I am saying is that we should not teach *reading* comprehension, we should teach *language* comprehension. Once the skills of decoding have been mastered and the complex lexicon and grammar of difficult texts have been taught, a student will understand what he or she reads, if his or her world knowledge is adequate. If that student does not bring sufficient knowledge to the reading task, he or she will have difficulty understanding and using reading to learn more. He or she will "take" from reading in proportion to what he or she "brings" to it. Teaching reading comprehension should start with the child's knowledge base.

> *Quote 11–5*
> *A fluent reader is most efficient when attending to the meaning of a sentence that he or she is decoding and when most component procedures of word recognition operate automatically. When word recognition procedures do not operate automatically (e.g. a new word is encountered), they must often be placed under metacognitive control. At this point, of course, reading is no longer fluent.*
>
> (MASSON, 1982, p. 40).

I believe that often teachers move too quickly from decoding to comprehension before the decoding skills at the phonological and grammatical level are mastered and reading decoding becomes automatic. If specialists wish to work on comprehension skills, they can do so at the oral level while teaching visual decoding, since the skills of constructing meaning and inference are similar in oral and written language.

DISORDERS OF ORAL AND WRITTEN LANGUAGE

If we study the ways oral and written language are alike and different, we may begin to understand the kinds of disorders children have in these domains. This approach will also help us to recognize why sometimes we find simultaneous problems in oral and written language and other times one is impaired and not the other. If we accept the assumption that both the cognitive/conceptual and basic linguistic knowledge systems are common to oral and written language, we can understand how problems in these two components may affect both domains of language performance simultaneously. If we also recognize the differences between oral and written language performance—the decoding processes—or differences in text, format, and context, we can then comprehend why it is possible to have difficulty in one domain in the face of normal performance in the other. Kirk (1983) believes that at the performance level, reading and speaking, and listening and writing are examples of skilled behavior and each makes specific but different demands on the learner. She says, "mastery in one domain is no guarantee of mastery in another" (p. 15).

INTEGRATIVE ASSESSMENT OF ORAL AND WRITTEN LANGUAGE

It appears obvious that an adequate assessment of language necessitates a study of both oral and written domains. The areas of similarity need to be compared: How does the child comprehend both oral and written language when the text is the same—the same paragraph or

> *Quote 11–6*
> The data show considerable similarity in the types of deficiencies these children [developmental language impaired (LI) and poor readers (RI)] present . . . . Although it is important to recognize that children with developmental language and reading impairments might demonstrate similarity on certain tasks, it is equally important to recognize that these children do not represent a homogeneous group.
>
> Although it might be best to maintain a categorical distinction between LI and RI children, it might be that these children are best viewed on a continuum or as subgroups of the general group of learning-disabled children.
>
> (KAMHI & CATTS, 1986, pp. 344, 345).

story? How well can the child identify the main idea of what is heard or read if the passages are the same? How well does the child remember the details of these passages in both oral and written language? How does the child produce the basic oral and written grammatical form of language—the syntax and morphology? How does the child's performance on vocabulary measures, including synonyms, antonyms, and analogies, compare in oral and written form using the same or similar items? How well can the child tell a story, following the basic story format, in both oral and written language?

What is the child's nonverbal conceptual level—that world knowledge that the child brings to both oral and written language? How can the child use his or her conceptual knowledge and memory for the purpose of inference and understanding and using figurative language, jokes, and so on? How do the perceptual and memory systems handle both auditory and visual forms and both spoken and written language sequences?

The areas of difference between oral and written language also need to be assessed: What is the skill level of the child's decoding of written language, that is, how well does he or she recognize or figure out nonsense and real words? How well does the child recognize (visually) basic syntactic constructions and what kind of grammatical closure can he or she bring to the reading task? What is the child's level of knowledge of the rules governing phoneme-letter correspondence? How well can the child construct meaning from complex embedded sentences of the type usually not available in oral language? How well does the child attend to and remember the basic points of long complicated paragraphs and stories? How well does a child write complex constructions of the type not ordinarily used in oral language? How does the child handle new vocabulary in reading and how developed is his or her vocabulary of the type found in written language but very seldom in oral language? How does the child mark pauses and propositions with punctuation in written language? How well does the child spell? How legible is the child's handwriting?

It would be impractical if not impossible to assess all of these areas in every child with a language disorder. If a child is in school, however, I believe the specialist should try to determine to what extent a language disorder is related to both oral and written codes. The whole intervention process would make more sense if this type of information were available.

INTEGRATING ORAL AND WRITTEN LANGUAGE INTERVENTION

Let me start this section by stating that after more than 30 years of teaching from elementary school level to graduate level and of concern with the language-disordered student throughout most of this period, I have come to the position that there are three basic kinds of language learners with respect to the acquisition of the rules and basic performance of language. This categorization applies both to learning *oral* and *written* language. (This assumes sensory, conceptual, and environmental adequacy.)

The first kind of learner is one who possesses extraordinary induction ability. Members of this group of learners need only to be exposed to one or two exemplars of a rule and they have already mastered it operationally. It probably happens in oral language but is more easily observed in teaching reading. For example, you show them one or two words beginning with the letter *p*, say the words, and almost before you can flash a third word with an initial *p*, their mouth is positioned to make the /p/ sound. These children do not really need to be taught to read or decode. They learn from exposure. They may not be the brightest children either, just the ones who have a good linguistic-learning ability. In fact, we have evidence of hyperlexia in which children who have little or no understanding of language can learn to "read" or decode even complex material easily without understanding any of it (Mehegan & Dreifuss, 1972).

A second group of learners need extra time or extra exemplars for the decoding skills to be acquired. Whether their induction skills are not as efficient as the first type of learner or whether there is lack of readiness in the system, these children acquire the language task more slowly. Because we provide a considerable span of time for oral language development, these children eventually learn to talk without needing special help. However, they are not given this time for learning to read at school. Children are required to pass through the same curricular steps regardless of age (sometimes there is as much as a 1-year age difference among first grade children) or language level or general learning style or ability. In order to learn, these children need the type of

> *Quote 11–7*
> *Whereas in the natural world appearances are by and large what they appear to be, when signaling systems are involved the signals always convey double messages—about their physical characteristics, and about their referential value. Both with spoken and with written speech, one has to attend selectively to the meaning of the message, rather than to the message as physical pattern. Insofar as the physical characteristics of the message may, particularly for the young child, be salient, an act of selective attention is called for—the adoption of a verbal (semantic) set.*
>
> (KINSBOURNE, 1982, p. 207).

sequential steps for teaching reading that are provided in the school. They also need a large number of exemplars and frequent exposure to reading. These types of children learn the decoding rules by induction, as do those in the first group, but the process needs to be broken down into smaller units with more practice in order for the induction to take place. If the school is flexible in allowing these children to proceed at their own rate, they will learn to read without great difficulty. A systematic prereading and reading program that helps them prepare for rule induction will be of great help. Their problem is not with comprehension, but with decoding.

A third group of children, the minority, have considerable difficulty with the inductive process. Even when breaking the process down to its basic sound/letter units or providing them with numerous exemplars, they seem to be unable to induce the rules and use them automatically. Presentation of a letter does not elicit the corresponding sound, nor, of course, does presentation of a series of letters produce a word. Almost every time the child sees (or hears) the same word it is as if he or she has never seen it before. These children need extra help in learning to read and to speak, and the approach needs to be at a metalinguistic or "metareading" level. The rules underlying sound-letter correspondence need to be made explicit as in teaching phonics. The grammatical rules of oral language need to be made explicit. The visual code in reading needs to be broken down and put back together artificially (through blending practice) with explanation regarding the rules. These children have as a primary characteristic the dependence on teaching and repetition for learning. They do not appear able to acquire new learning by means of their own inductive processes.

I believe that instead of teaching beginning reading decoding as a process of providing sounds for letters (a phonic method), it should be thought of as a process of attaching letters to sounds (phonemic method [Carrow-Woolfolk, 1980]). Once a child perceives a specific phoneme auditorially and can identify its position in words, a letter is associated with the phoneme. In this way the teacher starts with what the child already knows, the phoneme system, the oral language system. The response to groups of letters or syllables with appropriate sounds and vice versa, which is made possible by learning the sound-letter correspondence rules, needs to be made an automatic skill. If reading can be made to be automatic by using frequent and salient exemplars, it is more effective than by using the metalinguistic approach of teaching the rules artificially (phonic method). The phonic method teaches the verbal statement of a rule. The child needs to know the rules operationally. The knowledge should be one of knowing how to do and doing efficiently. There is nothing so conducive to learning to read as to read—the same thing over and over if necessary. Time and practice may be needed by many children, but if given those two ingredients, without making them face any failure, most of them should learn. The ultimate focus of the child should be on meaning, not on decoding. This can be accomplished, however, only if the decoding skills are induced through practice and become automatic early in learning to read.

In addition to the knowledge of the phonemic system, the language specialist also needs to make sure the child understands the grammatical system. We assume that because a child has mastered the basic forms of language, all he or she needs to be taught in reading decoding is the sound-letter correspondence. On the contrary, the child needs to recognize basic syntactic constructions visually. We need to provide the child with visual envelopes of frequently used sentence types. The child should be repeatedly exposed visually to the basic grammatical structures such as "The _____ is _____ing" until the syntactic envelope is recognized visually and the child does not need to sound out the phonetic elements of each word. The child's visual and auditory systems will join to supply the expected grammatical parts so that his or her attention can be given to the substantive words in the sentence. This means that the child needs to be taught to read syntax as well as to read words.

Related to this last idea is the need to teach complex language structures in teaching reading. Children should not be expected to understand conjoined and embedded sentence types that they have never heard in oral language. At the time they begin to read, most children have not had experience in locating the basic proposition and its modifying elements in a long and complex construction. How can they bring their meaning to a form with which they have no experience? We cannot expect them to understand everything they read once they have learned to decode. They need time to learn to comprehend the text of written language just as they have had time to learn to comprehend the basic text of spoken language. Poor comprehension can result from an inability to decode the complex syntax found in written language.

The reading curricula should also provide systematic instruction in the variety of textual forms. Most simple narratives have a "story grammar" that, once recognized by children as forming a frame for the story, will help them understand the stories they read. As children progress in elementary school, they encounter new styles of writing such as expository writing in history or figurative language in literature. These students should be taught explicitly how to understand these various text forms. I have found that many students' problems in a subject such as physics are not in comprehending the principles of physics but in understanding the encoding style of a teacher or textbook.

I have suggested in an early reading program (Carrow-Woolfolk, TRAM II, unpublished) that beginning reading should be based on communicative tasks rather than on reading stories. The use of reading to inform, direct, and communicate with children more closely resembles their accustomed use of language. The transition to reading becomes one of changing the mode of input but not the style and format. Children who have never been read to are disadvantaged in situations where the story format is used at the onset of reading instruction.

We cannot underestimate the role of conceptual development in reading comprehension for all three groups of children. A child cannot get meaning from words if he or she does not bring some meaning to them. In Chapter 9, I discussed the interrelationship of concept development, memory, and oral language comprehension. Once a child begins reading, he or she has an additional task to interrelate to the first three. The ability to infer, to generalize, and to expand comes from successfully learning to integrate oral language, memory, and concepts. The early stages of reading teaching must be accompanied by development of concepts as well as of oral language. In fact, one of the best preparations for reading is providing the child with real, vicarious, and verbal experiences and helping the child learn to relate these by exploring commonalities and differences in events and objects and by talking about them. One of the reasons, I believe, that children have so much difficulty with various aspects of language is because our systems, educational and social, demand so little of them in the way of expressing ideas and concepts. Once children have mastered the basic tools of decoding written language, it is possible to integrate reading, writing, listening, and speaking so that improvement in one will produce improvement in the others. At the primary grades, reading becomes the main source of new vocabulary or new knowledge of the world. If children have a decoding problem in reading, they will experience a relative decline in this knowledge.

It is my belief that language specialists can play a role in teaching all three groups of children, but particularly the last group because of their understanding of the phonemic and grammatical systems of language. It is obvious that the teaching approach for each of these groups should be different. Perhaps the different intervention techniques described in Chapter 5 can be selectively applied to the different kinds of problems described here.

SUGGESTIONS FOR IMPROVING READING

What we can do to help our children learn to read:

1. We can stop setting up uniform and artificial goals for them to reach. We know the goals are unrealistic for some children.
2. We can stop expecting all the children to respond to a single teaching method—we know children have different learning styles. (When something is not working for everyone, we replace it with something else that again does not work for everyone.)
3. We can stop expecting our children to reach goals at the same time—we know that children progress at different rates, particularly since such a wide age range is represented in each class.
4. We can give time for children to learn to decode before we place other burdens on the reading task.
5. We can remember that the conceptual knowledge that results from early experiences is not the same for all children and we should not expect them to understand what they read in the same way.
6. We should not forget that the best preparation for reading is oral language and that children have different early language experiences that may cause differences in their basic readiness to transfer from an oral to a written code.
7. We should know that if our children are allowed to develop at their own rate, if they are given much practice in an encouraging and accepting environment, if we permit them to learn in the way that is best for them according to their learning style, and if we provide a wealth of experience of all kinds, even verbal experience—talking with them, explaining, inferring—we will find that they will learn to read. Some may need some extra help, but not the large numbers that are presently receiving it.

SECTION III

Concluding Thoughts About Theory and Practice

As I pointed out in the first chapter of this book, the specialist in language disorders must be concerned with the totality of language in theory because he or she is concerned with the totality of language in practice—in the language system of individuals who need the help. For this reason, it is important to identify the necessary components of a broad theory of language and to integrate the existing theories to the best of our ability, particularly because the ideas essential to each theory are rarely mutually exclusive. In the first chapter of this final section, I will try to describe what I consider to be the necessary elements of a complete theory of language. In this following chapter, Chapter 13, I will make some suggestions, in the form of a summary of the first 11 chapters, for the reconciliation at a theoretical level of discrepant concepts in the various theories. Chapter 14 will attempt to pull together principles on the practical aspects of language assessment and intervention as these relate to theory. A last chapter will integrate theory and instructional methods in intervention. Together, the four chapters serve as summary and conclusions and hopefully as a stimulus to others to join in the integrative process if they are not yet doing so.

INTEGRATING THEORY AT THE THEORETICAL LEVEL: NECESSARY ELEMENTS OF A THEORY

The discussions in the preceding chapters have illustrated that the various theories of language have more commonalities than differences. Perhaps the differences have occurred because theorists have chosen to restrict the scope of their theories. This restriction results from efforts to remain within disciplinary boundaries. We find that the definitions of language generated within disciplinary circles address only those aspects of language that are within the scholarly realm of the participants in the discipline and omit those aspects outside of it. We also recognize, however, that we cannot limit a theory of language if we want to understand individuals with language disorders.

This chapter will state some theoretical assumptions that I believe need to be accepted before we can have a complete understanding of language and that can serve as necessary elements for the development of a full-blown theory. These assumptions have evolved from attempts to integrate the material presented in earlier chapter.

THEORY, ASSESSMENT AND INTERVENTION
IN LANGUAGE DISORDERS: © 1988 by Grune & Stratton
AN INTEGRATIVE APPROACH

ISBN   0-8089-1918-0

1. *To consider language in its totality, we should define the relationship between the cognitive and linguistic aspects of language.* The linguistic code *is not* language. The phonemes, morphemes, and sentence structures are combinations of sounds that are uttered and heard but are empty unless understood. When we hear a foreign language that we do not know, we hear the sounds but we do not understand the language. The code, therefore, is but one part of language.

The ideas and concepts we have of the world of events, things, and persons *are not* language. The cognitive system is not language. Children who have been deaf from infancy can relate to people and objects meaningfully—they drink from a glass, they sit on a chair, they attempt to influence their environment. Until they are taught the linguistic code or a substitute code, they do not have language. The cognitive system is a part of language, equal to the linguistic part—there would be no language without it.

When the linguistic code or form and the cognitive system of ideas and thoughts and concepts come together so that they are associated in a manner in which one elicits the other, then there is language. The association between the two is called semantics. If we refer to the code or form as *linguistic* and to the ideas and concepts as *cognitive*, we can reserve the term *language* to refer to the association between the two. If we do this, cognition and the activities associated with it will not be considered nonlinguistic in the sense that they are outside the purview of language but only in the sense that they do not address the computational aspects of language, the structure of the code. Semantics is not considered part of the form—the linguistic—aspect. It is used to refer to the association between these two parts, linguistic and cognitive.

The implications of this description of language for language disorders are significant. It places on the language specialists the responsibility of both the linguistic and cognitive aspects of language at the development level as well as at the assessment and intervention levels. Problems in each of the areas—in the linguistic area (linguistic problems), in the cognitive area (cognitive problems) or in the relations between the two (linguistic/cognitive or semantic problems)—will be problems of language and therefore the concern of the language specialist.

Other aspects of the cognitive system that need to be integrated into a theory of language are those of perception and memory, together with the related strategies of access and retrieval. A theory of language that is used to understand disordered language must include all aspects of knowledge and performance, even though the role or function of specific parts is not clear.

2. *To consider language in its totality, a theory of language must include as part of its descriptive responsibilities, the integration between knowledge and performance.* By performance, I mean (as in other

chapters) the internal processing by which a stream of language is taken into the human system and is translated into forms that are comprehended, stored, retrieved, reformulated, and performed. A dead language, existing in books, described in terms of rules governing the lexicon, phonemes, grammar, and suprasegmental phonemes and meaning, is a language. But we must distinguish between "a language" and "language." When a language becomes operational in the human being, it is called language—the individual performs it, so to speak. To do so he or she must internalize the rules that form the knowledge of the language and also accomplish with speed and accuracy (1) the decoding of the input, which involves grouping the input into structural units, searching the data banks for the rules governing its grammar and meaning, and comprehending it; and (2) the retrieval, sequencing, organizing, and formulating of the grammatical units needed to express meaning. The implication is that it is possible to have the knowledge of the rules and yet perform poorly in language due to problems in the processing system.

Acceptance of the position that there is a distinction between knowledge and performance permits the explanation of language acquisition in terms of a dual process. On the one hand, there is the process of inducing the rules by a self-regulating internal system, a process that may need little help from the environment except exposure and facilitation. On the other hand, there is the process of learning to perform language efficiently, accurately, and automatically, a process that needs teaching, repetition, and practice. For this, interaction with the environment is essential for refining and reinforcing and, in the case of disorders, for instructing.

This dual aspect of language will also be the basis for practices in assessment and intervention. The language specialist will need to "tease out" and separate problems that are related to lack of knowledge of the linguistic rules and those that are problems in performance. Some indicators that help to distinguish these two areas of problem are: (1) if comprehension is within normal limits but expression is not, the problem is probably one of performance, whereas if both comprehension and expression are involved, the problem is probably one of knowledge; (2) if there is inconsistency in performance where the linguistic and situational environments are constant, the problem is more likely one of performance, while if the inconsistency is related to linguistic complexity or environmental factors, the problem is more likely one of knowledge; (3) if retrieval, speed, and automaticity are the main problems, the disorder is likely one of performance; (4) if there is an ability to recognize the error in either or both the instructor's speech or the student's own speech, the problem is probably one of performance; conversely, if the error is not recognized, the problem is probably one of knowledge.

3. *To consider language in its totality, a theory of language must incorporate the concept of language use and context.* To describe language in terms of form and content only is to omit its most important aspect in humanity, the purpose it serves in society and the function it serves for humans. As stated before, the purpose of language in the broad sense of the term involves the intent of the speaker, which in turn usually involves the transmission of a message to a listener. Because such a transmission usually occurs in an interpersonal or social situation, the context of the communication becomes a part of the interchange. To be able to interpret context is a cognitive function, as is the ability to interpret events and concepts. This ability can be termed *social perception.* Language therefore cannot be viewed in terms of the behavior of a single individual but must be viewed within a relationship, the listener and his or her ability being as integral a part of the relationship as the speaker's ability since both change primary roles. The effectiveness of the communication is based to a great extent on the social perception of those involved in message transmission and their ability to modify and revise messages on the basis of this perception. The more closely the information communicated in the message conforms to the intent of the speaker, the more effective will be the communication.

The assessment of language, in addition to including information about the child's knowledge of the linguistic system and its rules and the ability of the child to perform this knowledge in an efficient and automatic manner, must include information about the child's social perception and ability to interact with and adapt his or her language to the environment and the persons in it.

Including the concepts of language intent and function within an interactive paradigm in the description of language will help to specify the intervention agendas and protocols that will take into account the function that language serves for the child.

4. *To consider language in its totality, a theory of language must clearly describe the components of language and their interrelationship.* If we consider language as having two basic components, the linguistic and the cognitive, we can then describe the other components on the basis of the relationship between these two. The linguistic component is viewed as a module that has unique characteristics that are distinct from the cognitive component both in terms of development as well as in performance. The linguistic module (Chomsky, 1980) includes the computational aspects of language, the phonemic and grammatical aspects together with their own input and storage processes. The cognitive module (conceptual and pragmatic) includes the concepts, ideas, social perceptions, interaction abilities, and self-perceptions that form the various meanings that are associated with the linguistic code. This module also includes reasoning, determining cause and effect, solving problems, etc.

The semantic component is the result of the association between the above two modules. This association occurs at many levels, for example:

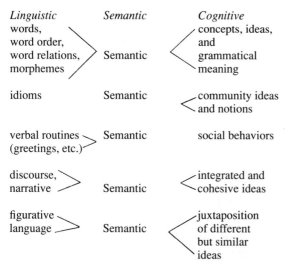

Linguistic	*Semantic*	*Cognitive*
words, word order, word relations, morphemes	Semantic	concepts, ideas, and grammatical meaning
idioms	Semantic	community ideas and notions
verbal routines (greetings, etc.)	Semantic	social behaviors
discourse, narrative	Semantic	integrated and cohesive ideas
figurative language	Semantic	juxtaposition of different but similar ideas

Many of the above relations between form and meaning are usually invariable, that is, there are dictionary meanings or community and socially accepted meanings within a social group and as such are accepted by all members of the group. When the surface structure is connected to social meanings, the associations are said to fall within the realm of pragmatics. In fact, because Foster's (1984b) data indicate that topic maintenance is a cognitive not a linguistic skill and since it could be said that turn-taking and other interpersonal behaviors are also cognitive, it can be hypothesized that pragmatics is primarily a cognitive skill that describes social interactions and that the relation between these social interactions and the linguistic code is semantic just as other relations between the form and cognition are. The semantic task, *to mean*, includes to indicate, refer, connote, infer, connect, and so on, and it is these functions that the linguistic form as a symbolic process has in relation to ideas, concepts, and thoughts.

Meanings that are variable such as in similes and metaphors are a function of the cognitive process recognizing similarities between ideas and using their corresponding words interchangeably. To understand these types of linguistic structures, there must be a complete understanding of the meanings of each of the words and the circumstances within which they are used, and an understanding of the threads of commonality in the meaning and the creative ability to use or exchange one for the other. Again the cognitive and linguistic components intermingle.

If we accept the distinction between grammar and semantics (discussed in Chapters 6 and 7) and if we accept both the cognitive and linguistic components as equal parts of language we can propose the system illustrated in Figure 12–1 as a way for classifying the kinds of disorders of language.

Semantic problems of knowledge can be due to either the cognitive or linguistic components. Pragmatics would be classified as part of the semantic component that relates the linguistic form to social situation and could be due to a cognitive problem in which the social perception or situational meaning is impaired, to a failure to form a match between the linguistic form and the social behavior or meaning (knowledge), or to a failure to generate the appropriate form at the appropriate time due to memory or retrieval problems (performance).

5. *To consider language in its totality, a theory of language must describe the relation between comprehension and expression.* If comprehension and expression have a common knowledge base and have some common access mechanisms, it accounts for the fact that many children with language disorders exhibit both comprehension and expression problems —problems of language knowledge. If comprehension and expression differ at the extremities of performance—in the processes of input and output that may include some of the retrieval mechanisms as well as the searching and encoding/decoding functions, it accounts for the fact that some children may have ongoing comprehension problems even after they have mastered the basic structure of the language or may have problems in formulation and production of language in the face of good comprehension. These are problems in the performance system.

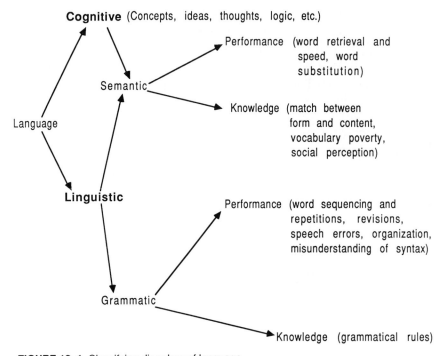

FIGURE 12–1. Classifying disorders of language.

If a problem is one of semantic or grammatical knowledge, the problem would be evident in comprehension and expression. Inadequacy of the common knowledge base would influence both. A performance problem in comprehension would influence production primarily during the years of language development. Once the rules are mastered, it is theoretically possible to have a continuing disorder of comprehension, one in which the auditory processing system functions inadequately, but have intact production. The reverse is also true. It is possible to have a performance disorder of production, with comprehension intact.

From the standpoint of language development, a theory that describes language as both knowledge and performance has implications for comprehension and expression. Comprehension performance is essentially a more simple process than expression. Whereas comprehension processing requires a search of the storage system, to select recognition and match internal entries with an input, expression requires a search without a model. In expression, the stimulus for the search is a concept or idea and what needs to be retrieved is not only words, but grammar and word order rules. It would indeed be difficult to comprehend or express grammar and lexicon that are not yet in the storage system. In language acquisition, knowledge of the rules of the language is induced and stored. The check of their presence is usually more easily identified through the comprehension system since, as stated previously, the process of comprehending is a more simple process than that of expressing. In other words, the acquisition of the knowledge of the rules of language affects comprehension and expression simultaneously. The presence of the knowledge is more easily identified through comprehension, therefore comprehension is "said" to develop earlier than expression.

Expression, on the other hand, demands greater knowledge of specifics of grammatical usage and greater accuracy in performance than comprehension. A message can often be understood without knowledge of every element in the input, but a message can rarely be communicated effectively if the utterance of the speaker has errors in grammar or vocabulary. It is for this reason that it is suggested that, from the standpoint of grammatical development, intervention should be focused on production.

With reference to the identification of disorders of language, comprehension testing should identify more accurately the adequacy of the knowledge of the language *if* one can use techniques that will provide such information. If production alone is used, it would be difficult to distinguish between knowledge and performance problems. The identification of knowledge and performance problems would be helped by testing both comprehension and expression. We could describe the following problems:

1. If a child has difficulty comprehending but has mastery of the expressive system, the disorder is one of the comprehension performance system. (During development, the expressive system is also impaired.)
2. If the problem is about equal in both comprehension and expression, the disorder is one of language knowledge.
3. If comprehension is good but expression is disordered or delayed relative to other systems, the problem is one of expressive performance.

If there are both comprehension and expression problems, we need to include both in the assessment procedure of language-disordered children. If we include only analysis of expressive functions, we may miss some children with comprehension problems or we may provide inappropriate intervention procedures for such children.

6. *To consider language in its totality, there should be integration of the roles of the organism and the environment in language development.* An accurate view of the developmental process in language would describe the role of the self-directed inductive system in the child that permits him or her to be selective in the aspects of the language environment for which he or she internalizes and formulates rules and the role of the environment itself. It appears obvious that the environment does not select rules for the child nor does it teach the child how to internalize them. In this sense, the environment acts only to trigger the language rule-learning mechanism in the child. However, there are aspects of language learning in which the environment is not only important, but critical. The quality, extensiveness, and quantity of language in the environment affects the quality of the language that the child induces and the efficiency with which it is induced. It provides props, pointers, and formats for learning. To learn rules, the child must be exposed to numerous exemplars. The variant and invariant aspects of each rule must be observed to be distinguished.

7. *To consider language in its totality, the dimension of the desire for communicating must be made an integral part of a theory.* Specialists who have worked with language-delayed children are aware that a child must have a need to talk. If the environment supplies all of the child's desires without effort on the part of the child to communicate them, the child may function without language. The response of the environment to the child's language is a way of ensuring the continuation of using effective language for communication. Language is more than the learning of rules, and so it must be described in a way that encompasses the broader framework of communication.

Language is not utilized in a vacuum; it is spoken by human beings for specific purposes, ordinarily for communicating with other human beings. Specialists who deal with disorders of language recognize that such disorders can arise from the lack of desire to communicate—where communication has no purpose or is not needed. It is useful to separate this aspect of pragmatics from those dealing with rules governing social routines and interpersonal exchanges because these two problems arise out of different dynamics of the language system.

Related to the desire to communicate is the desire to change when communication is ineffective. Change is related to motivation, and so any process that attempts to bring about change must first address itself to factors that are motivating to the individual who needs to change. The word *needs* is an important one because motivation is most stimulative when the individual experiences a need—in this case a need to be understood and to understand. The aspect of desire needs to play an important role in intervention.

8. *To consider language in its totality, we need to develop a classification system for language components that will include all aspects and all dimensions of language.* In such a classification system we should attempt to place similar functions within a category and not lump together the apples and oranges of language, for example, turn-taking, retrieval, narratives, and syntax.

A classification of language may theoretically have three major parts: (1) the code itself, (2) the child's cognitive system with its operational knowledge of the code and its unique processing capabilities, and (3) the unique aspects of an actual performance of language by an individual or individuals (the speech act) and the context within which this performance takes place. Each of these merits some discussion. See Figure 12–2 for a proposed classification system of language.

The linguistic code is the sum of the phonological, semantic, syntactic, paralinguistic, and pragmatic rules that govern a language. If language is viewed in a broad sense, extralinguistic components (facial expression, etc.) are also considered to be part of the code. When the code is used, either verbally or in writing, to accomplish specific purposes such as narration, description, exposition, and instruction there are additional rules that govern its use. These rules govern the use of cohesion, sequence, logic, inference, figurative language, and so on, or whatever is needed to make the form effective for its purpose. When the code is used in a social context, there are rules governing the forms of language to use based on the age, sex, and role of the speakers as well as factors related to the type of verbal interchange. For example, in a dialogue of a conversational nature, there are rules governing turn-taking, topic maintenance, talking-time, and so on. All in all, the above forms the knowledge base of the language, the rules that can be identified, described, and set down and against which individual performance is judged.

The second component in language is the child's system, which includes a knowledge base and cognitive processing capabilities for acquiring the knowledge and using it adequately. The child's cognitive

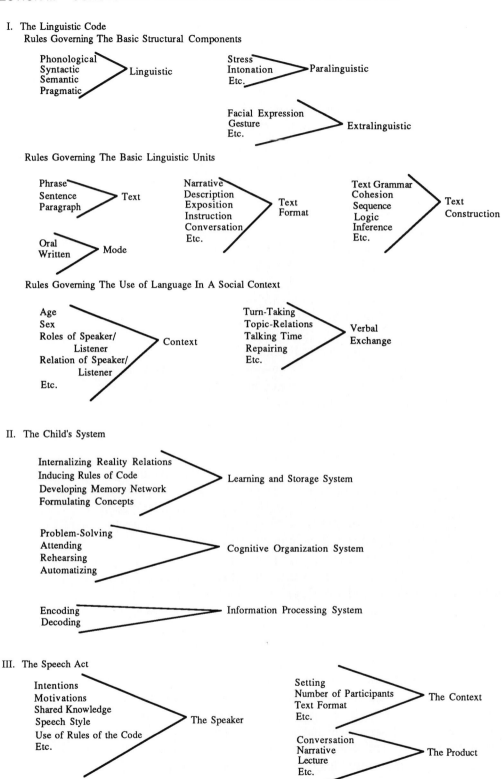

I. The Linguistic Code
   Rules Governing The Basic Structural Components

   Phonological
   Syntactic   } Linguistic
   Semantic
   Pragmatic

   Stress
   Intonation   } Paralinguistic
   Etc.

   Facial Expression
   Gesture   } Extralinguistic
   Etc.

   Rules Governing The Basic Linguistic Units

   Phrase
   Sentence   } Text
   Paragraph

   Oral
   Written   } Mode

   Narrative
   Description
   Exposition   } Text
   Instruction   Format
   Conversation
   Etc.

   Text Grammar
   Cohesion
   Sequence   } Text
   Logic   Construction
   Inference
   Etc.

   Rules Governing The Use of Language In A Social Context

   Age
   Sex
   Roles of Speaker/
      Listener   } Context
   Relation of Speaker/
      Listener
   Etc.

   Turn-Taking
   Topic-Relations
   Talking Time   } Verbal
   Repairing   Exchange
   Etc.

II. The Child's System

   Internalizing Reality Relations
   Inducing Rules of Code   } Learning and Storage System
   Developing Memory Network
   Formulating Concepts

   Problem-Solving
   Attending   } Cognitive Organization System
   Rehearsing
   Automatizing

   Encoding   } Information Processing System
   Decoding

III. The Speech Act

   Intentions
   Motivations
   Shared Knowledge   } The Speaker
   Speech Style
   Use of Rules of the Code
   Etc.

   Setting
   Number of Participants } The Context
   Text Format
   Etc.

   Conversation
   Narrative   } The Product
   Lecture
   Etc.

FIGURE 12–2. Classification of the kinds of language disorders.

system is what makes possible his or her inducing the linguistic, pragmatic, and other rules of the language code just described, thereby
forming a knowledge base that permits the generation of language. In
addition to storing the rules of the language, the knowledge base stores
the concepts about persons, events, objects, and social relationships that
provide material for the meanings of the language. The development of
these concepts and their association with the code is also a function of
the cognitive system of the child. The child's unique processing
capabilities govern the manner in which language input in any linguistic event is guided through appropriate channels in the system to
the point where it is understood or the manner in which an idea is
guided through the system to emerge as an utterance. The effectiveness
of processing influences the effectiveness of language. In addition to
the transmission of language signals through the systems, cognitive
processing also provides the general strategies by which all cognitive
behavior takes place, such as induction strategies, problem-solving, and
inference (see II in Fig. 12–2).

The third component of language is related to the acts of speaking
and listening in a particular setting on a particular day. This component
describes (1) the internal conditions of the speakers, their intentions,
their inferences regarding shared knowledge, their chosen manner or
style of speaking (e.g., indirect/direct messages, figurative/explicit
usage), their use of feedback and repair and the effectiveness with which
they use all the language rules they know—the rules involving the code,
the social interaction, and the particular form of the code (narrative,
conversation) they are using; and (2) the external conditions, the setting,
the station, sex, relationship, and other variables of the persons involved
in the interaction, as well as the response and feedback of all the individuals involved in message exchange.

If we have a good classification system, we will not need to evolve
a new theory every time we are confronted with a new aspect of
language; we can just integrate new insights about and aspects of language into the classification system.

9. *To consider language in its totality, we need to integrate
language disorders and the facts about such disorders into our theoretical descriptions of language.* It is important to recognize on both
theoretical and clinical levels that we cannot extrapolate from normal to
disordered language. When we study and describe normal language, we
are concerned only with language output or behavior because we assume that the internal processes of the children we study fall within the
range of normal variations. We cannot make this assumption with
language-disordered children. Therefore, we cannot direct our attention
exclusively to language output behavior. We must also be concerned
with the cognitive and social systems of the child in both assessment
and intervention.

To assist our understanding of disordered language and to aid in the development of a paradigm for dealing with such disorders, we need to seek answers to questions such as the following: (1) What are the subtypes of language disorders? (2) Do the profiles of language-disordered children change with age and, if so, how? (3) Is one of the basic difficulties in language disorders one of learning? (4) Why is exposure to language not sufficient for some children? (5) Why do some language-disordered children have difficulty in generalizing new information? (6) Why do some language-disordered children, even after basic structures are learned and tools such as reading are mastered, still have trouble understanding and using language? (7) Is the problem with some language-disordered children one of access to the knowledge base—one of deficient strategies for learning—one of proficiency? (8) What accounts for changes in the children's profiles with age?

In view of the complex system of language, we can no longer simply classify all language-disordered children into one category. Clinical experience, neurological findings, as well as recent empirical studies (Aram & Nation, 1975; Wolfus et al., 1980; Rapin & Allen, 1983) show that there are a number of syndromes of disordered language, each involving a different combination of cognitive, processing, and linguistic difficulties. This is true even within the pragmatic subset of language disorders (Fey & Leonard, 1983). Research and practice should reflect the heterogeneity of language disorders. Perhaps one of the reasons that research findings regarding language-disordered children have been so inconsistent is that we have grouped all these children together on the assumption that all language-disordered children are alike.

The different syndromes of language disorders may be related in part to the age at which we test individuals who have such problems. It may be that each specific age, with the corresponding task that needs to be learned at that level, demonstrates new and different aspects of the problem. Clinical experience certainly shows that a preschool child with a language problem frequently will have learning disabilities when he or she reaches school-age. Theories need to reckon with this fact.

10. *To consider language in its totality, we must integrate into our theoretical and practical descriptions of language, the four processes of reading, writing, speaking, and listening.* We must not allow professional and academic divisions to influence the manner in which we view the relationship between oral and written language.

Written and oral language have a common data base; they both deal with the basic structure of the linguistic code. Each also has rules that are specific to the performance in their respective domain, and each makes specific but different demands on the learner. In other words, oral and written language have similarities and differences: what children have to learn and know, how they go about learning it, how they store it, and how they access it and use it.

Studies on the interrelationship of oral and written language when these domains are both defective or when one is unilaterally defective will aid in understanding the nature of the language process. If the peripheral (modality based) systems differ, then a disorder in both systems might indicate a problem in a more general cognitive function or in the language data base.

If we integrate oral and written language, we help to describe the relationship between language disorders and learning disabilities. The integration of cognitive processes (auditory memory, perception, retrieval) and language will further explicate how language and learning disorders either overlap or are essentially one and the same thing. We cannot just say they are the same; we must show, at a theoretical and empirical level, how in fact they are.

11. *To evolve a theory of language that is a valid as well as useful base for understanding language disorders, we must consider the totality of language.*

13

INTEGRATING THEORY AT A THEORETICAL LEVEL: INTEGRATING THE ISSUES

KNOWLEDGE AND PERFORMANCE

COGNITIVE AND LINGUISTIC DOMAINS

COMPREHENSION AND PRODUCTION

SEMANTICS AND SYNTAX

PRAGMATICS AND LINGUISTICS

EXTERNAL AND INTERNAL DESCRIPTIONS OF LANGUAGE

In the Introduction of this book and in the first part of this chapter, I have listed specific areas that a theory of language needs to explain. If we match the theories of language to the areas that need to be addressed in defining language, a clear picture of the scope of each theory emerges:

1. The *substance and structure* of language—the knowledge about the syntactic, semantic, and pragmatic structures of a language, the underlying rules that exist in the abstract and that an individual acquires in the development process—is the general concern of *linguistic theory*.

THEORY, ASSESSMENT AND INTERVENTION
IN LANGUAGE DISORDERS: © 1988 by Grune & Stratton
AN INTEGRATIVE APPROACH

ISBN   0-8089-1918-0

2. The *performance* of language—the internal processes involved in performing language, how the processes function in such tasks as word retrieval, transmission through the perceptual system, strategies for execution of language, storage, automaticity, and so on—is the general concern of the two cognitive theories, *information process* and *cognitive organization theories.*

3. The *use* of language—the intent and motivations of the user, the social interaction and context factors that contribute to effective messages and cause variation in the selection of the language form—is the general concern of *pragmatic theory.*

4. The *individual who develops* language—the quality of the neurological system involved, the relation between language structure and the brain—is the general concern of *neuropsychological theory.*

5. The *modification* of language—the ways of changing language, the ingredients of a program for improvement—is at least to some extent the general concern of learning theory and the specific concern of *behaviorism.*

If it is true, as it appears to be, that each theory addresses a different aspect of language, can we simply use them all, allowing each theory to explain a different domain of language? In the form that they presently exist in the literature, the theories cannot be used simultaneously. Because each is used to explain development and some to explain disorders, assessment, and intervention in addition to explaining the general nature of language or learning, we find, at these levels especially, some ideas that are incompatible. We find also that some of these theories do not account for the evidence we have about disordered language. The fit has to be especially good in relating theory to disorder. Perhaps the place to start in the integration process is at the level of language disorders.

Language specialists' experience as well as the literature in language disorders has demonstrated that language-disordered children do not form one homogeneous group. There are differences in the kinds of problems children have in language. It is possible to identify specific combinations of problems that can be called *patterns* of language disorders. Specific difficulties within these patterns may be problems in, for example, retrieving a word, knowing a rule for a morphological construction, understanding specific sentence construction, or in discriminating spoken speech. If we accept these descriptions of language problems, we cannot accept a theory of language that describes language in terms of its rules *only* as a total explanation of the language process. If we cannot accept a theory's explanation of language because it cannot account for disorders, we cannot accept its explanation of acquisition and intervention.

KNOWLEDGE AND PERFORMANCE

Linguistic theory explains language in terms of its form, context, and use rules. The competence a child develops is a function of his or her induction of the rules of the language from exposure to exemplars of rule use in the environment. A disorder is a problem in rule development, and therefore intervention is a process by which the rule induction is facilitated. Since rule induction is an internally directed selective process by which a child takes in, sorts, organizes, stores, and uses rules, the specialist has little other duty than to provide "material" for this process.

I have attempted to illustrate in this book, Chapter 6 in particular, that language is not solely a function of correct application of rules. Examples abound in support of this position from the disorder perspective. A personal example may help illustrate this position. I know the Spanish language. I understand 98 percent of what I hear in any context at any level; I know the rules of the language. I have had little opportunity to speak Spanish throughout my life, however. A few short trips to Mexico and occasional conversations with Latin American friends, domestics, gardeners, and others is the extent of my production experience. Consequently, I have difficulty in expressing abstract ideas, not only in retrieving vocabulary (which I can understand), but in constructing complex sentences. Of particular difficulty for me is the use of informal and formal pronouns and their corresponding verb endings. I have trouble shifting pronouns, depending on the person to whom I'm speaking. I know the rules but I use the pronouns incorrectly in specific situations and I recognize my errors immediately. This "problem" I have in Spanish is not a rule-based problem; it is a problem of performance, one that would improve with increased use of the language.

In my opinion, the process of performing language must be included in a definition of language. If performance is included at a theoretical level, it can be integrated with the application of the theory at a practical level and it will help us differentiate between performance and knowledge problems in language disorders. If we attempt to integrate linguistic theory with cognitive organization theory, we may be able to account for both. As described in Chapter 1, cognitive organization theory includes within its theoretical framework both the learning of rules and the performance of them, learning something and learning how to do it. It includes the concepts of performance accuracy, efficiency, and automaticity. The linguistic theory approach could be used to describe the induction of rules, and the cognitive organization theory the acquisition of strategies for performing.

Linguists might object to the fact that cognitive organization theory considers language as a parallel and equal skill to that of other cognitive skills. Linguistic theory considers language to be unique, to develop in specific and unique sequences. As Chomsky proposed (1980; see Chapter 7), the linguistic module has its own characteristics that are different from the characteristics of other cognitive behaviors. A theory could be evolved that would separate the linguistic rule-learning aspects of language (the computational aspect of language—the rules—that form the syntactic construction and phonological or semantic patterns) from the performance aspect (the internal processes such as word retrieval, storage, transmission, not the performance of behavior as in a speech act). The linguistic aspect and rules would be acquired by the child in much the same way as described by linguistic theory, and the disorders and corresponding assessment and intervention procedure with its concept of facilitation for those types of problems would be derived accordingly. The performance aspect of language would be described similarly to that of cognitive organization and information process theories. This approach would describe the performance of language to be learned rather than "unfolded." Such a position would also allow for the description of performance problems in language-disordered children and would permit intervention to include more direct teaching of performance skills in cases where these are needed. Language intervention techniques would not be limited to facilitation activities. A child may have either a knowledge-of-rules–based problem or a performance problem, or both.

Distinguishing between the knowledge and performance aspects of language may also clarify the relationship between reading, writing, speaking, and listening. It helps to explain how deficiency in one does not necessarily mean deficiency in any of the others. If language were the knowledge of rules only, then a failure to induce the rules correctly would simultaneously affect all of the skills that are based on the knowledge of the rules. In fact, when all the above skills are uniformly impaired, there is validity to the conclusion that the problem is one of language knowledge or knowledge of the rules. We know from experience that reading, writing, speaking, and listening can be differentially impaired. Therefore, a description of language as knowledge of rules is inadequate to describe these differences. The differences can, however, be explained in terms of performance differences among these domains. Differences in the factors involved in the perceptual transmission, access to storage and retrieval, and so on may explain the differences among the domains.

The study of the performance component in language will lead to further clarification of the levels of performance, the voluntary and automatic levels that were first described in neuropsychological theory and further explained in information process theory. It will give a theoretical perspective to behaviors of autistic children who can mimic and even use correct grammar in nonmeaningful utterances or to the semantically empty but grammatically accurate utterances of the aphasic.

COGNITIVE AND LINGUISTIC DOMAINS

A second issue, discussed in Chapter 7, is the relationship between cognition and language. We know that cognitive problems can affect the development of the linguistic aspects of language, as in mental retardation, and vice versa; linguistic disorders caused by hearing impairments can influence to some extent the conceptual development of the child. Both conceptual and linguistic components are integral to language. As I have previously suggested, even to state the problem questioning the relationship is to imply that cognition and language are separate entities. However, language has both linguistic and cognitive components, so if we say cognition and language interact, we are saying that cognition and cognition interact. If we specify the grammar of language—the syntax, morphology, and phonology—as the linguistic component, then we can more accurately state the question: How do the conceptual and linguistic components of language interact? The term *nonlinguistic* will mean nonform; it will not mean nonlanguage. This position allows the components of language, the conceptual and the linguistic (the grammar), to *develop* integratively but independently. Instead of asking which comes first, language or cognition, we should ask: How do the conceptual and linguistic aspects of language interact in its development? How does the development of the form for a concept help refine and crystalize the concept, and how does the emergence of a concept prepare the way for understanding the form?

The view of the conceptual and the linguistic aspects of language as parallel and equally important parts of language leads to study of language through each of the components, not only study of one through the other. When we refer to "the content of the form" we infer that the form has a content that is invariable and definable. To some extent, this is true; there are specific, acceptable dictionary definitions for specific forms of the language and, for the most part, when the speakers of the language use these forms, the listeners understand. There are, however, meanings of the forms that are not in the dictionary, nor do the forms mean the same things in unique and figurative contexts. The variations in meaning from individual to individual depend on their particular experiences with specific concepts. The word "truth" will vary in meaning from person to person depending on the persons' experiences with truthfulness. Individuals bring their own meaning to the form. We cannot, therefore, label only a portion of our world knowledge as the meanings of language and therefore the semantic portion. Any and all parts of our world knowledge and concepts have the potential of serving as the meaning of the linguistic (form) part of language at any time. The semantics of the language are the accepted meanings of the forms of the language as well as the idiosyncratic meanings of any individual when using the linguistic form. From this it follows that to examine the content of language by studying its form is not a valid way of evaluating the conceptual base of language. To do so would give a biased picture of the quality of the conceptual development of an individual.

Another benefit of viewing cognitive and linguistic components as equal partners in language is the manner in which this relationship lends itself to understanding the role each plays in tasks such as inference, reasoning, and problem-solving. These tasks are not purely linguistic activities, but they can be purely cognitive activities. Such cognitive skills can and often should be developed outside the framework of linguistic elements. When the linguistic component is used to improve and strengthen basically cognitive tasks, the ability to use language improves as does the ability to use the cognitive functions themselves.

If attention to linguistic relations becomes the exclusive function of intervention, the child's improvement may be limited to a narrow linguistic skill and there will be no general improvement in the overall conceptual framework for using the skill. An example of this may be instruction in analogies. On the one hand, specific instruction in verbal analogies might reap the benefit of improving performance on analogy tests. However, attention to such a specific activity probably has little influence on the child's understanding the relationship within and between concepts and the words that symbolize them. Precision in understanding the meanings of words and in discriminating among them comes both from general enrichment at the conceptual level and from increased specificity of the meaning of words. The ability to "do" analogies will improve as the child both widens his or her understanding of the world and of the meanings of words and also narrows those meanings so that they are clearly distinct from other similar words. In other words, there needs to be an ever-increasing specificity of correspondence between meaning and form.

COMPREHENSION AND PRODUCTION

Another issue that separates theories is that of the relation between comprehension and production. I have argued in earlier chapters (9 and 12) that comprehension and production are common at the basic level of rule knowledge but different at some point in the performance process. Both language disorders data (Carrow-Woolfolk, 1985) and neuropsychological theory support this position. As I have stated previously (Carrow-Woolfolk & Lynch, 1982), a theoretical description of the relationship between comprehension and production needs to clearly define what is meant by comprehension.

By distinguishing language knowledge and language performance, it is possible to identify two aspects of comprehension. At the knowledge level is the association between a form and the meaning it has for the listener. This association is not the S-R type as described in behavioral theory. It describes a much more complex response on the part of the child. When a child comprehends, he or she has been able to "understand" the form (word, sentence, etc.). The child brings his or her conceptual information and world knowledge to the meaning. If a linguistic stimulus is received by a child and it fails to elicit appropriate meaning because the relationship between the form and meaning either has not been developed or has been learned incorrectly, the child does not comprehend. If we say that comprehension does not precede expression, we say that the ability to respond to a form meaningfully does not precede the use of the form in speech. In other words, children use words that they may not understand. This interpretation may be accurate in some instances. Even adults use words they do not fully understand. I would dare say, however, that most of the words children use in development are words for which they have at least some rudimentary meaning. Using words they do not understand in contexts that they do understand may assist in developing their meaning.

A second interpretation of comprehension relates to the "on-line" performance domain. Failure to understand in the presence of adequate rule knowledge may be due to a breakdown in the processing system that may deliver inaccurate messages. Individuals who have auditory discrimination disorders because of a central auditory disorder experience difficulty in accurate message reception.

A theory of language needs to account for the two types of comprehension and to define clearly the similarities and differences between comprehension and production in order to use effective intervention procedures. Acceptance of the position that comprehending involves understanding at the rule-knowledge level as well as understanding at the performance-process transmission level helps us understand how it is possible to have a comprehension disorder without a production one (performance problem) and how if we have a comprehension disorder of knowledge (between the form and meaning), such a disorder will automatically affect production. This latter problem is the kind that we find in echolalia and is one that improves with direct work on comprehension; in this type of disorder, direct intervention in production is the most reasonable.

SEMANTICS AND SYNTAX

The psychoneurological literature has provided us with examples of aphasics whose difficulty relates to open/closed class differentiation in words and morphemes. The open classes are those that continually admit new members, such as nouns, adjectives, and adverbs. The closed classes are those whose membership is finite, for example, pronouns, plurals, and interrogatives. We refer to the open classes as having lexical meaning and the closed classes as having grammatical meaning. It appears, then, that some aphasics have difficulty with semantics (open classes), and others have difficulty with syntax or grammar (closed classes), and the difficulty relates to the type of lesion.

Chomsky (1980), in his description of modular organization theory, suggests that semantics, the system of "object reference," may be, from a modular standpoint, separate from grammar. The findings from aphasia corroborate this position. This view is compatible with one that considers the linguistic system (grammatical system) to be unique and different from other cognitive systems and acquired through rule induction by the child's own selective self-driven procedures of internalization. Placing semantics in the conceptual module frees the specialist from the concept of "facilitating" the acquisition of semantics and places the improvement of semantic skills with those of cognitive skills under the umbrella of more direct participation of the specialist in the intervention process.

PRAGMATICS AND LINGUISTICS

If we apply the term *linguistics* to the rule-based knowledge of the grammar of the language, the term *cognition* to the conceptual and parallel partner of linguistics, and *semantics* to the relation between the two, how do we classify *pragmatics*? The major notions in pragmatics involve a purpose for action and a context (person or situation) in which the action occurs and which influences the action. Pragmatics can be used to describe both language and nonlanguage behavior. Therefore, it is not exclusively tied to language. It is a specific aspect of cognition and probably those aspects of pragmatics that deal with interaction should be thought of as separate from cognition regardless of whether they actually are. It may be useful to propose a pragmatic module that comprises behaviors of a social or interactional nature.

The tie between the conceptual module and the linguistic module is called *semantics*. Perhaps we need a special term to refer to the tie between the pragmatic module and the linguistic module, the rules that govern the use of grammar for pragmatic ends, the act of speaking. Perhaps *pragmatic-semantics* or *linguistic-pragmatics* would be appropriate. Distinguishing between general pragmatic behavior and linguistic pragmatic behavior has practical value. The recognition that pragmatic behavior exists outside of language encourages specialists to work with pragmatic skills before language emerges or when it is severely impaired. It is possible to have pragmatic behavior in the absence of language. It is not conceivable to have true language behavior in the absence of pragmatic behavior.

Such a distinction would also clarify the use of pragmatic theory in intervention. If we separate pragmatic *content* from pragmatic *procedures*, we can develop a realistic rationale for including pragmatics at all stages of intervention. Pragmatic content may be considered to be analogous to syntactic content or cognitive content in an additive fashion. Pragmatic procedures, on the other hand, can be integral to every intervention approach and to every intervention session because the notions of intentions, function, messages, and interaction are basic to communication competence.

As stated in Chapter 12, the classification of the components of language helps to understand the nature of the disorder of language. Intervention-wise I believe it is important to know if a disorder is one of pragmatics in general, a problem in social awareness and interaction, or if the disorder is one of difficulty in attaching the appropriate linguistic form to the pragmatic action. If an inappropriate linguistic surface structure is used in the face of adequate pragmatic behavior, is it because of the failure to relate semantically the form to the social meaning or because of a lack in the knowledge of grammatical rules, or because of a difficulty in the process of retrieving with accuracy and facility the particular sequence of morphemes that constitute the appropriate and acceptable routine?

EXTERNAL AND INTERNAL DESCRIPTIONS OF LANGUAGE

One of the basic dichotomies among theories is the distinction between an internal and external focus. The external aspects of language deal with such factors as the input, the stimulus, language production, the environment, and the context. The internal aspects of language deal with such factors as the knowledge induction, the process, decoding, encoding, retrieval, and inference. As was illustrated in Chapter 2, the major theories focus on either one or the other. The extreme position of theories that describe the external factors of language is that of behaviorism, whereas the extreme position regarding internal factors is called *mentalism*. The information processing and cognitive organization theories are primarily mentalistic.

If in our work with language disorders we choose one position to the exclusion of the others, we will neglect significant aspects of language. It is important to remember that the language-disordered child's language-learning system may not function like that of a child without such a problem. We must be concerned with the differences in the child's system in order to adapt to that difference. Furthermore, the environment may not react to the language-disordered child in the same way it does to other children. We must be concerned with these environmental differences. In work with the language-disordered, we need a theory that integrates the internal and external aspects of language. Perhaps our problem has been that we want a partial theory to explain the totality of language and it cannot do so. But each of the theories we have discussed appears to describe a different part of language. If this is true, we might begin theory integration by showing how they fit together.

The essence of behavior theory is to consider only those issues as significant that are within the reach of empirical investigation in order to explain external phenomena on a behavioral level rather than on a mental level. This means that there is and can be no explanation for language at all, simply a description of events. Therefore, language and language learning cannot and should not be, in my opinion, explained by a behavioral model.

Aspects of behaviorism may be useful, however, in the modification of language in work with some of the language-disordered. Strict adherence to behavioristic methodology is most effective when teaching individuals who have impaired cognitive behavior such as the mentally retarded or the autistic. The response to conditioning is greatest when there is little rational resistance to the process. However, the best results are obtained if the procedure is functionally directed. The greater the personal motivation of an individual to learn, the less the specialist needs to rely on the formal principles espoused by behaviorism.

I also believe that the concept of reinforcement is a valid one, one that is inherent in all social learning. Response of any kind by its very nature has an influence on the individual who is the object of the response. All intervention needs to include even in a subtle way the concept of reinforcement, the natural response to good communication being the best. If we use some of the principles of behaviorism to bring about change in some children with disorders, the concepts described in this theory will be useful.

This then is our task: to integrate theories by describing how each addresses a different aspect of language and to identify those aspects in which theories differ and attempt to reconcile them. If we keep as a frame of reference, disorders of language, we will not be satisfied with theories that cannot accommodate the known facts about such problems.

INTEGRATING THEORY AT THE PRACTICAL LEVEL: PRINCIPLES OF ASSESSMENT AND INTERVENTION

INTEGRATING LANGUAGE DISORDER
   DEFINITIONS

FROM THEORY TO ASSESSMENT
   Issues That Separate Assessment Approaches
     Language Components
     Knowledge and Performance
     Comprehension and Expression
   Factors Influencing Assessment Approaches
   Integrative Assessment

THEORIES AND INTERVENTION PROCEDURES
   Age and Intervention
   Development and Remedial Approaches
   Intervention and Types of Disorders
   The Intervention Setting
   The Referral Problem
   Compensatory Teaching

THE LANGUAGE SPECIALIST

Thus far, this book has presented various positions about language on which specialists in language disorders base much of their practices in assessment and intervention. I have pointed out that although some specialists who espouse specific theories consider them to be autonomous and inclusive, these theories are in fact partial theories that explain some aspects of the language system but not all of it. If there

THEORY, ASSESSMENT AND INTERVENTION
IN LANGUAGE DISORDERS: © 1988 by Grune & Stratton
AN INTEGRATIVE APPROACH

ISBN   0-8089-1918-0

> *Quote 14–1*
> The data demonstrate that children with language disorders generally do not present disorders confined only to oral language or present only during childhood. Rather, even when retarded children are eliminated, the majority continue to present broadly based language-learning problems with educational and social consequences for years to come.
> (ARAM, EKELMAN, & NATION, 1984, p. 243).

were no attempt to stretch each theory to make it account for the totality of language, we would find it possible to live with a theoretical marriage among these positions in all but a few issues. What occurs, for example, is that a theory is constructed to explain grammar and is then extrapolated to explain language development. A theory is constructed around pragmatic behaviors and because pragmatics by its very nature encompasses interactional language, it may ignore internal processes; the proponents often act as if there are no internal processes that are part of the language behavior system. This is acceptable as long as the theory explanation remains at a theoretical level. When individuals begin to apply the constructs to practice and particularly when they move out of the realm of normal to the area of disordered language, the extrapolative process cannot be accepted. We cannot omit from the total framework of language any aspect of it simply because we cannot find a place to fit it into a model.

A few years ago, a colleague and I were discussing our current activities and I mentioned that I was designing a perceptual/memory test. In horror, she exclaimed, "Why, didn't you know that perception is passé?" I guess I had not yet been informed that we no longer need to discriminate or remember in using language or in learning to talk. At some later period it was explained to me that syntax was irrelevant in describing disorders of language. Somehow, I had failed to notice that we no longer use syntactic structure when we speak. I eagerly await the time when pragmatics, cohesion, and narratives have been buried in the dusty volumes on the shelf. For at that time, the only means of communication left will be mental telepathy.

There is also some confusion that arises when an individual who is associated with a specific theory, for example, linguistic or pragmatic, presents points of view about assessment or intervention. Aspects of their philosophy and procedures of assessment or intervention may not relate to their general theory. Unfortunately, by association, these unrelated philosophical and procedural statements are accepted as part of the theory even though the methods and procedures are found to be contrary to the espoused theory. This makes it appear that the theories are mutually exclusive on many practical points when, in fact, they are not.

In this section, I would like to describe some principles of assessment and intervention that influence the decisions that are made by the specialist and discuss how the various theories can be integrated within these philosophical boundaries. I would like to begin with a word about disordered language.

INTEGRATING LANGUAGE DISORDER DEFINITIONS

One of the major tasks of a language specialist is to determine whether a child has a language disorder. The task is made difficult for the specialist because there are few definitions in the literature of disordered language other than the statement that a child has a language disorder when his or her language is delayed or different. Because as a profession we have borrowed theories describing normal language and applied these to disordered language, we have shackled ourselves with constructs that do not accommodate well the data that we have about disorders. As was stated in the previous chapter, only a theory that encompasses the entire spectrum of language can be used to explicate its disorders.

Because we are lacking such a theory, the specialist is left with the problem of making a decision about children. Such specialists need to develop an operational definition of disordered language that will serve their needs in a professional setting. Such an operational definition must take into account both qualitative and quantitative differences with reference to external criteria such as language behaviors of normal children and social environment and internal criteria such as intelligence and other social and cognitive functions.

Ultimately, the decision to classify a child as language-disordered is just that, a decision. No test, no language sample, no history information can make that classification for the specialist. I am often asked to give the cut-off point (in standard deviations units, for example) of test performance that can be used to determine if a child is language-disordered. Some specialists have a difficult time understanding that a test cannot make the decision for them. A test or any other index tells us how a child has performed in a specific task, and some tell us how other representative children have performed at that age. *The specialist has to decide*, given other data regarding environment, intelligence, motivation, standards, and so on, whether a difference in performance between the child tested and the normal population is in fact a disorder.

Although the concept of language disorder needs to include the condition of the neurological system as a part of its breadth, the notion of neurological involvement cannot be a constant in the definition of the problem, since there are disorders without such evidence. The only solution, as I see it, is to think of language behaviors along a continuum and each behavior in each individual's performance charted at some point on the continuum from exceptional to very poor. When an individual's per-

> *Quote 14–2*
> *An attempt to formulate a diagnostic approach which applies theories and concepts from various fields to the solution of practical problems presents certain dangers. It is possible to oversimplify a theory which was not intended for application and to draw conclusions which are not warranted. However, if these risks are not taken, we are faced with the task of solving speech and language problems without a sequential approach and rationale, which may be even more dangerous.*
> (CARROW, 1972, p. 54).

formance on one or more behaviors reaches a point along the continuum that he or she is significantly different either quantitatively or qualitatively from normal or presents a pattern of differences that is abnormal and when normal is interpreted to mean normal for the child's age, stage, social environment, or intelligence, then the clinician *decides* to call the child language-disordered if that label will help in assessment and intervention decisions. It is important to the profession that some uniform definition of language disorders be used even if at an operational level. Research will have no meaning unless this is done. I believe the only way in which this can be accomplished is to redefine language itself, taking into account all facets of the knowledge and performance of language. If we describe the cognitive, linguistic, and pragmatic contributions to language, if we characterize the knowledge and performance components, if we delineate the similarities and differences between comprehension and expression and if we relate these to psychoneurological concerns about language, and if we recognize the educational and social implications of the disorders, we may begin to understand disordered language.

If we could arrive at an integrated description of the nature of language, we could possibly describe better the patterns of language disorder. A broad-based theory would allow us to describe seven major problem sources and an interrelationship between certain types of patterns: (1) sensory-based disorders, (2) cognitive-based disorders, (3) linguistic (rule)-based disorders, (4) performance-based disorders, (5) pragmatic-based disorders, (6) connection problems, and (7) environmentally based disorders. Viewed within the broad theoretical boundaries described in the last few chapters, we may be able to differentiate among these patterns. (For a detailed discussion of these disorders, see Carrow-Woolfolk & Lynch, 1982, pp. 212–225.)

A broad-based theory would also provide for the heterogeneity of disorders, recognizing that because cognitive, social, and linguistic aspects are interrelated in different ways in each individual, they are also interrelated in different ways in each language-impaired individual.

Therefore, it is important to recognize that the following classification is theoretical, generated on a logical basis from an integrated theory

> *Quote 14–3*
> *The diversity of explanations, however, suggest a diversity of contributing factors as well; some children's problems may be a consequence of one limitation whereas other limits operate in other cases; or different patterns may be involved across children. Such possibilities would focus on the heterogeneity of language-disordered children instead of the assumption of homogeneity, and would move theoretical formulations toward clinical reality.*
>
> (RICE, 1983, p. 355).

of the components of language. Children's problems are not so easily distinguished and for the most part have signs of combined characteristics. The reality of patterns of disorders has been presented in earlier sections of this book.

Sensory-based disorders such as those found in hearing impairment have certain characteristics that, if taken as a whole, may distinguish this type of problem from others. A sensory-based disorder impairs that aspect of language that is sensory-dependent with relation to the input. Since linguistic code development is auditory-dependent, an auditory impairment in infancy will delay the acquisition of language. If the sensory impairment is moderate, the resulting linguistic impairment will be in the form of generalized linguistic delay. Since the closed classes (grammatical morphemes, etc.) are finite, the child with a sensory loss will at some point in development and after frequent input master these forms. The open classes, however, will continue to be delayed, as the child will miss parts of the ongoing steam of language in the environment. Because the cognitive system is unimpaired (unless there are multiple problems), there is discrepancy between cognitive and linguistic development. If the cognitive system is measured without language, it should not display any delay. However, the refinement and expansion of concepts occur with the aid of the linguistic code, and therefore some children with sensory impairment may exhibit some cognitive delay. Because production is dependent on reception and storage of the auditory input, production will often reflect the level of auditory impairment. A problem in the input performance system will thus create a problem in the knowledge system of language.

In *cognitive-based disorders*, the problem lies in the inadequate development of concepts and concept-schema, in difficulties in learning the procedures of learning such as generalizing, problem-solving, induction, seeing relationships among concepts, and/or the ability to represent reality by means of symbols. What is observed is a generalized delay in all aspects of development and difficulty in organizing at any level. With respect to language, the delay is exhibited in both the form of language and in its meaning. The child with such a problem often has not developed the conceptual framework needed to bring meaning to language. The linguistic form may be taught or conditioned, but its use is often without complete understanding. There is particular difficulty with figurative language.

There are children who have not developed concepts or learned to symbolize, but who use phonological sequences in imitation. There is, however, little connection between the linguistic and the conceptual. The child perceives the speech adequately but does not understand it. His or her intonation and rhythm patterns are good, but his or her voluntary speech consists of phrases and words that appear to be "lifted" from the environment and used inappropriately. Our theory needs to account for the ability of some children and brain-injured adults to manipulate and exploit automatically the rules of language in speaking or in orthography without understanding what they speak or read.

Linguistic (rule)-based disorders can be characterized by difficulty with inducing the rules of grammar—the phonology, morphology, and syntax and semantic rules. Because of this difficulty, children with linguistic-based disorders exhibit comprehension and production problems related to grammar; in fact, where a rule-based problem exists, results on expressive and receptive tests are similar. One would expect the child's language to be discrepant, that is, show difficulty with specific types of structures and not others. There may be difficulty with earlier-learned structures in the face of adequacy with later-learned structures. Since the disorder is rule-based, the specific structural problem is consistent throughout all the language domains—comprehending, speaking, reading, and writing. It may affect either or both closed and open language systems, although the closed systems are the most usually impaired. There is ordinarily no discrimination or recognition on the part of the language-disordered child of the errors he or she makes.

Performance-based disorders appear to be related to perceptual, storage, access, and retrieval strategies and abilities. Because performance channels differ in reading, comprehending, speaking, and writing, the problem may be exhibited in one but not necessarily the other modalities: for example, comprehension but not expression. Where there are common performance strategies, there will be simultaneous problems in all modalities. In production the disorder is one of execution, which may occur conditionally depending on the linguistic context or speed of utterance. The difficulty may occur only in complex contexts or in rapid speech. It may be a problem of word retrieval or of difficulty in accurately producing certain morphemes. The individual ordinarily recognizes his or her errors, but finds fluid and automatic speech difficult. The comprehension problem may occur in transmitting the input through the child's system for decoding oral input. A problem in discrimination will produce garbled messages and therefore interfere with message understanding.

The primary characteristic of *pragmatic-based disorders* is one of difficulty with producing clear and/or appropriate exchanges and messages in order to accomplish the intended purpose. There may be lack of perception of the nature of the social situation or lack of knowledge of the verbal messages that accurately and adequately communicate what is desired. The language-disordered individual may not be perceptive of the social cues that indicate when a message has been received or the listener is no longer interested. The child may have difficulties in generalizing social situations or in recognizing and remembering appropriate behaviors.

Connection-based disorders have to do with the interaction among all aspects of language. A child must not only perceive and store concepts, social events, and linguistic rules but must recognize and remember the relations among them. In a way, semantic disorders are connection-based disorders since the problem is one of relating words and morphemes to meaning. Similarly, pragmatic disorders, when viewed within the framework of relating linguistics to interactive and social events and behaviors, can be seen as connection-based disorders. The relation between the event and its corresponding linguistic form is either not established or remembered.

The last type of language disorder may not be classified by some as a disorder because it is a function of the environment in which a child learns language. Lack of *environmental feedback* or excessive response to a child's needs without requiring language may reduce the child's motivation to communicate. Deprivation of language in the environment will cause language deprivation in the child.

As we attempt to understand a theoretical description of the kinds of language problems children and adults may have, we need to recognize that these do not occur in unitary form. The categories just provided describe different levels and types of functions and domains, a number of which can interact in producing a problem. We must continue to search for patterns of disability. To do so, we must not exclude any aspect of language from our concern. As we combine information regarding neuropsychological factors, cognitive functions, and linguistic and pragmatic behaviors, we may be able to tease out subtle deficits that may help us provide better assessment and intervention.

FROM THEORY TO ASSESSMENT

As I have repeatedly stated throughout this book, the theoretical framework within which specialists describe language influences the basic assessment and intervention approach that they use. There are four main areas in which theory has a definite influence on practice in language disorders. These are (1) the domains included as components

> *Quote 14–4*
> *With regard to the semantic/pragmatic language disorders . . .*
> *severity is based on the distinction between delay and disorder*
> *as well as on the amount of deviation from a child's normative*
> *expectation. But more importantly, the severity should also be*
> *determined by the degree of academic and social effects that*
> *can only be assessed by a thorough language evaluation.*
>
> (LUCAS, 1980, p. 75).

of language, (2) the knowledge/performance distinction, (3) the comprehension/expression relationship, and (4) the nature of language acquisition. These issues were summarized and integrated as they apply to language theory and language disorder theory in the previous chapter. I would like to review them again briefly with special note of their application to assessment and intervention.

Issues That Separate Assessment Approaches

Language Components

If the definition of language is limited to its *linguistic* component, the emphasis in assessment will be on analysis and description of the child's language product, the sentence, the text, the story, the conversation—the language behavior in terms of form, content, and use. This does not, in my opinion, give an accurate picture of the child's functioning. Looking at conceptual behaviors by analyzing linguistic form is the same as making a diagnosis of an illness by looking at a single symptom. Ironically, a theory that is far removed from a medical model describes assessment by analysis of behavior symptomatology; deficiencies of use, content, and form are diagnosed by studying the child's production. Correspondingly, emphasis on the linguistic component in production leads to intervention emphasis on the *linguistic* elements alone. For example, if a child has difficulty in understanding figurative language, the emphasis in intervention will be on teaching this relationship at the surface level of structure rather than at the cognitive level of exploring commonalities among ideas. If, on the other hand, *cognition* is considered an integral part of language, the level of cognitive behavior, the description of conceptual schemata, the skills of problem-solving, inference, and language creativity, and the relation between linguistic and cognitive behaviors will be included as an essential part of assessment. If cognition is considered an integral part of language (as in the cognitive theory) not only in the early stages of acquisition but throughout life, it must be an integral part of assessment and intervention.

Specialists might choose to address cognitive problems through language, a legitimate way of addressing the problem, but they need to recognize that problems in language inference, for example, may be related to general problems of inference and may be found within the broader framework of a child's cognitive behavior.

A definition of language that considers language *function* and *use* as central will provide assessment procedures that are concerned with children's needs, their motivation to speak, their interaction with the environment, their responsiveness to social cues and events, and their ability to match linguistic and social behaviors. A language description that integrates the cognitive, linguistic, and pragmatic systems but that also views them in terms of their uniqueness and distinctiveness will best serve the individual with disordered language. This description cannot be formulated from the analysis of a language sample only. Rice (1983) supported a need for independent measures of cognitive and linguistic knowledge in view of the fact that the relationship between linguistics and cognition is not one-to-one. Inferences about cognition therefore should not be based on the analysis of the linguistic form only.

Knowledge and Performance

The importance of considering both knowledge and performance as separate but interrelated aspects of language has been defended in Chapter 6 and other chapters of this book. Acceptance of this distinction in language as theoretically sound requires that both language knowledge and language performance be objects of study and change in assessment and intervention. I concur with Kirk's (1983) belief that production (behavior) is not the only measure that can provide information about a child's level of learning. We need to observe that manner in which children approach a task as well as analyzing the errors in the task. We need to understand the strategies the child uses in task execution.

Analysis of language knowledge will be directed to study of the level of rule acquisition in the linguistic code, study of the level of semantic knowledge, and study of the level of conceptual development. Intervention directed toward language knowledge will be in the facilitation of rule-development and concepts. Study of the performance aspects of language will include the processing system, visual and auditory, perceptual and memory, retrieval, access, and automaticity. Except for increased opportunities for practice, intervention will not be directed toward this aspect of processing; awareness of a child's deficiencies in these areas will help in planning general strategies for intervening and will assist the specialists in understanding and predicting the kinds of life problems the child will experience in adolescent and adult language situations.

Also in the area of performance, assessment and intervention should include study of the child's ability in learning to learn, problem-solving strategies, generalization ability, and so on. Unless a child can be helped in learning language and other information using language within the framework of his or her own performance system, unless we look beyond facilitating rules, we will not be providing the kind of assistance the child or adolescent needs. In general, theory and intervention that is solely knowledge-based focuses on rule discovery and facilitation. Theory and intervention that includes the domain of the performance aspect of language in addition to the knowledge aspect includes practice and skill-learning as an important ingredient of language. In the latter type of problem, intervention is more structured, direct, and focused in the acquisition of skilled automatic behavior.

Comprehension and Expression

In various parts of this book and in other publications, I have attempted to show the importance of distinguishing between comprehension and expression from both a theoretical and practical perspective (Carrow-Woolfolk & Lynch, 1982; Carrow-Woolfolk, 1985). This distinction is not essentially contradictory with any of the six theoretical positions described here. However, those theories that focus on the development and analysis of surface structure and that emphasize production in intervention do not emphasize the role of comprehension in their description of language. Behavioral theory is opposed to the idea of describing comprehension, whereas linguistic theory prefers to address comprehension indirectly by attending primarily to expression. Other positions recognize a distinction between comprehension and production strategies, although recognizing common knowledge between them. This latter view holds that there may be disorders of one in the face of normal performance in the other. Measurement of comprehension helps to determine the level of the child's semantic or grammatical knowledge. Production problems will demonstrate the same level of knowledge as comprehension but may in addition exhibit a problem of language performance. Comparison of the results of comprehension and expression analysis will help identify the nature of the disorder. As stated in the previous chapter, if they are similar, the child probably has a rule-based problem; if they differ, the most probable reason is that the child has a performance disorder.

Because it is difficult to measure comprehension directly and as a consequence there are limited data on the development of comprehension, some specialists believe that comprehension is best served by direct intervention on production, particularly if the input is paired with meaning. My own clinical experience has taught me that there are children who echo language and who appear to have little or no comprehension. Work on production would simply reinforce the echoic behavior they already have. The development of concepts and their association with surface structure has been a much more productive approach in these cases. What I am saying is that I believe that we need to try to understand both the comprehension and expressive states of the child. We may need to learn to measure comprehension more completely and more accurately than we have in the past. Perhaps we need to experiment with assessing comprehension by requiring retelling, synopsis, or discussion of what is heard in free or structured production or by using recall procedures in which we ask questions of different kinds—fact questions, inference questions, and others—about what the child has heard, in addition to continuing to explore recognition procedures of the type already utilized in comprehension testing.

Factors Influencing Assessment Approaches

If we break down the assessment process with language-disordered children, we find that there are at least six factors that help to determine the assessment approach and procedures in addition to that of theory. In practice, they often play a more important role than that of theory. They are the specialist's education and experience, the purpose of assessment, the setting in which the assessment takes place, the type and severity of the problem, the reason for referral, and the accepted level of professional responsibility of the specialist (see Fig. 14–1). Since the first factor, the specialist's education and experience, is a variable over which there is no control, we will not discuss it here. The others, however, merit discussion. The factors that influence assessment are interrelated and so I will need to discuss them in that manner.

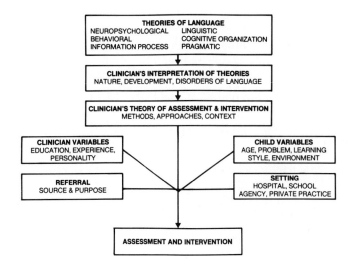

FIGURE 14–1. Variables other than theory that influence assessment and intervention choice.

Probably the most influential factor with respect to assessment is the setting in which the assessment takes place. Setting-dependent variables include the amount of time provided for assessment, the area of specialization associated with the setting (cerebral palsy center, neurology clinic at a medical school), the number and type of professional disciplines who participate, and the general focus of the agency, research or service.

If the language specialist works in a service-oriented clinic for children, for example, his or her purposes for assessment will need to be integrated with those of the clinic, and the particular areas the specialist assesses will depend on the other disciplines that are represented on the clinic team. More than likely, the problems of the children referred to such a clinic will be multiple and complex, so the philosophy of the clinic will probably be to determine the nature and cause of the problem. The language specialist's assessment purpose should be to do likewise.

A general approach to evaluating cognitive processes in addition to a complete analysis of language behaviors (neuropsychology and information process theories) will be the most useful for providing information on the child's learning strengths, related learning difficulties, compensatory needs, and prognosis for improvement. The particular areas of cognitive processing that are the responsibility of the language specialist may vary depending on the areas of assessment responsibility of individuals from other disciplines. The evaluation of the total spectrum of language behaviors (even behaviors of reading and writing if no other specialist assumes this responsibility) is always the responsibility of the language specialist. (For the past 30 years, I have included academic and perceptual/cognitive assessment as a part of language evaluations.) The important task is that all processes involved in the language system be assessed.

In such a center, adequate time is usually provided for a complete evaluation and for providing assistance to the family and school in all areas of concern. The language specialist's professional responsibility for the child's linguistic and academic future is only one part of the responsibility of the total clinical team, so the burden of anticipating future problems and of planning is not borne by the language specialist alone.

In the service center the language specialist selects for evaluation only those areas that appear to be significant on the basis of the case history and the evaluation results from other specialists. A key to understanding the child's problem is the integration of the findings from the various disciplines. Such integration takes considerable study of the assessment results, but it yields insights about the pattern of language disorder in the child, the factors that exacerbate or minimize it, and the best avenues of learning for the child. A comprehensive evaluation that includes perceptual as well as linguistic information, academic as well as

> *Quote 14–5*
> *Thus, what is suggested is that the initial categorization need involve only the term* **language disordered**. *Any co-existing problems such as mental retardation should be identified as secondary categories. For the purpose of establishing training goals, a thorough determination of the child's language and related skills must be made. In addition, evaluation of the child's neurologic functioning should be routinely conducted to determine both his readiness for learning and appropriate procedures to be used in therapy, particularly the possible need for training through alternative modalities of communication.*
>
> (WARYAS & CROWE, 1982, p. 775).

intellectual and neurological, will provide the best basis for planning for the child's future. Specialists with years of clinical experience know, as Rapin and Allen (1983) have stated, that the symptoms of children with language and learning problems change with time. When one problem appears to be eliminated, another seems to arise. What happens is that children face new linguistic and learning tasks as they proceed through school and as adolescents they appear to have a whole new set of deficits. Adequate assessment can assist specialists in predicting these problems and make them aware of the necessity of following children throughout their school history even though they are not enrolled in intervention.

A similar procedure of assessment occurs in a specialty center devoted to *research*. One major difference is that the general approach to assessment in a research center compared with a service center is one of planned measurement of specific cognitive and linguistic areas. The same tests may be given to each child. Research agencies do not need to have a practical purpose for studies of a child's problem. Therefore, the evaluation task is much more detailed and complex. Its main purpose is to identify relations among skills as they relate to each other and to central functioning.

Often the language specialist works in a setting in which language services form a separate and semiautonomous unit. This may occur in a school, hospital, or similar institution. The type of assessment provided will depend, to a great extent, on the reason for referral. In a hospital, for example, the request from a physician may be for an evaluation of language. The physician's concern usually is whether there is indeed a problem in language and, if so, how severe and what can be done about it. The language specialist should provide just that information along with recommendations. There may be no need at this point to do a complete language analysis together with language samples and detailed pragmatic studies unless there is someone who needs this information in order to carry out intervention. Frequently, language specialists get so involved in doing what they do best they forget to keep the reason for referral in mind and to focus on the particular referral questions. This is

---

Quote 14–6

Although theoretical orientations may vary, it is important for diagnosticians to have a plan that will yield data for planning intervention. Without a set of questions or hypotheses, the assessment battery may be little more than a series of tests. Therefore the clinician should ask questions such as: What do I want to know? Why? What are the best ways to obtain the information? How will I use the information after it is collected?

(JOHNSON, 1981, p. 16).

---

unfortunate since the reason for referral is related to the actual problems the child experiences in everyday life. The specialist's task is to find the relationship between the child's functioning in everyday situations and the disorders found when assessing the child. Finding areas of deviancy is easy, finding how these areas of deviancy relate to the child's functioning is not so easy. If we tested every child in a classroom we would probably find all sorts of syntax and pragmatic differences. If these differences do not make a difference, we should not use them as context for intervention.

The age of the child to be assessed interacts with the setting, type, and severity of the problem, the assessment purpose, and the reason for referral. The study of a very young child may need to be in the form of a broad-based evaluation of a number of language and language-related components. The predictive and planning value of such an approach cannot be overestimated. With older students, the evaluation of the many factors that contribute to a problem and their interrelationship may be difficult, if not impossible. We may need to settle for assessing those areas that seem to be causing the student difficulty in real-life situations, particularly in language/academic and communicative/social areas.

If assessment is to be followed by intervention of any kind at any location, the language specialist's own agency or school or at another agency or school, the focus of assessment should be on the language behaviors. An analysis of the dimensions of the linguistic system with specific suggestions for intervention should be the basis of assessment. If intervention is to follow assessment and is the main purpose of referral, analysis of linguistic and pragmatic behaviors may be the only behaviors assessed. This occurs particularly in schools where there may

---

Quote 14–7

Total agreement [between clinical judgment and objective tests] is not necessary for a valid language assessment. The critical factor is for clinicians to consider carefully both their subjective evaluation and the more objective test data. This final decision concerning the language status of a child should be made upon the careful review of the information from both sources.

(ALLEN, BLISS, & TIMMONS, 1981, p. 68).

> *Quote 14–8*
> *Language is complex. It entails complex underlying cognitive-linguistic-communicative systems and processes. The extent to which the clinical fields vest assessment in various short profiles is the extent to which misrepresentation and distortion contribute to the enterprise . . . . One rather vacuous argument is that the clinical fields must deal with large numbers of clients and therefore they need simple, quick, and easy tests.*
> (MUMA, 1983, p. 197).

be a limitation in assessment time. The task is to discover the existence of a language disorder, the language needs of a child, and the identification of strategies for addressing these language needs, not the nature and cause of the problem. Other disciplines will probably already have assessed the child's problem. Language assessment becomes a way of planning for intervention. In these cases, assessment should be limited to language analysis.

In current language-disorder literature, we find the observation that a valid and complete language assessment, which includes structural analysis, pragmatics, morphology, semantics, and other factors, would be difficult to complete within a 2-hour period. According to Lund and Duchan, "Our hope that we can measure a child's language ability in one context in a two-hour diagnostic session will be demolished as results from the research in pragmatics become known to us" (1983, p. 6). Criticism is leveled at assessment procedures that do not provide detailed analysis of language samples that are not carried out with naturalistic methods and in naturalistic settings (Muma, 1986). It appears obvious that anyone familiar with the work places for helping language-disordered children (other than the university clinic) should recognize the impossibility of such a task. There simply is not time for such a procedure in most settings for the number of children involved. The proponents of lengthy naturalistic assessment might suggest that we not assess at all if we cannot complete a detailed analysis in a number of contexts, and they may be right, although I doubt that all the details obtained in such an analysis are used in bringing about change in a child's language. Ultimately, the final judgment in selection of approaches should be based on efficacy in intervention. I believe that the question should not be "How much information about language can we obtain in the assessment process?" but "How much information is needed to improve the child's language?" Many of us who functioned prior to the detailed naturalistic approaches to assessment were successful clinicians, effective in changing language.

I am not saying that the detailed naturalistic assessment approach has no value. Where it can be carried out in its entirety, it can serve to provide significant information about the language of children with disorders. I only caution that we not imply that assessment is worthless unless we use this approach. If we do, we will find clinicians frustrated at not having the time to accomplish it and ending up with piecemeal data that may have less validity and reliability than what they used previously. Idealism is praiseworthy but not always effective in real-life settings, such as a school or private practice setting. If the clinician uses probes, it appears to be better to use probes that have been carefully designed for obtaining data (even if they happen to be standardized) than to try to develop their own probes that have not been studied for their effectiveness or for their representativeness. We need to continue to study ways to provide methods for naturalistic or equivalent assessment that are also reliable, valid, and economic in time. Whatever normative data we develop must have descriptions of variability to be truly useful.

If the language specialist is the only specialist to see a child, as in the case of a parent's self-referral, the specialist cannot abdicate the responsibility of identifying broad-based problems that may need referrals to other specialists and of indicating to the parents future problems that they may need to be concerned about, particularly with young children. In some cases, academic testing may be needed to determine the effect of the language disorder on school functioning and perceptual testing to predict future academic problems in addition to those of language. Compensatory behaviors cannot be taught unless the language specialist understands the role of the child's cognitive system in his or her learning—whether of oral or written language. Cognitive skills of problem-solving, perceptive/learning strategies (cognitive organization theory), response latency time, and others are important skills to understand in relation to language learning. The child needs to understand his or her own learning style so that he or she can use compensatory techniques throughout a lifetime of learning. Unless someone understands the total problem of the child, the child will never understand it himself.

There are assessment issues that are not explicitly related to general language theory. One of these is the use of tests versus naturalistic methods for obtaining data about the language-disordered child. This is a theoretical issue about the validity and reliability of judgments and decisions and not one about language *per se*. This is an issue on which I believe the jury is still out. My position is that both the naturalistic and testing methods provide information and both have limitations. We should learn to use both within the boundaries of their usefulness and within the settings where they can provide the most reliable data.

Integrative Assessment

Integrative assessment is not a uniform or set procedure. It must be *adaptive* to the situation, age, and type of problem of the individual

> *Quote 14–9*
> Guidelines for developing formal and informal assessment:
> 1. *Utilize normative data to provide inter-individual comparisons (skill levels of child compared with age peers).*
> 2. *Utilize a comprehensive normative test to provide an overview of the child's strengths and weaknesses.*
> 3. *Utilize normative assessment to provide direction for further testing.*
> 4. *Keep the assessment plan flexible, so that assessments can be added or deleted as necessary.*
> 5. *Utilize criterion referenced data to supplement normative data and to provide intra-individual comparison (specific skill levels of an individual child compared).*
> 6. *Develop new CRT's as needed for individual children.*
> 7. *Consider any biases the test may have when given under standardized conditions, and supplement the assessment with instruments designed to show maximum performance levels.*
> (LINDER, 1983, pp. 110–111).

being assessed, as just described. To be adaptive, it must be *functional*; it must take place for reasons that will assist the child in life experiences. Good assessment is also *dimensional* and *balanced*. An evaluation of all aspects or dimensions of language (such as those described in this book) should at least be considered and then rejected for valid reasons, for example, those of assessment purpose or setting. The balance of assessment is achieved by evaluating at each step of assessment, the relation between what we chose to measure or describe, the overall goal or purpose of assessing, and the child's problem. Assessment that is restricted to one area of language or to one procedure for obtaining data is not balanced assessment. Assessment should be *selective*; the means for obtaining data should be purposefully selected from a wide variety of possible procedures. Uncritical use of many procedures or the use of a single procedure makes assessment meaningless and invalid. Assessment should be *predictive*; the breadth of evaluation should permit the projection of findings into the classroom and to later school years so that assistance can be provided to the classroom teacher, the parents, and the child regarding the child's learning and language style. The theory that is selected by the specialist as a basis for assessment should allow for integrative assessment.

If time does not permit adequate integrative assessment, then perhaps there should be no asessment at all. An estimate of the child's performance can be obtained by some criterion-referenced procedures in the skills necessary for adequate academic and social functioning. Specific evaluation in the area of concern to the teacher or parent is another alternative. Informal analysis can provide sufficient information for beginning intervention. These procedures, however, do not comprise a true assessment. The output of an integrative assessment on which serious decisions are made about children should have demonstrable validity and objectivity, as well as an estimate of the probability that the findings are indicative of a real difference from the normal population. This can be accomplished in any manner the specialist chooses, formal or informal, structured or unstructured, but it cannot ignore the importance of the normal distributional characteristics of the population in the categories under study, nor can it be limited to procedures with which the specialist feels comfortable.

THEORIES AND INTERVENTION PROCEDURES

As with assessment practices, intervention procedures are also influenced by factors other than that of theory. The age of the child, the type of problem, the setting, the purpose of intervention, and even the personality of the specialist influence some of the choices made about intervention. These factors are so important that reference to them should be made whenever intervention procedures are discussed.

Age and Intervention

Age influences the content, goals, and methods of intervention as it interacts with theory. In choosing the content of intervention, the specialist who is working with very young children will consider the social function or pragmatics of language as the highest priority and the cognitive and linguistic aspects as secondary goals. This focus means it is much more important for a child to want to communicate and to make attempts to do so than to use perfectly correct utterances. With older children, however, this procedure may be reversed. The correction of "fossilized" or residual syntax or articulation errors may be a greater need for the child than working on what the specialist considers to be a difficulty with taking turns, particularly if the syntactic errors also occur in written language.

Developmental and Remedial Approaches

The developmental and *nurturant-naturalistic* approaches associated with the linguistic and pragmatic theories are more properly used in working with very young children than with older children. Very young children usually have a broad range of structures and behaviors over which they do not have mastery. They need input to all areas simultaneously. The intervention environment that follows language development sequences and "facilitates" the learning of these sequences in a naturalistic setting (linguistic theory) is appropriate for the child whose organism is still internalizing language in learning stages and is still learning rules. The use of developmental sequences for intervention does not need to be limited to a naturalistic or semistructured approach; developmental content can and has been combined effectively with a structured behavioral approach (Stremel & Waryas, 1974) for some children.

The importance of using a development approach with very young children who have barely crossed the threshold into oral communication is borne out by a study by Bishop and Edmundson (1987). They conducted a prospective, longitudinal study of 87 language-disordered children who were assessed at the ages of 4, 4½, and 5½ years and found that the language delay of 44 percent of the children with nonverbal ability had been resolved. This finding may be interpreted to mean that a developmental approach with children 4 years of age and younger whose language appears to be disordered will probably be all that is needed to "boost" many of them into the normal category. However, if the rate of development over a period of a year is not normal (the child does not make progress equivalent to a year or more within a year's time) and the child's language is slow to begin with, a more structured approach may be warranted.

For the child who has essentially mastered language but who exhibits residual or fossilized errors in either language rules or language performance, a more didactic approach (direct language instruction) than is used in naturalistic intervention may be effective; simply making available the correct input for the child to internalize may not be sufficient. The older student has probably been exposed to the correct behaviors and structures an infinite number of times without effect. This latter student might need *teaching* rather than *facilitation* and may need *practice* to improve performance rather than *rule discovery* to develop knowledge. Even some type of traditional ear-training may help the child become aware of his or her own errors in grammar, for example, and may make the process of generalization easier. With the adolescent, his or her own *organism* may be the most important aspect of learning; with the younger child, the *environment* and the organism are the most *influential*. Whether facilitating or teaching, intervention techniques should always be functional and should focus on messages rather than on static nonmeaningful strings of words and drills.

The developmental approach may also be effective with children who can induce language rules but who do so slowly, needing large numbers of exemplars before they master the rules. Increasing the saliency and frequency of exemplars for these children may be all that a specialist need do. Other children, however, have great difficulty inducing the rules because their induction mechanism functions ineffectively. Still others do not have a rule-based problem but a performance problem. With these two latter types of children, a more direct approach,

> *Quote 14–10*
> The argument as to whether the home or the clinic is the best teaching environment for the language-impaired child is not readily resolved, and it may be that a more sophisticated understanding will find a different solution depending on the characteristics of the child, the nature of the problem, and the resources that are available in the environment.
>
> (SPRADLIN & SIEGEL, 1982, p. 5).

which brings language to a metalinguistic level for the child, may be the most effective. Factors that may lead to choosing content other than on a developmental basis are the particular need a child may have for learning a particular structure, the frequency of occurrence of the structure in language, the comparative ease or difficulty with which a particular structure can be taught, and the level of approximation to mastery that a child has reached with respect to the structure.

Intervention and Types of Disorders

The type of problem also influences the choice of intervention procedures used. A severely hearing-impaired child needs the broad-based language facilitation procedures used with the young hearing language-disordered child. The emphasis should be on naturalistic procedures that are based on language developmental data. The primary goals are functional language and rule discovery. The severely autistic child, on the other hand, might not profit from a naturalistic setting, insofar as detachment from environmental stimuli is a characteristic of such children. Broad-based language stimulation will fall upon "deaf" ears. Instead, a systematic, structured approach may be the most effective. Functional language is the goal, but it may need to be taught via operant techniques. The choice of content for these children should be based on functional needs rather than on developmental sequences. As with age, the intervention approaches used with different types of problems are essentially (and theoretically) different.

The Intervention Setting

Intervention is also affected by the setting in which it takes place. In some settings, for example, a hospital, it may be difficult to arrange for a group of children to come at one time or space may not be available for group work. This may also be true in a school setting. A naturalistic environment may be the ideal for language stimulation, but it may be impossible to meet that requirement. Specialists should not force the setting to meet a theoretical demand. It is possible to simulate, however imperfectly, the requirements of social interchange, even if only two persons are involved. If the essential aspects of good exchange and the child's intent and sense of the event (Duchan, 1986b) are kept in mind, the specialist can construct an adequate setting for effective communication.

In working with adolescents, particularly those with pragmatic disorders, in a school setting, there may be a need to work with groups on general skills of communication. Good communication skills include those of turn-taking, repairing communication breakdowns, alternating forms on the basis of the context or person to whom one is speaking, and so on. These skills can be taught effectively at a metalinguistic level, and it is at the middle and high school years when these skills are most needed. Convincing an administrator of the need for a course that teaches students about their own learning and communicating styles and how to improve them may be difficult, but if it can be done, it will be a true victory and the best thing that can happen to get the students involved.

The Referral Problem

One of the most important aspects of intervention is its purpose. I am not referring here to the purpose of the specialist, but to the purpose or goal of the persons referring the child. A child is referred for a reason; perhaps he or she is not using the past form of verbs consistently. The specialist assesses the child's language and finds what he or she considers to be a problem in topic maintenance. The choice for intervention should be based to a large extent on what is a problem for the child and the persons in his or her environment and the communication skills needed for the child to succeed in his or her worlds. We can find many behaviors among "normal language" individuals that we could classify as problem language, but it is unrealistic at best to consider them candidates for intervention. Language differences are problems when they are life problems, when they interfere with an individual's functioning at home, in the classroom, at work, or in social situations.

I cannot stress enough the need to focus on "real-life" problems. An example comes to mind of a child I assessed on the request of his physician father who wanted a second opinion. This child was 12 years old and had been in intervention for 8 years. Although I found minor problems in the ability to understand analogies and in motor functioning, I was curious about the effects of these problems on his everyday world. I asked him, "How do you get along in school?" "Fine," was the answer. What kinds of grades do you make? "A's and B's," he responded. I went on in this vein asking about friends, extracurricular activities, and every aspect of life that I could. I did learn that he used a typewriter because his penmanship was poor. I then asked the father why he was still receiving help and he told me that the clinician said he still had some problems. And I would say now that he probably always will have some problems. In fact, everyone we know would probably have a problem or two if we assessed them. I have friends that have significant pragmatic problems. Just because individuals have problems does not mean we have to do something about the problems. We cannot make everyone function at maximum capacity. As my daughter says, "Nobody's perfect." If something is not a problem for them or for the parents, teachers, or others in their environment, and it will not truly interfere with their real world, we must think twice before intervening and creating a greater problem in the family because of it. A final illustration of inappropriate intervention of this type is that of a child who had severe behavior problems—his mother was at the point of breakdown—and he was being taught turn-taking skills in intervention!

A last point in this regard relates to the need to clarify the classification of different types of pragmatic behaviors. When we say that pragmatic factors should take precedence over others in intervention, we mean that the functional aspects of communication are more important than other aspects and therefore should always be the top priority in intervention. Other behaviors, also classified as pragmatic, such as turn-taking and using shared information, are not of the same level as functional language and need not receive the same priority ranking.

Compensatory Teaching

If the specialist accepts the basic positions of the neuropsychological theory regarding language and its relation to the brain and of the information process and cognitive organization theories regarding the involvement of cognitive, perceptual, and memory processes in language, the specialist will recognize that the basic language disorder cannot be "cured" and the individual with such a disorder will continue to have difficulty with some parameter or other of language throughout life. A very important role of the specialist within the framework of these theories is to teach compensatory techniques to the language-disordered child.

Once the language-disordered child is sufficiently mature to understand, he or she will need to recognize the facts of his or her own problem. The child, or adolescent as the case may be, needs to understand his or her learning style, how difficulties in the language components are related to academic problems, social relations, and life goals, the strategies he uses to remember, to understand, and to discover which strategies are the most effective ones for his or her learning (e.g., clustering, reauditorizing, rhyming, association, imagery, etc.). Rule-

> *Quote 14–11*
> *Metalinguistic awareness . . . is assumed to be a product of adolescent thinking rather than childhood thinking. The ability to step back and consider one's own thought (or language) as itself an object of thought and to use the subsequent conceptualization to direct and redirect one's cognitive theories is currently believed to be late developing.*
>
> (BROWN & PALENCSAR, 1982, p. 3).

learning at this level involves the metafunctions of learning the rules at a verbal level in order to learn them at an operational level. The child also needs to learn to inform his or her teachers about the way he or she learns best and when he or she needs rephrasing or extra help.

The specialist also must play a role in helping teachers help the language-disordered children in the classroom. For example, test formats can be altered so that instead of needing to retrieve a specific word or words, a student can indicate the answer by a "yes" or "no" or by a multiple choice response. Teachers can provide outlines covering the basic information to be covered in a class for students who have trouble processing and understanding a rapid flow of speech. Taking a test orally rather than in written form may help a student who has difficulty expressing ideas in writing.

The language problems at the adolescent level are numerous. The degree of interaction among listening, speaking, reading, and writing in academic and social situations is complex and so is the difficulty the young students have in language. Attempting to isolate and describe disordered language is virtually impossible. Intervention is best directed to the improvement of everyday communication and social and academic skills: how to listen better, what to do when you do not understand, how to carry on a conversation, make introductions, study better, improve vocabulary, and so on.

THE LANGUAGE SPECIALIST

Most studies of the teaching/learning paradigm have concluded that the single most important factor in learning is the teacher. The personality of the specialist often dictates which intervention approach will be most effective for the individual teacher. Some individuals find the organization and execution of group intervention difficult. They do not have the internal structure necessary to effectively carry out specific language goals for specific children in an informal naturalistic setting. What results is often called "chaos." Specialists need to function in the manner in which they perform best. This can be done to some extent by selecting a work environment that provides certain age groups or types of problems. The important objective to meet is one of change for the

> *Quote 14–12*
> *If our knowledge of language intervention is abstract, or theoretic, in nature, we can be productive and creative therapists. No longer stuck with formulas, no longer hopeful imitators, we can use our intervention "rules" to generate activities that are thoroughly responsive to the client and the moment.*
> (JOHNSTON, 1983, p. 56).

child so as to help him or her function better in his or her language world and to bring about this change in a way that is interesting to the child and satisfying to the specialist.

A specialist who is competent, well-prepared, and organized and who functions within an integrated theoretical position will be effective. The specialist needs to understand the relative effectiveness of specific theoretical approaches for use within age, setting, and problem constraints. The specialist needs to understand which aspects of theories can be combined in intervention, which are incompatible, and at what point or within what framework they are incompatible.

The language specialist also needs to remember that theories are theories. We do not yet have evidence to prove or disprove any one approach to language and language disorder. We can, however, choose for ourselves those theories that seem to account for all the data we have about language and our observations in language-disordered individuals. Uncritical acceptance of a single theory is one way of putting blinders on our insight, particularly if the theory is a narrow one that does not integrate well with other theories or with our experience. Undiscriminating acceptance and use of all the theories is not the answer either. What results is a hodgepodge of unrelated ideas and a consequent hodgepodge of assessment and intervention techniques. We must be able to select from positions that are compatible the specific ones that best suit our particular setting and situation and best fit the overall theoretical framework we have chosen. Since many of the issues among the theories are compatible, we have considerable leeway for choice. Our choices should be reasoned rather than random. Once we have a basic framework we can accept, we can easily integrate new ideas and positions into it. The integrated position in language and disorders is like a main road. There are many detours—new ideas—that eventually lead back to the main road. The rider may benefit from having gone on the detours, but too many get stuck in the detours and never find their way back.

The good practitioner has discovered the rules governing good clinical intervention, has recognized the variability among language-disordered children, and has developed strategies and adapted techniques to meet the needs of children. Many books on intervention provide a rich source of examples and suggestions from which to choose. The

276 SECTION III CONCLUDING THOUGHT ABOUT THEORY AND PRACTICE

lack is not so much in specific intervention techniques but in the principles governing their choice for particular children. The problem has been with the theorists who have not provided the practitioner with a sufficiently comprehensive set of principles and theory of disordered language, the patterns of disorder, the components of disorder, the basis for decision-making, and the best means of change. This then is the task. We cannot afford to just look at the pieces of language—we must look at the whole because the child who uses language is a whole and what has gone into his or her ability is complex.

15

THEORY-DERIVED INTEGRATIVE INTERVENTION PROCEDURES

THEORY, ASSESSMENT AND INTERVENTION
IN LANGUAGE DISORDERS: © 1988 by Grune & Stratton
AN INTEGRATIVE APPROACH

ISBN   0-8089-1918-0

In the last three chapters, I have attempted to integrate the six language theories that have been the focus of this book with respect to selected theoretical issues. I have also presented principles of assessment and intervention that are compatible with an integrative theory approach. In this chapter, the translation of theory to practice will be most specific. How can intervention *procedures*, *strategies*, and *techniques* be developed to satisfy the requirements of an integrative theory, one that takes into account the needs and diversity of children with impaired language? At this level of discussion, the practical level, it is imperative that empirical data be included wherever possible to support specific propositions. Just as language theory cannot ignore data regarding language disorders in order to provide a valid underpinning to practice, language intervention theory cannot ignore research on intervention if the intervention theory is to be valid. It is at this point that theory and science come together.

When one begins to look at intervention from a theoretical position, it becomes obvious that some aspects of intervention may not be compatible with the theory and must be omitted from the intervention plans. More important, however, is the realization that theory-based intervention may require that some aspects of intervention *not* be left out. Once a theory has integrated certain issues in its basic construct, and these issues are directly involved with language and language learning, the issues must be addressed in an intervention program. Intervention can and should be faithful to theory, not because theory makes intervention work in changing specific problems and meeting specific goals (see Perkins, 1986), but because theory helps us view a language-impaired child's problems within a framework that takes into account all aspects of the disorder in the attempt to bring about change. A theory that encompasses the nature and process of language and an understanding of its disorders as well as methods for describing the observed language differences will assist us in predicting and understanding the multiplicity of problems the child has in learning the many aspects of language. Furthermore, such a theory will give us the bases for teaching the child a wide range of language skills simultaneously, instead of concentrating on one target form or behavior at a time. One of the reasons, I believe, that language-impaired children continue to have significant problems throughout their school career is that too much time is given to changing specific and sometimes irrelevant behaviors and not enough time on a generalized program of language improvement. An integrative program of intervention would avoid this pitfall.

If, as Perkins (1986) says, specialists have considerable success almost in spite of theory, it is because the experienced and/or gifted clinician intuitively knows what and how to perform in an intervention setting. If we were to observe such individuals, we would find their procedures to be theoretically sound for the most part. An intervention program that is completely contrary to sound and empirically-based theory would most probably not have continuing success. Siegel and Ingham (1987) have stated that "... it is costly in the long run to accept as a legitimate form of therapy anything that 'works'" (p.103). That there are many clinicians who do not perform in an integrative manner seems apparent from the literature that continues to criticize the sterile "across the table" pure S-R approach. Many of us who had worked with language-disordered children before the widespread adoption of S-R technology resisted the wholesale incorporation of this methodology into our practice (although I spent many hours debating this issue with colleagues) just as we had at an earlier time resisted the wholesale incorporation of John Dewey's pragmatic principles into our teaching. We recognized that we could not make choices on one principle of behavior only; we knew that many factors operated both within and outside the individual and to choose one exclusively over all the others was to err.

This chapter will consider intervention procedures that are integrative in nature. In some respects they are idealistic. I recognize the impossibility of carrying out the kinds of recommendations that are found in the literature, considering the time, space, and load constraints in practice. But the discussion may provide a rationale and therefore some security for intervention choices. I will begin the chapter by stating some assumptions that are based on the integrative theory issues presented in earlier chapters and then describe essentials of intervention derived from the assumptions. The second section will describe the skills that a specialist needs to develop in order to maximize the opportunities for functional communication with children and therefore to conduct effective intervention sessions. This section will suggest a description of intervention strategies by a classification of children using developmental stages, age, educational status, interests, and other factors as classification criteria. The next section of the chapter will identify some basic components that I believe should be a part of every intervention plan. Lastly, specific intervention strategies and suggestions for planning intervention will be described.

INTERVENTION PROCEDURES DERIVED FROM THEORY-BASED ASSUMPTIONS

Neither language theory, cognitive theory, nor language development theory are generated for the purpose of suggesting methods of improving or changing language behaviors. Language intervention theory does have this purpose. It is precisely for this reason that those who work with language-impaired children must be careful in basic theory selection. The basic theories should interface logically with a theory of disorders and intervention principles and procedures. This section will present some assumptions based on the integrated theoretical principles described earlier in this book and draw some conclusions on intervention procedures from these assumptions. The assumptions will be grouped in terms of the type of theoretical principle involved—the nature of language, language development, language disorders, and so on. The listing of assumptions is not meant to be all-inclusive. I have selected those that I consider to be most important and discuss them in the following sections.

The Nature of Language

Assumption 1: That the primary purpose of language is communication, therefore all intervention programs must have as their primary goal the establishment of communicative competence.

Assumption 2: That one aspect of language is its rules of syntax, semantics, and pragmatics, and a child must develop a data base of this rule knowledge in order to use the language effectively, therefore intervention must provide for the child's continuing development of these rules through opportunities for observing the rules under varying conditions and contexts.

Assumption 3: That one aspect of language is the process by which language is performed and this process involves the development of processing skills, therefore intervention should provide for the child's practice of language so that it can be performed accurately and efficiently and opportunities should be provided for frequent production and frequent decoding of specified linguistic targets.

Assumption 4: That because comprehension is an integral part of functional language use and its development is actually a means by which the child learns to represent the world through a network of memories of events and experiences matched with linguistic counterparts, comprehension intervention should be an integral part of every intervention plan, the type of comprehension training and the emphasis on comprehension varying with the age of the child and the type of language impairment.

Assumption 5: That because language expression is the primary means of establishing communication interactions and of stabilizing formal distinctions in semantic and pragmatic use, intervention should provide the language-impaired child with the means of communicating in interactive settings and for functional purposes, and therefore should have specific expressive goals to include semantic, syntactic, and pragmatic objectives for language production use.

Assumption 6: That because the theoretical and empirical support for a linguistic-specific module is sufficiently strong to suggest a distinction between the phonological and syntactic computational aspects of language from the cognitive, semantic, and pragmatic ones, intervention can legitimately take this distinction into account in language-impairment intervention for the purpose of either grouping children in intervention classes or for planning the intervention program. For example, the semantic, comprehension (understanding), and general pragamatic problems might have more in common with each other than with phonological, syntactic (primarily expressive), and comprehension (decoding) problems.

Assumption 7: That oral and written language use common elements such as the linguistic rules of the language and word meaning and may even have common lexical access procedures; therefore, at the appropriate ages, interrelating reading, writing, speaking, and comprehending in intervention should reciprocally benefit all processes.

Language Development

Assumption 8: That the combined and integrated social, cognitive, and linguistic input to the child during the first years provide the context within which language is learned; therefore the intervention program needs to recognize this and to include all three factors within its procedures, particularly in facilitating language development in the young child.

Assumption 9: That because pragmatic, semantic, and syntactic aspects of language are integrated during language development, they should also be integrated in the intervention plan and in the sessions.

Assumption 10: That the frames, routines, stories, scripts, and event structures used by the family have provided a sound and functional framework from which the child is able to construct his or her language; therefore, intervention should utilize these same means in helping the language-impaired child build on what he or she already knows and use what is functional for him or her.

Assumption 11: That children appear to learn language more efficiently in a meaningful context and in a situation that is natural for them; therefore intervention should be meaningful and naturally constructed.

Assumption 12: That children's language at different ages changes not only as a result of cognitive and linguistic growth, but also from the impact of outside factors such as school and social and family changes and demands; therefore intervention approaches should take these external factors into account in the relative emphasis placed on specific procedures and goals.

Assumption 13: That the general cognitive level of a child influences the level of language development, particularly the semantic development; therefore placement of a child in a particular intervention group and the expected language achievement levels of the child should take into account the child's general cognitive level.

Language Disorders

Assumption 14: That because language-impaired children form a heterogeneous group representing different patterns of disorder, intervention should not involve a standard approach that is expected to fit everyone.

Assumption 15: That each child with language impairment usually demonstrates a breadth of problems in the perceptual, linguistic, and pragmatic areas; therefore intervention programs should address a general program of language improvement as well as a specific program for improving specific skills or knowledge, that is, each intervention session should have semantic, syntactic, and pragmatic objectives.

Assumption 16: That intellectual information is useful in understanding the learning style of each language-impaired child; therefore this type of information should be available to the specialists for selecting the type of intervention approach to use.

Assumption 17: That perceptual and memory deficits appear to be a characteristic of many language-impaired children; therefore the type and frequency of input in intervention should be adjusted to the ability of the child to process input data and compensatory suggestions should be provided to the child for dealing with the problem in everyday situations.

Assumption 18: That language-impaired children exhibit comprehension and/or expression disorders; therefore both systems need to be studied in assessment in order to determine the major focus of intervention.

Assumption 19: That detailed descriptions of the comprehension and expression systems under controlled and naturalistic conditions are the best sources for planning for intervention; therefore such analysis should be provided for in assessment.

Assumption 20: That because the main goal of intervention is the development of competence in communication (see Assumption 1), opportunities for functional communication and interactive exchanges should be an integral part of any and all intervention plans or procedures.

PREREQUISITE CLINICIAN KNOWLEDGE AND SKILLS FOR INTERVENTION

While it is important for a clinician to provide for the components of intervention in planning, it is even more important, in order to be successful in intervention, for the clinician to have internalized certain kinds of knowledge and to have developed certain kinds of skills. This knowledge and these skills influence what the clinician does and how he or she acts in every intervention session regardless of the age, setting, or type of problem or the procedure used. The knowledge needs to become practical and the skills need to become automatic so that both are part of an art of intervening and bringing about change. They are used at any time within the intervention session.

What is this knowledge and what are these skills? The *knowledge* to be internalized has to do with (1) the ways in which the language-impaired child differ from the normal child with respect to language and language acquisition strategies, (2) the general approaches that parents use with normal developing language, (3) the approaches that have been found useful in helping the language-impaired child, and (4) the interaction of age, cognitive, social, and linguistic levels with intervention activities. The *skills* needed by a clincian are applications of the knowledge and pertain to ways for eliciting language and encouraging specific kinds of language behaviors to occur in others. These skills include also the eliminations in the clincian's own responses of those behaviors that are not conducive to good communication. The ability to apply this knowledge and these skills effectively will come from practice—perhaps practice prior to beginning intervention with language-impaired children.

The Language Problems of Language-Impaired Children

A clinician's knowledge and understanding of the breadth of language problems that occur within the population of language-impaired children will have an impact on his or her manner of conducting intervention for these children. Awareness of the considerable language needs of these children will cause the clinician to provide a language intervention environment that will allow the simultaneous enrichment of a variety of language skills as well as will focus on the specific needs and problems of the children in specific areas.

Early studies reported problems of the language-impaired in auditory perceptual (Tallal & Stark, 1976; Keir, 1977; Tallal & Piercy, 1978); auditory memory (Menyuk, 1964; Keir, 1977); symbolic behavior (Lovell, Hoyle, & Sidall, 1968; Inhelder, 1976; Johnston, 1978); syntax (Menyuk, 1964; Lee, 1966; Menyuk & Looney, 1972); and semantics (Morehead & Ingram, 1973; Leonard, Bolders, & Miller, 1976).

Studies reported in the 1980s provided further evidence of the breadth of the language impairment in children. A brief summary of a sample of these studies, presented in the following sections, indicates the enormous task facing the clinician in providing help for the language-impaired.

Cognitive Deficits

Johnston and Weismer (1983) reported findings that suggested an impairment of visual imagery and consequent representational deficits beyond those of language in language-disordered children. Weismer (1985), in studying the constructive comprehension abilities of language-disordered children, found these children less likely to correctly respond to inference items on both verbal and pictorial material as compared with controls. She suggested that this finding indicates a cognitive deficit in these children. Kamhi (1981) and Savich (1984) found language-impaired children to perform poorly on imagery and symbolic play.

Comprehension Deficits

Van der Lely and Dewart (1986) found that the comprehension strategies of language-impaired children relied heavily on semantic cues and on "probable events."

Verbal Recall and Inference

Language/learning-disordered children were found to perform more poorly on story recall and inferencing questions than age-matched controls (Ellis Weismer, 1985; Crais & Chapman,1987).

Verbal Rehearsal and Memory

Kirchner and Klatzky (1985) found evidence of a broad deficit in processes related to short-term memory in a language-disordered group. The deficits were described in terms of diminished verbal capacity.

Mothers' Interaction

Lasky and Klopp (1982) found that the interaction of mothers with their language-impaired children differed from that of mothers with normal-language children.

Requests and Questions for Clarification

Olswang, Kriegmann, and Mastergeorge (1982) found the language-impaired to have a low frequency and a limited variety of information requests. Donahue, Pearl, and Bryan (1980) reported that the language-impaired asked fewer questions for clarification than their normal counterparts.

Responses to Requests

According to Brinton and Fujiki (1982) the language-impaired ignored or responded inappropriately to requests.

Repair Strategies

Brinton, Fujiki, Winkler, and Loeb (1986) found that language-impaired children had inappropriate repair strategies in response to requests for clarification.These children appeared to know the response needed but lacked the persistence to repeat a repair or the flexibility to try a new strategy.

Narrative Cohesion

Liles (1985) reported differences between normal and language-disordered subjects in their manner of cohesive organization, their cohesive adequacy, and their story comprehension.

Narratives

Language-impaired children produced less detailed story descriptions and used props and activities less frequently than their nondisordered peers (Sleight & Prinz, 1985).

These findings concerning the language-impaired child's problems in such a wide variety of language tasks underscore the need for the clinician to plan intervention using a broad focus in addition to attempting to meet specific objectives. Furthermore, the intervention procedures that are chosen must be constantly adjusted to the child's ability to initiate and respond to language, taking into account the deficits that impair this ability. It implies that the clinician be aware of each child's language needs as well as of those deficits that require adjustment in procedures on the part of the clinician. The clinician who learns to make every interaction moment one in which the child is learning something about language may ultimately be successful in helping the child cope in his or her language-dominated world. It is somewhat discouraging to recognize that a follow-up study on a group of 16 adolescents who were not mentally retarded and who were originally studied ten years earlier as preschool language-disordered children found that 69 percent of them had required special tutoring, grade retention, or language-disorder class placement (Aram, Ekelman, & Nation, 1984). Perhaps we need to recognize that work with the language-impaired is an ongoing process throughout the school years and that the changes in the demands at different academic levels will bring to light the varied deficits that seem to be present in the language-disordered population.

> *Quote 15–1*
> . . . *let us consider them [the features of adult speech] in functional interactional terms, that is to say in terms of the intentions that may be assumed to guide a person's behavior when they wish to succeed in communicating, particularly if their partner is a less skilled communicator.*
>
> *There seems to be four broad types of intention that are relevant:*
>
> 1. *to secure and maintain inter-subjectivity of attention;*
> 2. *to express one's own meaning intentions in a form that one's partner will find easy to understand;*
> 3. *to ensure that one has correctly understood the meaning intention of one's partner;*
> 4. *to provide positive responses in order to sustain the partner's desire to continue the present interaction and to engage in further interactions in the future;*
> 5. *to instruct one's partner so that he or she may become a more skilled performer.*
>
> (WELLS, 1985, p. 399).

Effective Strategies for Incidental Language Teaching

Within the framework of general planned intervention procedures, the effective clinician is constantly, and often incidentally, using strategies that assist the child in developing those skills of language that are essential to communicative competence at his or her age level. Just as a parent does not limit language teaching to a specific time, neither should the clinician think of intervention as only those activities that are planned and written into a lesson. Every interaction can be a learning opportunity for the child if the clinician learns to use the skills of becoming a good communication partner.

The skills that the clinician needs to learn are those that parents use to facilitate language development in children and those that language specialists have found to be helpful in improving the language of the language-impaired child. They are not the kinds of strategies that a clinician memorizes and then writes into an intervention plan as the approach to use; they are the skills that a clinician learns to perform and can do so at any appropriate time as part of or incidental to the intervention procedure. The kinds of suggestions that will be provided here will also be useful to the clinician in working with parents and helping them to function well in communication exchanges with their children. The changes suggested here relate to the adult behaviors—those adults that need to learn in order to facilitate language instead of constrain it (Hubbell, 1977; Olswang, Kriegsmann, & Mastergeorge, 1982).

I have selected from a wide variety of literature, suggestons that have been offered for the adult to become a good communication partner for the child. These suggestions have evolved from studies of the successful behaviors of parents of normal-language children in helping their children develop good communication skills and from the studies of techniques that appear helpful to children with language disorders in the improvement of their language functions.

Planning the Environment

Because certain kinds of environments appear to stimulate language, care should be taken to (1) select materials of interest to the child, (2) select toys with multiple components so as to encourage continuation of a topic, (3) choose activities for young children that can be completed quickly, and (4) choose activities that have repetitive actions and provide novelty for the child (Halle, 1984). If some desired materials are inaccessible but in view, there is increase in the need for a child to express what he or she wants and to use language (Klein, Wulz, Hall, Waldo, Carpenter, Rathan, Myers, Fox, & Marshall, 1981; Warren & Kaiser, 1986b). If the environment causes the child to signal an interest, select the topic, and thus initiate communication, the child controls the incidences in which teaching occurs, factors that have been found to be critical in learning (Hart & Risley, 1975).

Providing Adult Input

In general, the adult input is effective if the vocabulary, grammar, and cognitive complexity level of what is addressed to the child corresponds to the level at which the child responds most effectively (Owens, 1984; Wells, 1985; Conti-Ramsden & Friel-Patti, 1986). The input should also be adjusted to the child's learning style and whatever perceptual or memory constraints the child might have. Cues from the child's comprehension will determine the nature of the input. For improvement of production, some portion of the input should be in advance of the child's production (Wells, 1985). Owens (1984) also suggests that the input provide frequent repetitions and a slow rate of speech with long pauses between utterances and after content words. The pauses after the utterances provide the child with a turn at speaking (De Maio, 1984) and are effective if, while waiting for a response from the child, the wait is accompanied with eye contact and other body language to indicate that something is expected (Wulz, Hall, & Klein, 1983). Wells (1985) agrees that the quantity of conversations should, other things being equal, facilitate the task of communication development since the child requires evidence of how language works.

Other ways in which the adults' input can serve to assist the child's development are through (1) modeling—providing a linguistic model for what the child is trying to express; (2) expanding—interpreting what the child means to say and arriving at a mutual understanding (Rice &

Haight, 1986); Snyder-McLean and McLean (1978) say that a child's initiation followed by expansion of his or her utterance may serve as a
means for the child to rehearse the specific motor act in an appropriate
context and also get a confirmation from the adult; (3) paraphrasing; and
(4) emphasizing the here and now. (See Chapter 5 for other suggestions
of this type.)

Encouraging the Early Functions of Language

Halliday (1975) states that the first stage of language development
is that of mastering the basic functions of language, each having a
limited range of alternatives or "meaning potential" with which it is associated:

Instrumental:	"I want"
Regulatory:	"do as I tell you"
Personal:	"me and you"
Heuristic:	"tell me why"
Imaginative:	"let's pretend"
Informative:	"I've got something to tell you"

According to Halliday, these functional expressions appear ap-
proximately in the order listed and each expression has just one function. The children acquire descriptive functions of words before
determiner functions (Karmiloff-Smith, 1979). The basic functions of
a word, according to Karmiloff-Smith (1979), must be highly consolidated and automatic before competing functions are allowed. This
implies that a single most important feature of a word should be
stabilized before expanding its meaning to related but even slightly
different meanings. This is contrary to what is sometimes recommended in intervention regarding the simultaneous provision of a target in
many different contexts and illustrating numerous functions in which
a word can be used. Related to this idea is Blank's (1975b) recom-
mendation that polars not be taught simultaneously, for example, up
and down, red and blue. Instead we should teach "up" and "not up,"
and so on.

Children progress from the functional (interpersonal) phase (the
use of language to act) to the ideational phase (the use of language to
think) (Halliday, 1975). Language intervention with very young
children should be entirely on an interpersonal level. Naturalistic approaches, which include play and conversation, are the best means of
facilitating functional language. Howe (1981) goes so far as to state
that every acquisition must be tied to particular functions.

Selecting and Teaching Early Words

In selecting the early words for labeling, the adult should try to determine those words that are most functional for the child. Actually, Halliday (1975) says that many of the words that are learned first are called for by existing functions. Bruner (1975) and Snow (1972) suggest that the adult follow a child's line of vision or motor attention to an object in the environment. Then the adult can identify the critical features of the object and provide an appropriate verbal label within a linguistic structure that the child is capable of understanding. In addition to the communicative significance of the words, Weiss, Leonard, Rowan, and Chapman (1983) recommend that the word be composed of phonological features that are within the child's repertoire and be appropriate to the child's style of learning. A child who has a referential style will respond better to picture and object names, whereas a child with an expressive style would need social words for interacting with persons. Some children may respond better to pictures than objects and this preference can be identified (Olswang, Bain, Dunn, & Cooper, 1983). Olswang et al. also point out the importance of highlighting the relationship between nonlinguistic and linguistic cues and of making the nonlinguistic cues more salient if a child does not have receptive knowledge of the words.

When labeling is used, it should be inserted within the central dialogue (Ninio & Bruner, 1977). If the correct conversational setting is provided—asking "what" questions or allowing the child to initiate a request for labels—there is greater likelihood that a child will label. Ninio and Bruner (1977) say that providing the child with a model *for imitation* actually depresses the probability that the child will utter a word immediately.

Expanding Syntax and Semantic Behaviors

According to Leonard, Steckol, and Panther (1983), the expansion of semantic categories should be based on the positional patterns that are already operative in the child's productive language. Schlesinger (1981) suggests that semantic assimilation, a process of extending already existing semantic categories by the recategorization of semantic relational concepts, is a process that occurs in the development of semantic categories. It appears that the defining of semantic category features is an ongoing process, and the clinician should utilize known semantic categories for expanding the features and recategorizing them.

In moving from single-word to multiword productions, Schwartz, Chapman, Terrell, Prelock, and Rowan (1985) suggest a procedure that engages a child in vertical construction. For example, the adult and child are looking at a picture of a boy eating an apple:

> Adult: What's this?
> Child: Boy.
> Adult: What's the boy eating?
> Child: Apple.
> Adult: Yeah, the boy is eating the apple.

The impaired-language child can be helped by using some of the techniques that normal language children use in expanding their utterances in the natural process of learning. Some of these are described by Kuczaj (1983):

> Build-ups: Block → yellow block → look at the yellow block
> Breakdowns: Clock off → clock → off
> Completion
> (separation
>   by pause):   Anthony take the → (pause) → take the box
> Substitution: What color car? → what color glass?
> Imitation: Repeat another's preceding utterance
> Repetition: Repeat own preceding utterance

Kuczaj (1983) suggests that these processes develop best through play not only because children exert some control in play but also because through play children may simulate behavior, that is, create situations in which the normal consequences of activities are absent—they can make mistakes. Early in language acquisition play serves a practice function, whereas later it is engaged in for enjoyment (Kuczaj, 1983).

Nelson (1977) suggests recasting children's utterances to form tag questions (Child: "I'm big." Adult: "You're big, aren't you?") or to include complex forms (Child: "Where this piece [puzzle] go?" Adult: "Where *will* it go?").

Using Evoking and Facilitative Strategies

The purpose of evoking and facilitative strategies is to encourage the child to engage in spontaneous talking or to use oral expression for communicative purposes. Culatta and Horn (1982) list procedures they suggest for assisting children to move from rule knowledge to conversation.

1. Require the child to convey information
2. Request information by specifying the reason for the request (I can't find the soap).
3. Create a situation that stimulates a need to obtain an action or call attention to an event.
4. Create an unusual or novel event.
5. Provide inaccurate information regarding something the child needs or wants to know.

> *Quote 15–2*
> *When judging how well the clinician's response matches the child's intent, consistent potential mismatches can be found. They all emanate from the clinician's placing the child in an intentional state of wanting an object and then treating the child's verbalization as good talking rather than as a request for something.*
> (DUCHAN, 1986, p. 206).

Others have provided additional suggestions for encouraging spontaneous speech or for avoiding its constraints:

1. Encode the next action in a sequence of actions that the child is carrying out (Wells, 1985).
2. Comment on the child's verbal and nonverbal involvement during play (De Maio, 1984).
3. Increase questions that do not require yes/no answers (Warren, McQuarter, & Rogers-Warren, 1984) except in early language where direct requests appear to be more associated with progress than questions calling for comment. (Direct requests make it easier for the child to discover the relationship between form and meaning [Wells, 1985]. At later stages, direct requests have an inhibiting effect.) Duchan (1986a) suggests that if the adult asks questions, he or she should ask for information that he or she really wants to know and that the child cares about.
4. Minimize total number of utterances used by adults (De Maio, 1984).
5. Avoid verbally interrupting the child and be prepared to relinquish turn if the child interrupts (De Maio, 1984).
6. Avoid asking the child to talk or telling the child what to say. These serve as constraints. Without constraints (including physical limitations to play space), vocabulary increases and children talk for longer periods (Hubbell, 1977).
7. Follow child's lead and comment on child's activity.
8. Recognize that verbal interaction is more effective than verbal stimulation (Hubbell, 1977).

The preceding suggestions are for the evocation of spontaneous speech by the child. They may not serve as well for other types of language teaching purposes. Hubbell (1977) cautions that they may not meet the goals of structured training or be as successful with children with specific processing problems as they are with normal-language children.

Encouraging Conversational Discourse

Related to the evocation of spontaneous speech is that of facilitating conversational discourse, which occurs at a later stage of language development. Conversational discourse is built on a framework of social interaction. Early social interaction is supported by the adult's use of parallel talk and self-talk during periods of silence (De Maio, 1984). Even nonverbal imitations will establish and maintain contact with the child (De Maio, 1984). As the child begins to converse, the adult provides feedback regarding how the child's utterances are interpreted—this allows the child to evaluate the effectiveness of what he or she says in expressing his or her intentions. Recasting the child's utterance by changing the form but not the meaning is a way of checking the adult's understanding and verifying to the child that the message has been understood. Although back-channeling (saying, "Yeah, I know") on the part of the child can be a way of avoiding taking a turn or contributing to the exchange (De Maio, 1984), *adult* back-channeling can serve the purpose of maintaining the child's adherence to the topic.

When responding to the child's message, priority is given to the intent. Reinforcement will be provided naturally if the message is understood. Correction should be minimized. Artificial reinforcement should be avoided as well as comments on the manner or form in which the child expresses intent. The child's improvement will come more naturally if it is in response to a problem in being understood in a functional situation.

If a child's messages are not clear to the adult, the child needs to learn how to repair his or her utterances so that they become clear. Brinton, Fujiki, Winkler, & Loeb, (1986) suggest a series of requests for clarification that can be used by the adult in order to engage the child in repair strategies:

1. Provide a neutral or nonspecific response like "Huh?" or "What?"
2. Request conformation by repeating the last portion with an interrogative inflection.
3. Request the repetition of a particular constituent: "To a what?" "Who saw the ball?"

These principles concerning ways of becoming a good communication partner apply to adolescents as well as to young children. The essence of language growth is language use in functional activities. Recommendations have been made that the clinician become a facilitator by manipulating the environment and providing "creatively systematized, linguistically enhancing experiences" (Friel-Patti & Lougeay-Mattinger, 1986). The clinician is also responsible for becoming a good communication partner for the child or adolescent. It is in the process of interacting with them in a manner that brings about changes in their language behavior that communication competence develops. Furthermore, the selection opportunities for increasing the frequency of language use that are functional and motivating and in which the student wishes to succeed is also part of the clinical role. Good teaching has always been made up of these factors. It is unfortunate that the term *teaching* has become associated with training and operant techniques and has been rendered meaningless. We are all teachers of each other and we all learn from each other. The process is most successful when the process is less didactic and more functional.

Encouraging Abstract Thinking

Blank (1975b) provided suggestions for fostering abstract thinking in young children. Some of her suggestions are as follows:

1. Techniques for encouraging children to observe all perceptual qualities of objects rather than those that are most salient by (1) reducing the physical salience; (2) requesting the child to search for objects on the basis of a specified characteristic; (3) eliminating competing cues (e.g., eliminating visual cues in order to focus on auditory or tactual ones, etc.).
2. Techniques to reduce egocentric perspective by having the child assume the role of another thereby creating psychological distancing behavior. Another way of encouraging the child to separate him or herself from the ongoing observable field is via representation and language (Sigel & McGillicuddy-Delise, 1984). These authors suggest that the level of requests made of the child provides the distancing opportunities. Low-level requests—label, produce, describe, define—require little distancing. Medium-level requests—sequence, reproduce, describe similarities, estimate, classify—provide greater distancing and high-level requests— evaluate consequences, infer effect, generalize, transform, plan, conclude, propose alternatives—provide the greatest distancing.
3. Techniques to teach recognition of the tangential from germane (Blank, unpublished) by questions that cause the child to identify relevant factors from those that are irrelevant—"Would it matter if the coat were red or blue?" as opposed to "Would it matter if the coat were heavy or light?"
4. Techniques for providing rationale for behavior and events: (1) seeing a picture of a girl crying and asking, "How do you know she is sad?"; (2) looking at a box and asking, "What makes you think that the box will be heavy?"
5. Techniques for helping the child cope with complex cognitive situations by having him or her respond to the unexpected request—"Draw something that is not a circle."
6. Techniques to teach recognition that labels are not arbitrary by exploring how the parts of objects have similar functions (wings of a bird and of a plane, skin of a fruit and of the body).

Increasing Motivation and Interest

One of the most important ingredients of intervention is the motivation and interest of the child. It is also an ingredient over which the specialist has very little control. However, there are general guidelines for increasing motivation on the part of the child. These are ways of encouraging *attention* and *intention*, which are elements essential to learning. If the theory that a child uses his or her own system to induce the rules of language from the language input he or she receives (and it appears to be a logical proposal), the child must select from the environment those features that are needed for specific rule formation. Selection is based on attention or focus—a readiness to receive the input —and particularly, the intention to do so. The importance of perceptual salience for assisting the child in the selective process has already been discussed. Attention and intention may be increased if tasks are motivating to the child. A review of some of these with examples from other areas might be of help.

1. For a child to be motivated, it helps if the child is actively and directly involved in the task or event. Regardless of the theoretical orientation of and approaches to intervention, the specialist should endeavor to have the child be an active rather than a passive participant in the process. The effect of action is dramatic. Example: Many of us have had the experience of being a passenger in a car while traversing a particular route numerous times and then, after being asked to drive to the same destination, saying, "I don't know how to get there." In other words, the attention needed for learning is called on primarily when an individual is responsible for executing a task. It is for this reason that the topic, situation, and message orientation used in pragmatic theory have been found effective. These force involvement on the child's part.

2. For a child to be motivated it helps to create for the child a specific purpose or need for behaving in a specific manner. Example: In which situation is a student most likely to learn a poem—one in which the teacher assigns it for homework or one in which the teacher indicates that the student will present and explain it to the class? The intervention specialist who creates situations in which a child needs to use his or her skills for a real and interesting purpose will most likely succeed in motivating the child.

3. For a child to be motivated, the child's own knowledge and interest should be exploited in intervention. Example: Every day hundreds of cars are seen in the streets and yet few individuals can accurately classify each car by the company where it's made, its name, and style. (The only one I can recognize is the Jaguar!) However, when an individual is in the market for a car, the distinctions among cars and their unique characteristics are noted, and classifying the cars as

they pass is accomplished without effort. The interest and purpose have made the difference.

4. For a child to be motivated, the child should have joint responsibility with the specialist for his or her own change. Every individual knows how easy it is to avoid something we are not responsible for. Example: We are asked to be on a committee but the responsibility for the execution of its function belongs to someone else. How hard do we work? Do we just do what we're asked? What happens if we are chairperson or cochairperson?

5. For a child to be motivated, the child's emotion should be charged. An event charged with great happiness, excitement, competition, or even a little anxiety will be remembered over others. An intervention experience should be just that—an experience. To make it so, the specialist should also be excited about the intervention event. Example: Try to remember the earliest event of your childhood. How specifically do you remember it? Do you recall any other things that happened at the same time? Do you remember those charged with emotion better than the others?

To find that which truly motivates a child, the specialist needs to learn to "read" the child. In fact, "ability to read" the child is a more accurate way to describe an effective clinician than his or her "teaching ability." When we "read" a child, we are in tune with that child, we observe his or her natural responsiveness, reticence, and behavior under various conditions. We do not force the child to play the clinical game our way; we adapt our way to get the maximum responsiveness from the child. The most effective techniques are those that take into account the child and his or her learning style.

Age Adaptation of Intervention Procedures

Our concern about language may direct us to select intervention procedures and activities on the basis of the language level of the child. There are other factors, however, both within and external to the child that need to be considered also. Along with language development, the child changes in cognitive, social, and motor areas. In addition to this growth, the child is placed in situations that provide new experiences and make new demands. The school experience of course alters the child's life in a most dramatic way. New cognitive and social demands are made upon him or her. Other children stimulate new interests. The child begins to learn how to learn and subsequently uses the tools of learning to learn about the world. Intervention procedures need to take into account the changes within the child and the context, home or school, in which the child interacts.

If the factors that produce change and the changes that actually occur in the child are considered in planning intervention, it is unlikely that a clinician will utilize a single methodology for all children. For example, play may be an effective means of interaction at the beginning preschool stages of language, but not during the elementary grades. The use of groups may be naturalistic for middle-school children, but not for the 3-year-old. The kind of play that children engage in changes with age and so should the type of play used in intervention. Narrative styles of children and their knowledge of story grammar change with age (Klecan-Aker & Swank, 1987a), and so should our expectations and demands in intervention. Play, routines, narratives, event structure, and other strategies are all useful frameworks within which to build intervention, but their usefulness is age-dependent and their structure should increase in difficulty and breadth as age increases. Effective intervention is built on the child's interests, abilities, and needs. Procedures that under- or overestimate the abilities of the child or do not include aspects of his or her environment that are meaningful will not achieve the same results as those that do. Even if a child's language is delayed, that child should be taught in a manner that suits his or her age unless, of course, there is also cognitive and/or social delay.

Table 15–1 provides a list of selected abilities and interests of children classified by age groups. These particular age groups were used because they correspond in general to the classification by grades used in schools. From age 2 to ages 3–11 are the preschool or nursery years; from age 4 to ages 5–11 are the prekindergarten and kindergarten years; from age 6 to ages 8–11 are the primary years; from age 9 to ages 10–11 are the elementary years; and from age 11 on up are middle and high school years. The items listed within an age category may apply to the lower or upper end of the category, and therefore the clinician needs to observe the responses of children in intervention to the activities he or she chooses. The list does provide a general guideline to the type of procedures that may be most effective with children of a specific age.

The use of school classifications for grouping skills and activities was chosen because if there is integration between intervention and what is happening in the classroom, there is greater likelihood that the intervention process will be successful. Word meanings and syntactic structures chosen for intervention should be those the child needs to know in spelling, reading, history, or science. The pragmatic skills selected for intervention should be those the child uses in everyday classroom situations. Both the child's specific deficits and needs and the demands made on the child in his or her environment provide input for choosing procedures.

When reading the literature on intervention, the clinician should note if the application of suggested procedures is to the developmental stages of language or to children whose basic structures and pragmatic

TABLE 15–1. SELECTED COGNITIVE, SOCIAL, LINGUISTIC, AND METALINGUISTIC ABILITIES AND INTERESTS OF CHILDREN CLASSIFIED BY AGE GROUPS*

YEARS: 2 to 3-11

LINGUISTIC

Syntactic

1. uses three- to five-word sentences
2. develops basic transformations
3. develops 14 grammatical morphemes
4. overregularizes
5. uses S + V sentences mostly
6. begins asking questions
7. relies on word order for interpretation
8. uses limited coordination
9. understands negation
10. understands some contractions
11. uses -ing and -ed verb endings

Semantic

1. uses stages I and II basic semantic relations
2. uses intonation for meaning
3. earliest vocabulary, expressive or referential
4. vocabulary up to 1500 words
5. shifts from purely pragmatic comprehension to semantic comprehension
6. understands compound sentences
7. learns language of environment
8. remarks on possession, location, recurrence, and nonrecurrence
9. uses functionally-tied language
10. understands color and size words

Pragmatic

1. comments on actions and names/objects
2. utterances begin to have communicative intent
3. appears to understand almost everything
4. learns communicative strategies of environment
5. uses nonverbal strategies to persuade
6. interaction skills of expressing a wish, refusing, complying, requesting information
7. uses simple greetings
8. will repeat an utterance when not understood
9. likes to ask *why* questions
10. uses and understands the language functions of labeling and describing
11. exchanges primitive conversations

SOCIAL/EMOTIONAL

1. plays egocenteredly
2. uses parallel play—one partner
3. talks while playing
4. takes turns
5. uses disconnected play action
6. uses joint action routines
7. recognizes self distinct from others
8. uses appropriate eye control
9. socially responsive to maternal stimulation

TABLE 15–1.   *(Continued)*

COGNITIVE

1. draws representational art
2. matches primary colors
3. has concept of two
4. counts rotely to 4/5
5. recognizes three-dimensional shapes
6. holds two or three chunks of information in memory
7. reasons from particular to particular, syncretic
8. juxtaposes elements
9. utterances represent here and now
10. begins to use metamemory
11. distinguishes play from nonplay

METALINGUISTIC

1. begins word play—rhyming
2. corrects others
3. is aware of print
4. plays "routine" games
5. enjoys being read to

ACTIVITIES

1. plays with toys
2. looks at pictures
3. "draws" with a crayola
4. swings
5. plays in water/sand/clay

YEARS: 4 to 5-11

LINGUISTIC

Syntactic

1. masters major syntactic forms
2. uses major transformations
3. uses irregular past tense of common verbs
4. future tense model "will" used where context requires
5. limited use of conjunctions
6. some use of relative pronouns in embedded structures
7. some use of infinitives, gerunds, and participles
8. responds to active/passive constructions
9. uses morphological rules to express inflectional changes
10. can rely on syntactically conveyed information to respond in adult form

Semantic

1. referential communication limited to child's own familiar language and familiar objects
2. uses words to symbolize fantasies, images, thoughts, and feelings
3. vocabulary about 2100 words
4. word definitions lack fullness of adult meanings
5. understands two adjective modifiers
6. understands some conjoined sentences
7. understands the concept of *like* and *different*
8. understands demonstrative and personal pronouns
9. can carry out sequences of actions consistent with topics
10. begins to understand verbal and perceptual analogies

TABLE 15–1. *(Continued)*

Pragmatic

1. talk centered on activity with toys
2. talk primary focus of attention
3. uses strategies for engaging others in conversations
4. begins to topic-associate for lengthening conversations
5. utterances mutually responsive and adapted to partner
6. uses evidence and opinions to support claims
7. awareness of rules of interaction
8. uses "listener" responses—nodding, "umm," etc.
9. has ability to identify emotional response
10. speaks differently to adults and 2-year-olds
11. uses talk related to listeners' activity
12. conversation skills follow conventionalized routines
13. can revise utterances when not understood
14. participates successfully in verbal turn-taking
15. settles agreements through negotiation
16. tells stories in sequences of unintegrated actions

SOCIAL/EMOTIONAL

1. facial expression culturally appropriate
2. is interested in group activities
3. uses associative and cooperative play
4. shares toys
5. participates in role playing
6. sustains interaction with peer
7. has egocentric perspective in identifying emotions
8. has ability to resolve disagreements
9. employs me-too behavior
10. employs psychological tactics to manage others
11. tries on roles of others

COGNITIVE

1. knows own right and left
2. counts to 10/13
3. develops time concept—yesterday, today, and tomorrow
4. remembers and repeats three digits
5. matches color, size, shape
6. pretends
7. uses constructive play
8. carries a rule through a series of activities
9. draws head, arms, legs (no body)
10. has image-like representations
11. uses riddles of logical relations
12. integrates verbal and nonverbal strategies
13. uses intuitive thought

METALINGUISTIC

1. has a budding sense of humor for simple jokes
2. recognizes letters
3. identifies sounds in words
4. learns to read
5. uses language creatively—novel words

ACTIVITIES

1. plays dolls, market, family
2. begins sports—swimming

TABLE 15–1. *(Continued)*

3. does jig-saw puzzles
4. does simple crafts
5. plays hide and seek
6. enjoys birthday parties

YEARS: 6 to 9-11

LINGUISTIC
Syntactic

1. has complete basic syntactic development
2. uses infinite number of well-formed complete sentences
3. uses complex syntactic structures
4. understands embedded sentences
5. uses relative clauses in embedded sentences
6. distinguishes direct/indirect objects

Semantic

1. recognizes semantic nuance as well as denotation
2. can identify synonyms and antonyms
3. expressive vocabulary of 2600 words
4. receptive vocabulary of 14,000 to 24,000 words
5. begins to acquire multiple word meanings
6. literal interpretation of what others say
7. use global terms to describe others
8. demonstrates little difficulty with comparative relationships
9. begins to understand special vocabulary of school subjects
10. vocabulary begins to increase rapidly through reading and instruction
11. understands words of amount and quantity: some, many, most

Pragmatic

1. expresses affection and hostility to peers
2. is able to carry on conversation
3. asks and answers questions
4. follows and gives instruction
5. speaks alone in presence of group
6. boasts and brags
7. uses slang
8. can make assumptions about the level of knowledge of the listener and adjusts the conversation accordingly
9. repairs language
10. manipulates and influences others through language
11. can tell a simple short story using initiating events and consequences

SOCIAL/EMOTIONAL

1. sensitive to context and situation
2. gets attention in socially accepted ways
3. uses adults as resources
4. leads and follows peers
5. expresses affection and hostility to peers
6. enjoys an audience
7. may become part of a "clique"
8. engages in making things with others
9. identifies with adult of own sex
10. overt behavior less reliable index of feelings
11. perceives incongruous facial expressions
12. demonstrates ability to empathize

TABLE 15–1. *(Continued)*

COGNITIVE

1. understands conservation
2. knows left and right of others
3. recognizes differences and similarities
4. recognizes multiplicity of object properties
5. uses inference in nonverbal situation
6. recalls sequence of events in story
7. holds about five chunks of information in memory
8. understands concept of reversibility
9. appreciates humor
10. coordinates notions of time/distance/ speed
11. engages in syllogistic reasoning
12. can formulate hypothesis
13. infer others' thoughts and points of view
14. seriate systematically by searching for characteristic such as size
15. make abstract (paradigmatic) or concrete (syntagmatic) associations

METALINGUISTIC

1. judges grammatical acceptability of sentences
2. can invent a true narrative with two or more episodes
3. uses reading to learn
4. enjoys simple poetry
5. imitates others' speech

ACTIVITIES

1. plays board games
2. enjoys field trips
3. plays jump rope, jacks, marbles
4. watches television
5. plays with pets
6. sings simple songs

YEARS: 9 to 10-11

LINGUISTIC

Syntactic

1. has more complete and sophisticated use of subordination
2. can act out task given sentences made up of two clauses joined by connective
3. can produce reversible and nonreversible passives
4. develops an understanding of reversible and nonreversible passives
5. expresses complex syntactic structures in writing and speaking

Semantic

1. uses unambiguous references when telling and writing a story
2. understands complex verbal analogies
3. uses context to understand new and difficult vocabulary
4. uses cohesive devices in writing and speaking
5. goes beyond what is demanded in response to questions (elaborations)

Pragmatic

1. can use language to express a variety of speech acts
2. varies language depending on the age and sex of the listener
3. can introduce, maintain, and shift topics with ease
4. uses polite forms
5. handles telephone messages

TABLE 15–1. *(Continued)*

6. answers questions from a variety of perspectives
7. identifies differences of social dialect and perceives significance of differences
8. uses a variety of arguments in persuasion
9. tells complex stories with a number of episodes

SOCIAL/EMOTIONAL

1. has allegiance to "gang" but still needs strong adult support
2. discovers that self may be the object of someone else's perspective
3. explains social interaction in situational terms
4. uses peer persuasion
5. recognizes intentions of others
6. plays games with carefully prescribed rules and regulations
7. has awareness of personal space zones
8. perceives social significance of dialects

COGNITIVE

1. plans future actions
2. solves problems with only minimal physical input
3. becomes decentered in thinking
4. has some understanding of reversible mental operations
5. thinking not dominated by visual impressions
6. remembers and represents events in symbolic form
7. understands complex riddles and jokes
8. represents imagined objects symbolically

METALINGUISTIC

1. enjoys proverbs and fables
2. evaluates and classifies words and statements
3. can correct own writing
4. learns narrative rules

ACTIVITIES

1. has interest in the world
2. has interest in possessions—bicycles, watches
3. has interest in actors, actresses, and other stars
4. has interest in spectator sports
5. enjoys making things

YEARS: 11+

LINGUISTIC

Syntactic

1. continues expansion by conjoining and embedding
2. uses a variety of syntactic means to express an idea

Semantic

1. has a 50,000 word receptive vocabulary
2. uses adult definitions
3. uses and understands similies and metaphors

TABLE 15–1.   *(Continued)*

Pragmatic

1. uses code-switching does occur as social situation dictates
2. uses language that is generally appropriate regardless of age, sex, or cultural position of the listener
3. can use a variety of revision strategies when not understood
4. provides feedback regarding messages
5. evaluates a message critically

SOCIAL/EMOTIONAL

1. friendship based on shared activity and, later, loyalty
2. prefers time spent with friends than family
3. rebellion toward adults
4. problems with self-esteem
5. discusses self, sex, love, and friendships
6. discusses society, religion, and justice
7. examines possibilities of personal and collective action
8. takes perspective of others
9. uninterested in school and acquiring knowledge
10. sees relationships between physical and psychological closeness

COGNITIVE

1. thinks about future
2. uses inductive/reflective thinking
3. has ability to judge logical relationships of propositions
4. uses formal operations—abstraction and speculation
5. uses hypothetical thinking
6. imagines logical consequences of existing states
7. ability to sense dissonance and note discrepancies
8. anticipates consequences
9. plans and executes multistep activities
10. conceptualizes own thought and the thought of others

METALINGUISTIC

1. writes creatively
2. evaluates writing of peers
3. aware of the use of language
4. uses peer language style and usage

ACTIVITIES

1. has interest in contemporary music
2. has interest in dancing
3. plays competitive sports
4. has interest in clothes
5. has interest in looks
6. desires possessions—stereos, cars
7. watches video movies

*Prepared in conjunction with Joan Klecan-Aker. References used: Allen & Brown (1977), Applebee (1978), Bruner (1975), Dore (1976), Flores D'Arcais (1981), Galda (1984), Gardner (1980), Garvey (1974), Gillam & Johnston (1985), Howe (1981), Klecan-Aker (1985), Klecan-Aker & Swank (1987, 1988), Owens (1984), Piaget (1958), Roth & Clark (1987), and Sachs, Goldman, & Chaille (1984).

skills have already been acquired. So much of the literature applies to the developmental level, and, although some of the techniques can be used with older children, others may not be suitable.

BASIC COMPONENTS OF AN INTERVENTION PLAN

There are numerous ways in which the intervention plan can be divided. I have found that a simple general structure is the best; therefore, I believe that a plan should provide for (1) goals and objectives (I am using goals and objectives synonomously here although I recognize that there are situations in which a distinction is useful); (2) content, and (3) general and specific procedures.

The Goals

The goals and objectives for intervention refer to the desired outcome for both an extended period of time—a semester—and for each particular session. The long-term goals specify the desired accomplishment in the areas of syntax, semantics, and pragmatics in both comprehension and expression. The goals in syntax, semantics, and pragmatics are selected on the basis of two criteria: (1) what the typical child at the child's specific age, grade, social environment, and intellectual level knows and does, and (2) what the child's specific needs are. If a child's needs only are used for decision-making, a clinician may begin teaching skills for which a child at a particular age is not ready or for which the child has no use at that time in his or her home and school environment.

In the objectives statement, the pragmatics, syntax, and semantics goals should be ordered in some kind of sequence—developmental in the early years—in which they are to be introduced in intervention. The sequence is flexible and should be changed or modified as the child's needs change. The ability to be flexible is an outcome of the clinician's ability to internalize the goals for each child as well as to know the general language knowledge and abilities that children have at his or her age. A considerable amount of incidental teaching occurs as a result (Hart & Risley, 1986).

The goals for the individual lesson reflect the general goals and objectives, but the expected outcomes are more completely specified. It is helpful to set time limits (number of sessions to reach specific objectives) so that not too much time is given to one small part of a total program. Often, when a specific objective is not achieved and the intervention moves on to a subsequent one to return later to the early goal, the child responds the second time around.

> *Quote 15–3*
> *We acknowledge that all the language skills go hand in hand and that development in one medium drives development in another. We know that students learn pragmatic skills from oral language as they respond to listeners and talk to find out what they should know, for example. We also know that the basic for learning what writing should "look like," i.e., what the characteristics of written text structures are, comes from knowledge, not just of information, but of how that information fits into larger contexts beyond her/his own personal experiences.*
>
> (BEACH & BRIDWELL, 1984, p. 185).

The Content

I believe it is important to specify content objectives in terms of desired improvement in four basic areas: (1) in the knowledge of rules as well as in performance, (2) in the aspect of comprehension (to include basic concepts and meaning) as well as expression, (3) in the areas of pragmatics, semantics, syntax, and articulation, and (4) in metalinguistic areas where appropriate. In other words, I believe that an intervention plan should address all these areas to some extent. The relative importance of each of these and the consequent emphasis placed on them in intervention vary with the age, language stage, and needs of the child and even from session to session. For example, there may be sessions in which the syntax is the foreground and semantics and pragmatics are the background. After a few sessions the pragmatics becomes the foreground and the syntax and semantics that have been already mastered are background, for example, in the development of conversational skills. At very early ages, comprehension and basic concept development may be the foreground, whereas at later developmental stages expressive language is emphasized. But each category is targeted with reference to the others. General language improvement therefore should be the container in which specific intervention strategies are wrapped. While detail targets are taught, overall language skills develop.

In the selection of content for intervention, we need to focus on the complex skills that use language within the framework of interaction, the ability to converse, to understand and tell a story, to write, to debate, to describe events, to argue, and so on. Whereas many of these are means by which we learn language, they are also some of the goals of language teaching. These language activities are governed by rules, and the competent communicator knows and uses these rules well (Johnston, 1983; Sleight & Prinz, 1985; Duchan, 1986a). It is not my purpose in this chapter to describe the organization of story grammars or other texts. However, the need to include these as part of the content of intervention must be recognized.

The Procedures

Within the framework of the assumptions previously described and the principles underlying the goals and content selection, it is possible to identify at least seven major elements of an intervention plan: (1) theme, (2) contexture, (3) repetition, (4) envelope, (5) practice, (6) interaction, and (7) generalization. These are not mutually exclusive elements nor are they sequential, but by giving each a separate identity we underline the importance of each in the intervention plan.

Theme

A thematic approach in intervention is one in which the parts of the intervention process both within a session and from session to session are united by having a central topic serve as the core around which procedures are structured. Themes are chosen on the basis of the interests of children at particular ages and those of the specific children that the intervention is serving. They provide a means to build language by continuous expansion of related concepts and vocabulary. Themes give cohesiveness to the overall intervention program and to the varied specific strategies used in each session and also relate the total program to its parts.

The theme concept can be applied to all ages with a slightly different interpretation. For very young children the themes are in essence topics that are of interest to the child. The child actually selects the topic or selects an activity or object around which a topic can develop. Because young children usually have central interests—boys may like play cars while girls may like dolls—the topics develop in a thematic fashion as the specific cars or dolls change. Linguistic expansion of simple themes can be through expansion of the vocabulary—cars, tires, hood, steer, drive, and so on; classification—cars, trucks, station wagons; experience—riding in a pick-up, exploring a fire truck, and so on. Topics lead to conversation, and conversation involves an interplay of linguistic, general cognitive, and social factors (Foster, 1984b). In this sense they become topics of conversation that can be defined as anything that is communicated jointly as a result of specific attention-getting and attention-directing activities.

Themes for children in the 4- to 6-year range may have a broader framework, such as animals, community helpers, or holidays. At an even higher level, the themes become more narrow in scope but at the same time have greater depth and details such as the study of butterflies, their metamorphosis, their classification, and so on.

In addition to the intervention activities that can be built into themes, such as events, scripts, and stories which will be described later, themes can also provide bulletin board material and field trip opportunities. A thematic approach is possible even in a setting where children are seen twice a week for 30 minutes. The excitement of learning about a topic of interest and the experience of sharing with others provided by themes is one way that the functional framework for intervention can be achieved.

Contexture

Each intervention plan and particularly each intervention session must have a contexture or fabric within which it proceeds. Intervention is not independent from its background or environment. I do not use the terms *background* and *environment* literally but to designate an operational mode that encompasses the act, process, and manner of intervention as well as the setting. The absence of this operational mode is itself a background. In this case intervention proceeds in a contextual vacuum.

One type of contexture can be a naturalistic one. With very young children, the naturalistic intervention approach is often recommended. Although many interpret naturalistic to be synonomous with play, group conversational interaction, and teaching in the home, I do not believe this interpretation is correct. Naturalistic for most young children is usually individual (with Mother) and egocentric—playing alone with limited interaction. Actually interactive, cooperative play does not begin to emerge until the child is well into language development about the age of 5 years (Garvey, 1974; Ratner & Bruner, 1978; Yawkey & Miller, 1984). Even at that age, conversational strategies are still developing. The essence of the naturalistic approach has to do with the act, process, and manner of relating to the child and the extent to which it and the objects and environment of this relationship resemble what he or she experiences in every day life. The communicative circumstances particularly should be natural (Cullata & Horn, 1982).

The term *structure* is often used as an opposite to naturalistic (as it was used in early chapters of this book), and in one sense this is true. With young children, the greater the structure and the more external control on their actions, the less naturalistic the situation, because most situations for young children are not structured. For older children, however, a structured environment, as in school, can be a naturalistic environment. Perhaps better terms for describing the opposite of naturalistic are *artificial* or *contrived*. An artificial situation is one in which the act, process, or manner of relating do not resemble what occurs in any aspect of daily living and hence have no functional or meaningful purpose. The artificial situation is not conducive to learning. The contexture may be naturalistic and/or structured, but not artificial.

Repetition of Input

I believe that one element of successful intervention is that of repetition of input. I am not referring here to drill. I define *repetition of input* as the frequent use of targets (syntactic, semantic, and pragmatic) within natural language contexts and in social or learning situations that illustrate their social and cognitive meaning. Although in natural language situations it may appear in a particular instance that a child is repeating a word immediately after a parent says it, it is probable that many instances of parent repetition have preceded that utterance by the child.

Children want repetitious learning. I have sat in a waiting room next to a mother and her young child and watched as the child turns the pages of a magazine, points, says an unintelligible word, and looks to the mother for a label for the object. As far as the child is concerned, this activity can continue indefinitely. What is interesting is that the child requests labels for the same objects—over and over and over.

I believe that the frequent provision of language structure within meaningful pragmatic and semantic contexts is a necessary part of language learning, particularly for the development of language *comprehension*, and should take place before the child is expected to use the forms himself or herself. The repetition in varied contexts helps the child by providing many experiences and events that become part of his or her memory network of meanings (event structure representations) and sufficiently strong linguistic patterns to associate with the network of meaning. The three elements are essential—the accurate linguistic patterns, the meanings, to include specific lexical meanings as well as general world information, and the association between the two.

In trying to teach specific distinctions among lexical entries and to stabilize learning, the child's *production* of the linguistic structures may be more effective than input repetition. This is why modeling and related techniques are useful in teaching specific forms. But they cannot take the place of the general input to the child's system for providing him or her with the breadth of language and meaning that is needed. Language teaching should provide both general and specific language growth and both comprehension and expression strategies.

Repetition of input implies that the concern is more with verbal stimulation than verbal interaction. This is not true for the overall intervention plan. We must provide more opportunities for interaction than input time within the total plan. But we cannot neglect input completely—time given for input in as natural a format as possible will have a payoff. Interacting time is valuable in developing the child's spontaneous language and in the child's use of new words and structures. Both are needed.

When facilitating the acquisition of language by language-impaired children, it may be necessary to modify the input by increasing the saliency of certain aspects of the input over others so as to engage the child's awareness. The basic structure of the input structure is not changed; the critical element of that structure is put in a foreground position. The saliency of input may be increased by the following:

1. Changing the quality of the critical elements of the input. The intensity level or rate of occurrence of the stimulus may be changed (e.g., by sound amplification). Making the critical element softer or louder, slower or faster will draw the child's attention to that element. (Highly stressed words are more likely to be held in memory than unstressed words [Dodd & White, 1980]).
2. Increasing the frequency of occurrence of the critical element so that the child can distinguish between those features that are essential to the form and those that are variable. Frequency increase is best accomplished by structuring real situations that need verbal support.
3. Combining the linguistic or cognitive input with action—the child's action. If a verbal input accompanies an activity that the child is engaged in and enjoys, that verbal input will be endowed with saliency.
4. Providing markers for input—familiar sequences or routines that help a child cut in on the ongoing stream of language. These markers are signals to the child that something important is going to be said or done.
5. Decreasing the density of the input. A decrease in the amount of information provided in a unit of time or space helps a child focus on the critical elements of the input. Too many instructions or directions can overload the child.
6. Providing redundancy so that the same input is provided by more than one source.
7. Providing input simultaneously through different input modalities.
8. Pairing two different stimuli (form and content) in order to make their association a salient one.
9. Arranging linguistic input so that the target grammatical structure is essential to the comprehension of the utterance.
10. Presenting in groups, stimuli similar with respect to the rules by which each is governed—temporally juxtaposing them.

Because emphasis on input can imply to the clinician that he or she spend more time talking in intervention, certain cautions need to be listed: (1) repetitive input should take place within the natural framework of interactive structures; (2) the use of repetitive input is most necessary for the very young child who has not yet fully developed linguistic and nonlinguistic representation (although growth in language and meaning should continue throughout life); (3) there should be repetitive input as part of every intervention plan but not necessarily every intervention session and it should never predominate—if a plan covers a series of sessions, the amount of time given to input for specific language behaviors can be decreased with the last sessions devoted almost entirely to opportunities for the children's production; (4) repetitive input is most natural if provided within interactive structures familiar to the child such as play, events, and stories. The following section will describe these structures in greater detail.

Envelope

There are many structures that parents and teachers use as a means of interacting with and providing information to children. These structures allow exchanges to develop between the adult and child via a third device such as a game or a story. They permit indirect communication, which is a better mode of eliciting language than the direct approach. The structures can be viewed as envelopes or frames within which learning can take place. Social and linguistic aspects of communication are integral to each envelope, although the envelopes differ from each other with respect to basic characteristics. Following is a description of the major types of envelopes with reference to their use in intervention:

Routines. There are numerous types of routines that parents use and consequently in which the child participates during the early stages of communication. These routines may pertain to activities of daily life that become almost ritualized by unvarying procedures and language formulas. They include routines involved in activities such as getting dressed or going to bed. There are also routines associated with the early social exchange games such as peek-a-boo and patty-cake (Ratner & Bruner, 1978). The latter play routines are believed by Ratner and Bruner to give assistance to the child in the mastery of language forms in the following ways: (1) by limiting the semantic domain in which utterances are to be used and making it familiar; (2) by providing a predictable task structure and sequence and clear boundaries that permit insertion of intelligible utterances; (3) by encouraging the reversible role relationships between speaker and hearer; and (4) by providing a playful atmosphere that allows the child to separate or distance himself or herself from the task and therefore to be ready to innovate.

As with other types of envelopes, such as scripts, routines provide a framework for sequences of joint attention and action between the child and another person. Snyder-McLean, Solomonson, McLean, and Sack (1984) define a joint action routine as follows: "a ritualized interaction pattern, involving joint action, unified by a specific theme or goal, which follows a logical sequence, including a clear beginning point, and in which each participant plays a recognized role, with specific response expectancies that is essential to the successful completion of that sequence" (p. 214). These authors suggest that joint routines are useful in intervention in the home and in the classroom. The success of routines appeared to be related to the routine's ability to engage the interest and motivation of the child, to contain a unifying theme, to limit and clearly define the roles involved and allow for role reversibility, to include predictable nonarbitrary sequences as well as sequences for turn-taking, and to provide for planned repetition and controlled variation (Snyder-McLean et al., 1984).

Once routines become sufficiently elaborate to include the criteria just listed, they can probably be described as event structures, a type of structure that will be discussed later. Event structures do not necessarily include the prerequisite of unvarying action and word formulas. They can be routinized but do not need to be so.

Routines are particularly useful in the early stages of language development in which children need the scaffolding provided by the internalized language patterns associated with specific actions and things. I believe they are of special value in the development and expansion of syntax—word order, grammatical morphemes, and so on—and pragmatics. Once the child has mastery over basic syntactic forms, other envelopes such as event structure and dramatic play may be more useful in the development and expansion of word meaning.

Story-Reading. Story-reading can be treated as a type of routine, but one which the child can practice without need for a partner. This activity requires the clinician to select a series of pictures depicting persons (or animals) involved in a sequence of actions. Published picture books that tell a story can be used for this purpose. Beneath each picture the clinician writes words, phrases, or sentences that together make a story. The language should include those sentence frames that will help the child develop the scaffold in which to insert new forms. The story is read to the child two or three times and then the child is allowed to participate by (1) turning the page at the appropriate time; (2) filling in words at appropriate places; and (3) at the point where the child is able, by saying the entire text for each page. The child can "practice" by using an audio tape recording of the story. New stories and new language patterns can be added gradually to his or her repertoire of stories.

The use of stories for this purpose is different from the use of stories for learning the parts of the narrative or other structures. Story-reading has a very particular purpose, one that is similar to that of routines and so is most useful in the developmental stages of language, between 2 and 5 years of age. It has an advantage of allowing the child to take the book home and "read" to his or her parents. The fact that the child memorized the words on each page does not concern me. I believe that the internalization of written language should first be experienced in frames or patterns, and story-reading can provide these patterns, particularly if the stories change routinely. Another advantage to story-reading is that it can be used as a supplementary or supportive tool in intervention—one that provides practice in early language.

Play. Just as routines and story-reading are conducive to the development of syntax and early pragmatic exchanges, play is particularly suited to the improvement of conversation and interactional development. There are many kinds of play—formal and informal, pretend and realistic, social and nonsocial, rule-based and nonstructured. Each has special uses in the development of language. Routines are a form of structured play, although not all play is routinized. Rule-based games are also a form of play. Each type has its unique characteristics and therefore serves different purposes in language.

In routines, the verbal and action rituals encourage joint action and joint attention. In play, joint action and attention can be a stimulus to verbal interaction. With young children, such joint action—such as playing with trucks and cars—may not lead immediately to verbal interaction. Children often go through stages of nonsocial play and parallel play (nonverbal imitations) before engaging in any type of social interactive play (De Maio, 1984). De Maio suggests approaching each child at his or her level of play in order to create a comfortable environment and then gradually advancing the level of play. As mature play forms, the receptive and expressive language abilities of children advance, although the relation between language and play changes as a function of the demands of the play task and the developmental stage of the child (Roth & Clark, 1987). In working with language-impaired children, the clinician needs to be aware that these children may not exhibit the same type of stages in play as nonimpaired children (Terell, Schwartz, Prelock, & Messick, 1984; Roth & Clark, 1987) and this needs to be accounted for in intervention.

Of particular concern in using play in intervention is the need for defining a particular purpose and structure for its use. The environment of play is a natural one for the child and therefore can be very useful in the development of interaction and communication skills such as turn-taking, directing others, following rules, and giving information. However, it will be of limited value unless there is careful planning. It is also important to make sure that the level of play and the level of language are similar; otherwise the use of play will not be effective.

The procedures for using play in intervention are actually inherent in the skills of a clinician to be a good language partner for the child, to know when to speak and when not to, and to understand what he or she must do or not do to encourage the development of interaction and conversation. (These skills were described in a previous section of this chapter.) This implies that the clinician must learn how to interact and to structure his or her own responses while preserving the naturally occurring conversational demands in a play situation for the child (Craig, 1983).

Event Structure. Although in other literature the preceding envelopes have been classified under event structures (Duchan & Weitzner-Lin, 1987), I find it useful to give the term *event structure* a very specific characterization, one based on the work of Nelson and her colleagues (Nelson, 1986a). Events, as described by Nelson (1986b), involve people in purposeful activites—acting on objects and interacting with each other for the accomplishment of a goal. The event, for example, of grocery shopping is bounded by goal-defined activities and therefore does not include preparing the meal. The events are dynamic, holistic structures having internal variation; they proceed in a temporal-causal sequence and are hierarchically organized—embedded in each event are smaller segments of activities.

Nelson suggests that the kinds of mental representation that serve as content on which the cognitive processes operate are event representations, which are similar to the schema described in Chapter 7. Schemata were defined as generalized concepts that underlie situations, objects, events and actions, and sequences of actions and events. The generalized concepts that form a schema and the representation of events are similar constructs. Event representation appears to be a type of schema.

Event representations change with time as the child experiences more episodes of the event and analyzes these to yield more abstract cognitive structures. The abstractions allow the child to construct novel representations of events and other novel classifications (Nelson, 1986b). Events are the primary source of world knowledge for young children. Older children may learn through other means, such as narratives or instruction.

Events are differentiated from scripts (Nelson & Gruendel, 1986). Scripts specify the actors' actions and props; the script is made up of slots and specifies who or what can fill the slots (Nelson, 1986b). Scripts are general structures and as such may be a type of general event. Events and scripts may be used to designate one episode or specific occurrence, but the resulting structure in script knowledge is expected to apply to all episodes of that event. Both scripts and events are represented in children's memory; the general event representation may not correspond with the script itself, however. A scripted event has strong temporally invariant structure—getting dressed and eating lunch are typical. According to Nelson, scripts integrate knowledge about objects and their relations with knowledge about the world of people and their interactions together with verbal knowledge. Nelson says that scripts are learned; they are the product of experience.

Events and episodes are also different. A child experiences an episode of an event. He or she may have a memory for an episode but has a schema for an event. Single episodes are not sufficient for an event representation to be acquired. Episodes that are exactly alike do not permit the generalization of the essential aspects of the events; generalization occurs only if the episodes occur in varying conditions. The event structure is a generalization from many and varied episodes.

Event structures and routines also differ. Routines are unvarying rituals involving activities and/or language—the particular manner in which something is accomplished. Event structure refers to an internal representation of activities and episodes that have similar functions and goals and that include all essential aspects of these events. The general event structure representation, which includes verbal scripts, are the "old knowledge" that serves as a scaffold for new knowledge.

To form accurate general event representations, a child must experience numerous episodes of a particular event. The development of representation may begin with general scripts that are gradually filled in with detail, or a script might begin with the assembling of details and become more abstract with experiences. Scripts develop as a function of both increasing age and increasing experience with an event (Fivush & Slackman, 1986).

Event structure representation appears to be a valid description of the way in which the child learns about the world and about language. Scripts contain cognitive, linguistic, and social data, which are internalized in an integrated fashion as the elements of episodes are abstracted to form event structures. An intervention approach using episodes to develop scripts about activities in which children engage might have a significant impact on the development of language.

The intervention plan might be constructed around the development of event structures (see also Van Kleeck & Richardson, in press). Episodes of events—to include the actors, actions, props, and verbal scripts—can be repeatedly experienced by the children. For young children the episodes might be of basic functions such as dressing or eating. Children in the late nursery and kindergarten years can experience such events as birthday parties, eating at a fast-food restaurant, or going to the grocery story. Young school-age children can experience eating out or going to the post office and buying stamps. The experiences for older children can be simulated. With older children, the episodes can also be narrower in scope but have greater depth. Episodes can be developed around a general theme of animals, while specifically addressing narrow topics such as the metamorphosis of the butterfly or taking care of a pet fish. With young children the verbal script may be more consistent from episode to episode than that used with older children. The number of episodes needed to establish the event structure representation will also decrease with age.

The use of events in intervention implies that the clinician and children engage in some kind of action or sequences of actions that can be engaged in naturally, are of interest to the child, and can be repeated. Developing a session around "circus" is not an example of an event. "Circus" can be the theme of a series of lessons. A related event can be for the children to paint clown faces (on themselves) and dress in a clown suit.

As the children are learning the scripts for an event, they can participate in the episodes in different ways. At first the clinician provides most of the verbal script. Gradually the emphasis shifts to the children, so in subsequent episodes the children can play different roles. For example, in a restaurant script, one child can be the waiter, another the mother, another the child, another the cashier, and so on. Essential parts of the script can be identified and made salient by the teacher who asks questions about the roles and what each actor says.

A way of developing role reversal can be through the use of a video recorded episode of, for example, a restaurant event. The sound track for a particular role can be eliminated and the children, as a group or in turn, can fill in what the child on the tape says. The same can be done for other roles in the tape.

Specific language behaviors can be targeted within the procedures for developing event structure representation. The episode itself can be selected to give new experiences to the children. New vocabulary can be chosen for use within each episode and will contine to be used from episode to episode throughout the development of the event. Syntactic structures that target forms at a stage higher than that used by the child can be provided in the episodes' verbal script. Because the basic words and sentence structure are scripted for consistency from episode to episode, both will be learned with in a meaningful context.

The pragmatic aspects of language are the goal and primary activity of event structure development. The three aspects of language—syntax, semantics, and pragmatics—are therefore learned within an integrated framework. Events can be chosen to provide experiences in using more complex language skills—in solving problems (What shall we do with the fish while we are washing his bowl?), in providing information (Where is the nearest fast-food restaurant?), in sharing feelings (How did you feel at the birthday party?), to plan the future (Let's decide what we will make tomorrow), and so on.

Narratives. In the early section of this chapter, narratives were listed as one of the aspects of language that need to be included in the content of intervention, particularly in the school setting. Because considerable classroom time is given to narration of one form or other, children need to learn about story grammar and to formulate and comprehend stories. Narratives can also be a means of developing other aspects of language such as vocabulary, syntax, cohesion, inference, and figurative language. They can also be a means of integrating oral and written language and comprehension and expression. In this sense, narratives can be envelopes through which vicarious experiences can provide episodes of events.

Through narratives children can take the role of another person and express ideas that they may not be able to express for themselves as speaker. The narrative also teaches about linking ideas and the words through which these ideas are linked; it teaches about setting and characters, about central themes and sequences of events and about arriving at conclusions. Just as routines provide a means for internalizing sentences in wholes for later analysis by a child, narratives, if listened to or expressed frequently, can help a child abstract and understand the basic grammar of narration. This in turn will provide the foundations for writing.

Once a child understands the basic structure of narratives—their grammar—comprehension and production is made easier. In comprehension, knowledge of the structure permits the listener or reader to attend to the information presented rather than the framework on which the story is developed and even to predict unknown or missing information (Gordon & Braun, 1983). In writing or speaking, if the structural components of the story have been internalized by the child and their use is automatic, the child can attend to the novel aspects of the story and its execution.

The use of narratives as a means of language improvement can begin as early as the first grade. Although the complexity of the story, the vocabulary, and the number of story components used increases with increasing age (Klecan-Aker & Swank, 1987), it is possible to utilize storytelling or retelling with young school children.

The first step in using narratives as a means of instruction is to develop the child's ability to tell stories—to teach the story grammar. The best method is for the child to be frequently exposed to story-reading and storytelling both at home and at school. Some of the techniques suggested under story-reading in this chapter can be expanded for use in developing narrative ability. The child's narrative skills can be strengthened through questions by the adult. Questions directed at information that is communicated by the story grammar will cause the child to attend to those aspects of the story and will help in its reconstruction (Page & Stewart, 1985). Another way to develop storytelling ability is to first provide an experience, then make a list of questions to guide the retelling of the experience.

With young children, an experience can be broken down by photos taken during the event showing the sequences involved in the event—or each child in a group of children is asked to draw one aspect of the event. The photos or pictures are then used as stimuli for recalling the experience for one child to tell the entire story or for each child to tell one part. After each part is presented, the other children add details or vocabulary that they believe are necessary. Together, the group constructs the story. Reasons given for including or excluding information will become part of the learning process.

Galda (1984) suggests using dramatic play as a way of improving story interpretation and the memory for story sequences. Dramatic play provides props, role reversals, and peer interaction, which in turn highlight multiple aspects of persons, objects, and situations and thus engage the cognitive system. In a comparison of story interpretation through dramatic play, discussion, and drawing, kindergarten and first-grade children in the play condition scored significantly higher than those in the discussion condition. The drawing condition showed the least effect on performance. These differences were not found with second-grade children, although the second graders who "played" about the story retold qualitatively richer stories (Galda, 1984).

To bring the children's inferencing and creative abilities into play, a part of the story can be changed hypothetically and the children asked questions regarding the consequences of such a change. This change directs attention to cause/effect relationships that Page and Stewart (1985) believe are important in storytelling. Actually, unless the children understand the relationship among the parts of the event, the story itself will not be cohesive and sequential. In order for children to use stories to learn, they need first to have sufficient world knowledge and knowledge of story structure to understand them.

As with other types of intervention, use of narratives should ultimately have a functional purpose. Stories should be practiced for telling to other classes or parents; stories should be written for publication in a class newsletter. Finding an audience for the story is as important as finding a listener in conversation. Through storytelling and writing, students can learn pragmatic conventions and audience awareness as well as having an effective vehicle for integrating new knowledge with old. Skills of restating, recasting, and inventing are brought into play (Beach & Bridwell, 1984). In fact, the narrative approach can integrate numerous aspects of language: comprehension and expression, knowledge and performance, oral and written language and syntax, semantics, and pragmatics.

Dramatic Play. Dramatic play is used with young children by having them assume roles that reflect the real world, imitating the players' actual experience through actions and verbalization, by engaging in a fantasy play of their own creation or by participating in a play created by someone else (Galda, 1984). Any one of these activities provides for the child a means of using language in unique ways. Learning a script that includes the words and sentences that have been generated by someone else provides the child with the opportunity to use utterances that are novel and that may become a source of expansion of his or her own language skills.

Plays written by the clinician are helpful in stabilizing newly learned language skills. The dialogue of the play can be written to include the target structures for each child's part—syntactic, semantic, or pragmatic—in appropriate functional situations in the drama.

Discourse. The learning of discourse skills is one of the goals of intervention. But, as is true of narration, discourse or conversation can be used as a means to help the child develop other language skills (MacDonald & Gillette, 1984). In fact, one of the reasons that children have difficulty with discourse is their difficulty with asking and answering questions, repairs, failure to request clarification, and other deficits.

Moeller, Osberger, and Eccarius (1986) describe a method of developing skills essential to discourse processing in which semantic content, semantic complexity, context, and function are manipulated to provide increasing difficulty. They describe the following stages:

Stage 1: Through modeling (use of a third person) and use of multiple choice alternatives ("Do you want pop? Yes or no?") and using high interest materials, the focus of intervention is on establishing yes/no responses to questions.

Stage 2: Yes/no questions are used to prompt responses to *wh-* questions (*What is the boat made of? Is it made of metal?*")

Stage 3: The use of strength in reading is used to transfer to discourse situations. The printed questions and answers are matched.

Stage 4: *Wh-* forms having varied functions are used in conversation, at first with context support, then with reduced context support.

Stage 5: The semantic abstraction of targeted question forms is emphasized.

Practice

Just as is true of repetition earlier described, the word *practice* is often interpreted to mean drill, and that is unfortunate. There are few behaviors that we acquire that do not need to be practiced before mastering them. This certainly is true of language behaviors. But the manner of practice does not have to be artificial drill. Actually, some of the envelopes described in the previous section can be modified and used to provide practice for the child.

Although I believe practice should be part of every intervention plan, it does not need to be included in every intervention session. With young children, particularly, who need considerable input of a broad kind, the practice period for specific language skills may take place after

---

Quote 15–4
The intervention teaching process is interactive and involves, at some level, a form of metacognitive and/or metalinguistic awareness. This awareness, as stated before, may manifest itself with respect to either the child or the teacher. In either event, it exists as a part of the deliberate act of teaching and learning.
(KRETSCHMER, 1984, p. 221).

---

four or five intervention sessions. Routines, story-reading, and dramatic play can provide valuable practice experiences.

Older children probably need less practice than the younger child because they have already mastered the basic language skills and they have learned how to learn. Adolescents need to expand their experiences with language to provide them with the knowledge and skills needed in social and classroom situations. With these students, the knowing about and doing are part of the same process! On the one hand, instruction may be more direct and didactic, but on the other hand, the application to functional use occurs more quickly and can be monitored more easily than that with younger children.

Throughout my years of teaching I have believed that the accuracy, fluency, complexity, and richness of language are directly affected by the degree and level to which it is used in production, not only novel production, but also memorized production. Recitation of prose passages that utilize words and structures not in the repertoire of the speaker provides the scaffold for language growth. Writing can also be developed by memorizing passages that are then written. This process helps the learner to internalize the frames or slots for the insertion of novel words and phrases. Gradually the structures become the child's own and can be used interchangeably in novel constructions.

Interaction

The sixth component of an intervention plan is that of providing an opportunity for natural interaction in which the language that has been learned can be used in a functional manner. Although interaction should be an ongoing process throughout intervention, special time should be given for a child to converse with his or her peers (Fey, Leonard, & Wilcox, 1986). These interaction situations can be open to allow for free expression or can be structured to permit the clinician to plan for the use of specific language skills. Once the child is aware of his or her own purpose and can monitor his or her conversational skills, use repair strategies, and so on, the child is most likely to benefit from a free conversational situation.

Roth and Spekman (1984b) described structured communication tasks for assessment that I believe would be of value in intervention:

1. Use a referential communication task in which one child (the speaker) is responsible for describing something (pictures, geometric shapes) so that partner (listener) can either select the object described or construct the pattern.
   a. Alter communication roles—the speaker becomes the listener.
   b. Manipulate the topic of conversation by introducing different materials or problem-solving activities.
   c. Vary communication partners with respect to age, cognitive level, status, and other factors.
   d. Vary the channels available for communication comprehension. Provide barriers so that only part of the feed-in information is available.
2. Have the child retell a story, describe the location of an object, and so on.

Fey, Leonard, and Wilcox (1986) support the inclusion of relatively unstructured periods in intervention in which the language-impaired child can interact freely with children of similar or lower ages and linguistic skills. They believe that situations that are less constraining lead to more active participation by the child and therefore opportunities for practice are optimized.

Generalization

Whatever method is used, the focus of the intervention should be on the child, his or her needs, interests, and natural contexts for learning. This will be the primary factor in generalization. In each approach, there should be and usually is provision made for stabilization and generalization of new learning. For the goal of intervention of whatever kind is to have a child use effectively a new language skill, grammatical form, or whatever is taught in the setting where it is appropriate. In a purely naturalistic setting, responses are stabilized by the amount of input to the child and the number of opportunities the child has for using a behavior before it is mastered. In more structured settings, some attempt is made to provide direct opportunities for response stabilization. The following descriptions of generalization principles illustrate the relationship between the instructional components and those of generalization. The overlap shows that activities can serve multi-functions. A description of stabilization and generalization principles will serve as a summary of the ideas presented as components of an intervention lesson:

Response Repetition. Whether it is accomplished in a naturalistic setting or it is planned, repetition is considered necessary for the generalization and mastery of a behavior. Even if one considers

---

Quote 15–5
One of the main messages from the strategy training literature is to train explicitly for generalization rather than training only for strategy acquisitions . . .
Moreover, the value and purpose of generalizing trained strategies are explicitly discussed with the learner.
(Ryan, Ledger, Short, & Weed, 1982, p. 57).

---

language to be knowledge of rules only, it is necessary to "practice" language so that the use of the rules becomes automatic and can easily be modified to serve the variable situations that make variable demands on the generating mechanism. Practice provides the child with routines or envelopes of structure that can be used as a format for new information.

Repetition has greater applicability to the improvement of the production of language as contrasted with its comprehension. The old adage "You learn to do by doing" applies here. The child will never learn to talk if he or she does not talk. We need to recognize that repetition is best accomplished within a framework of as normal a communicative setting as possible and not in the form of drills. Practice for practice's sake will not suffice: it must serve a personal goal or intention so as to bind the elements of practice with the functionality of language (Cazden, 1973). A creative clinician can accomplish this by integrating formal techniques in a less formal situation.

Response Evaluation. Regardless of whether it is done consciously, the stabilization of a new behavior, except at early developmental stages, involves the process of self-evaluation and self-correction. To encourage this behavior, children must be aware of the specific and general goals specialists have for them (and hopefully they have for themselves). This requires a high level of metalinguistic skills. To do this, the child needs two kinds of exemplars, those associated with the target form and those not associated with it (red and not red). In this way the distinctive features of the target can be clearly identified. The child's awareness of a target structure and its context will help him or her to anticipate the occurrence of the structure in spontaneous speech and "correct" the error even before it is uttered.

Response Cohesiveness. Response-oriented approaches will have the greatest impact on the child's generalization and mastery of a target if the responses are tied together both with respect to content as well as to structure. As discussed in the previous section, grouping concepts or forms to be learned around a central theme will assist the learner in retaining and stabilizing them, particularly core concepts with which the child is familiar. Those of us who spent early years in the elementary

> *Quote 15–6*
> *Blind strategy training involves instructions concerning the use of the target strategy and often leads to improvements, which disappear when instructional prompts are removed. Informed training supplements specific strategy directions with explanations to the learner about why the strategy is useful and about the benefits one can expect to follow from its use. Self-instructional training goes beyond informed training by providing explicit guidance in self-monitoring skills, such as how to define one's goals in concrete terms, select a strategy, monitor its use, eevaluate its outcome, reinforce oneself for successes, and cope with failure.*
>
> (RYAN, LEDGER, SHORT, & WEED, 1982, p. 56).

classroom know the value of "units" of study. This type of situation corresponds with the tenets of pragmatic theory.

Response Variation. An effective way of ensuring stabilization and generalization (or, if one wishes, mastery) is to provide within the framework of intervention, variation in the context of input and response. The variations assist the child in discovering the invariant aspects and distinctive features of things. Rules are more accurately induced if the exemplars represent the full gamut of linguistic and context variations. Such variation can be provided by variations in topic, situations, and materials.

Response Automaticity. The importance of automaticity is related both to the theoretical position of language as knowledge of rules and to the position of language as both rule knowledge (linguistic theory) and performance efficiency (cognitive organization theory). It is important to generate language from rules in an automatic manner as well as to use the performance system rapidly and with ease so as to free the language formulation system from attentions to detail in language production. As the child communicates under conditions of excitement or other emotion, he or she will need to attend to the total communication experience rather than concentrate on the form. If situations are provided where the child gets involved in communication, he or she will be more likely to carry-over the newly-learned language than if the child is a mere passive responder. I can still recall the peals of laughter that would come from a therapy room where a clinician and the client were engaged in a competition to see who could talk the longest without making an error. The excitement and energy that went into the effort placed the child in as difficult a language situation as he or she would find anywhere. The use of his or her target structure became automatic quickly.

Response Reinforcement. Knowing an abstract rule does not ensure that it can be used accurately at all times. Again, the distinction be-

> *Quote 15–7*
> There are a number of reasons why the success a clinician seems to have in a controlled therapy situation may not transfer to the natural environment. In some instances, it is enough to observe that the behavior required in the two situations is radically different. . . The problem is not that the child hasn't generalized. Rather, what he has learned is simply not what he is now required to perform.
>
> (SPRADLIN & SIEGEL, 1982, p. 5).

tween knowing rules and performing them needs to be made if we are to encourage mastery in performance. Mastery is aided by refinement of the contexts in which rules are used, and refinement occurs when a rule is performed efficiently in numerous contexts. The repeated use of target rules will occur in situations where a child is motivated to speak. Reinforcement helps in providing this motivation. Although behavior theory is responsible for directing attention to a specific kind of reinforcement and this theory uses a high degree of structure in this task, I believe that all intervention should incorporate, to some degree, the concept of reinforcement for stabilization. Only those committed to the view that language change is totally a function of the child's action on the environment will ignore the need to have at least the natural reinforcers in the environment. In pragmatic theory, reinforcement is provided by the success of the communication act, for example, the understanding of the listener and his or her response. However, response of any kind by the environment—expansion, correction, feedback, action—is a form of reinforcement. Feedback (as in answering a question or commenting on a statement, not just saying "Good!"), in my opinion, is essential as a form of increasing awareness and shaping the correct response. Gibson (1971) believes that the reduction of uncertainty is reinforcement for all cognitive learning. She states that discovery of structure or an economical distinctive feature of a rule that describes an invariant reduces the "information load" and decreases the search for invariance. This is why, she states, that the desire to understand what others are saying appears to be basic for learning to comprehend language. Obviously, if a child has difficulty in discovering the structure, distinctive feature, or rule, that child will not have the reduction of uncertainty and the natural reinforcement. Formal reinforcement strategies and schedules, such as reward or payoff, may be helpful in certain situations with severely impaired children whose system is so deficient that the normal motivating methods are ineffective.

Linguistic Specificity. Warren and Kaiser (1986a) found that subjects failed to generalize forms that were longer than the subjects' typical sentences and those that contained adjective modifiers that the subjects may have found nonfunctional in free play. In general, generalization was related to the syntactic complexity of the target utterance relative to the subjects' current production and the functionality of the form in relation to the condition of the generalization setting.

One assumes that given the opportunity for using a behavior, there will be generalization of it, that is, performance using a particular linguistic behavior taught in a particular context will generalize to other linguistic contexts or other forms. In theoretical approaches that accept structure in intervention, there is a provision for generalization. This is done by providing varied situational opportunities for applications, by varying the linguistic contexts in which a desired form is embedded, by providing experiences in a variety of interactional situations—with different persons. Even with some structure, however, generalization occurs more naturally in intervention settings that replicate contexts that occur in everyday life. Some opportunities for language use in a naturalistic setting should be provided with any intervention approach.

The need for including generalization activities in intervention is as important for rule development as it is for accuracy of performance. The contexts in which rules occur are variable and therefore can be either under- or overextended. Hence the need to provide opportunities for generalizing.

PLANNING INTERVENTION

Reviewing and understanding the literature in intervention is a relatively easy task for the clinician compared with integrating it into a plan for action. The process of intervention is a dynamic one that is influenced by many variables. Clinicians cannot expect to be effective without spending considerable time in preparation. As many years as I have been engaged in intervention and teaching, I still spend significant amounts of time preparing for each session.

In this section, I will describe some planning procedures that have been helpful to me. As I pointed out in the previous chapter, every clinician differs not only with respect to theoretical positions, but also with respect to assumptions about intervention and style of intervening. There is no recipe for intervention. But for those who are still struggling with the whole process, a few suggestions may be of assistance. I discuss these with the caution that they should be modified and adapted to the clinician's situation. The clinician might only find aspects of them of value.

General and Specific Objectives

The process of planning is facilitated if an overall plan for a designated period is designed before planning specific units or sessions. If a child participates in an intervention session twice a week, I would design an overall plan for a semester—3 or 4 months—to include smaller units of 4-week periods. The overall plan would list *general objectives* or goals (written as outcomes, if desired) in the major areas of language: cognitive, pragmatic, semantic, and syntactic. These objectives would be group objectives (if a group is used) of the language improvement type, designed for children at the age level of the children in the group. Such objectives for a 7-year-old group might be as follows (see Table 15–1 for age-related data):

Cognitive

1. The children will recognize and describe animals and objects in terms of their multiple properties and functions.
2. Using cause-effect strategies and inference, the children will predict the next step in a sequence of events.
3. The children will develop distancing behavior—separate themselves in space and time from the ongoing observable field by evaluating consequences, proposing alternatives, and so on. (Sigel & McGillicuddy-Delise, 1984).

Pragmatic

1. The children will delay their verbal response or reaction until time for their turn.
2. The children will adjust language to fit the roles of a listener.
3. The children will respond to probe questions and recall the essential parts of a story.
4. The children will tell a story using the story grammar suitable for their age.

Semantic

1. The children will learn to understand and use advanced words that describe size, shape, quality, attitudes. (These can be specifically identified by review of the reader and speller for the grade level.)
2. The children will learn words that aid in providing cohesion to narratives—after, before, when, if.

Syntactic

1. The children will understand and use complex sentences.
2. The children will understand and use active/passive voice and direct/indirect object in sentences.

3. The children will use and respond to questions of the basic type: who, what, how, how many, etc.
4. The children will understand and use personal and demonstrative pronouns.

Some of these general objectives will be addressed in each of the individual lessons. All of them will be covered at some time during the semester. There will be no way of evaluating the extent of general learning for each child, but some idea of growth will be evident if some preliminary estimate of performance is gathered. The direct focus of intervention may need to be shifted up or down depending on the child's ability in each area.

Specific objectives for each of the areas (cognitive, pragmatic, etc.) should be developed for each child in terms of his or her needs. These specific objectives will identify particular skills that each child needs to develop. They may be within the framework of the general objectives or at a much lower level. (If the overall level of a child is below the general level for his or her age, that child should not be in the group.) Perhaps one child needs to improve plural formation in syntax and basic turn-taking skills in pragmatics and another child confuses pronouns, does not understand or use past tense, and cannot answer simple where, who, and what questions. Objectives for these skills need to be specified. Once both general and specific objectives are identified, both can be written into the lessons.

The overall plan should include the selected theme to be used for the semester as well as the subthemes for the 4-week units. For the age level in the example presented here, the overall theme could be on pets or animals. Unit themes could be, for example, caring for a fish, caring for a bird, or caring for a dog. The themes to be chosen should lend themselves to involvement and action within an intervention setting. If a unit is on taking care of a horse, it would difficult to think of functional activities that could be carried out in a room.

Planning a Unit

The unit plan that contains eight lessons more or less should be planned in terms of lesson emphases. For example, the first lessons could focus primarily on verbal and experiential input, using a form of tightly scripted event structures and permitting role reversals in event presentation. The next three lessons could emphasize related activities to include storytelling and retelling, group story-writing, dramatic play, or any other functional activity that provides practice in a variety of circumstances and therefore stabilizes and generalizes. The last two lessons can be devoted to field trips, conversation sessions, communicating experiences, and any other type of interaction that permits the children to use newly learned skills in an informal setting.

Throughout the entire eight lessons, the specific needs of the children could be built in. These targets—semantic and syntactic—could be specifically written into the script of the event structure, in the stories, and in the plays. The pragmatic targets could be built into the interactive opportunities that are associated with these envelopes for instruction. There should never be a time when the clinician is not modeling, expanding, and so forth as the need arises. The clinician's awareness of each child's needs should be such that opportunities that arise are never ignored.

Each unit should contain also those aspects of the semantic, syntactic, and pragmatic skills contained in the overall plan that will be emphasized in that unit. These skills can be distributed among the lessons in the unit, some lessons concentrating on semantics, others on pragmatics, and so on. But together, they will form a cohesive whole. Once a decision is made regarding what is to be included in each session, the actual planning of a lesson is facilitated.

Planning the Lesson

The individual lesson should include the specific objectives for the session, the topic, the content, the materials that will be used, the envelope of instruction for input, the specific sequence of procedures, the related activites for practice, supplementary materials, or activities for generalization.

For example, the first lesson on a unit called "Caring For Fish" might have as its specific topic, "Cleaning the Fishbowl." The goals for the first lesson might be to provide an experience in the form of an episode of an event (envelope) that is tightly scripted—props, action, and actors—and to have the children learn the script. Within this tight script, the clinician includes child-determined vocabulary, syntax, and pragmatic targets that have been selected from the overall plan, as well as the general ones for language enrichment.

The *procedures* can begin with the clinician first talking about fish and how they need care in feeding and in keeping their environment clean. At this point, the children will probably want to share their experiences with fish or fishing. Then the clinician says, "Today we are going to clean the fishbowl." Subsequently he or she goes through the tight script in which specific sentences are used to describe a five-stage sequence in cleaning the fish bowl. A child can be chosen to help with each stage of the cleaning process. Once the activity has been completed, the clinician asks: "What did I do *first*? What did I do *next*?"

Other steps might be to have the children identify the next activity in the sequence of events and have the children answer who and what questions regarding the episode, to predict the effects of changing the sequence in any of a number of ways by responding to questions beginning with *if*, or *what if*, or *when this—then what happens*, and so on, and to have each child describe one event in the series of events in the episode and, if possible, to have one child assume the role of the teacher and run through the episode and questions again. From there, each child can take a turn as teacher. The children can monitor the script provided by each child.

Within the framework of these procedures, the clinician can emphasize the targets for specific children. He or he can ask for words for describing the properties of the fish, such as long, flat, quick, slippery, and colorful. The clinician's questions can be worded so as to elicit past tense —"what did we do first?" He or she can emphasize taking turns at answering and taking turns at being teacher. Gradually the children will take over monitoring the group and in subsequent lessons the activities will center on the children instead of the teacher.

In the next lessons the clinician reviews the episode, particularly if all the children did not have a turn as teacher. Then, a good follow-up might be to read the children a fish story (an original one could include targeted forms, words, and behavior) and have individuals retell it again reviewing what happened first, second, next, and so on in the story. Or the group could develop a story with the fish being the main character— how he felt while his bowl was being cleaned. Each child could take a turn at contributing to the story. The children could be asked to look for a picture of a fish and then describe it for the class. The fish pictures can then be classified by fish type, color, size, or whatever category is suggested by the children.

Since the children at 7 years of age have begun to read, the names of different fish could be learned. To make this fun for the children, names of fish printed on cards that have an attached paper clip could be placed in a bowl. The children can go fishing by placing a magnet at the end of a string that is attached to a rod and using that to "catch" the fish. A form of the "barrier" games can be used in this activity—instead of the names of the fish, the pictures of different fish can be put in the fishbowl and each child describes what he or she has caught. The other children must identify the correct fish on the basis of the description alone. To build on the children's imagination and creativity, each child could be asked to tell a "fish story" (explain the nonliteral meaning). It can be funny and full of make-believe. This provides an opportunity for considerable interaction among the children. The fish story can be open-ended or the clinician can have requirements: certain words need to be used (write them on chalkboard) or it must be told as if it happened in the past.

At some point toward the end of the eight-lesson period the children could be taken on a field trip—to an aquarium, a marine-world park, or even a fishing hole. This can provide a source of review of everything that has been studied in the unit. Snapshots of the field trip can be an additional means of sequencing, using past tense, taking turns, and emphasizing all the targeted behaviors. Such experiences also provide a valuable means for conversational interaction among the children.

The clinician cannot forget the goals of each lesson and each activity. He or she should constantly evaluate the activity in terms of the goals. The children should also know what the objectives are for the group and for themselves. They should know what they are working on. I have asked children in intervention sessions what they are learning, and many of them have not been able to tell me. As the children get older, the goals should be more explicit, particularly if less didactic methods of intervention are used.

Clinicians might ask how they can possibly plan in such detail for all the groups with which they work. I suggest that clinicians work together to develop the scaffold—the envelopes and activities, the themes, and the units that can be used at the different age levels. Published stories and plays can be found or original ones written, and pictures can be shared. The script that needs to be designed for each child in each group can be added by the clinician.

The suggestions provided here are just that—suggestions. These will not fit every clinician or every session and certainly not every age. The format for younger and older children will be adapted to their environment and needs. But what a format like the one described above does do is provide for language learning in an integrated way as it integrates the many components of language—comprehension/expression, knowledge/performance, cognition/pragmatics/semantics/syntax, and oral/written language.

REFERENCES

LANGUAGE THEORIES

General Language Theory

Craig, H. K. (1983). Applications of pragmatic language models for intervention. In T. M. Gallagher, & C. A. Prutting (Eds.), *Pragmatic assessment and intervention issues in language* (pp. 101–127). San Diego, CA: College-Hill Press.

Dale, P. S. (1976). *Language development, structure and function.* New York: Holt, Rinehart and Winston.

Johnston, J. R. (1978). Language disorders: What are they and who has them? Mini-seminar presented at ASHA Convention. San Francisco.

Johnston, J. R. (1983). What is language intervention: The role of theory. In J. Miller, D. E. Yoder, & R. Schiefelbusch (Eds.), *Contemporary issues in language intervention. ASHA Reports, 12*, 52–57. Rockville, MD: The American Speech and Hearing Association.

Kuhn, T. S. (1974). *The structure of scientific revolutions.* Chicago: The University of Chicago Press.

McLean, J. E. (1983). Historical perspectives on the content of child language programs. In J. Miller, D. E. Yoder, & R. Schiefelbusch (Eds.), *Contemporary issues in language intervention. ASHA Reports, 12*, 115–126, Rockville, MD. The American Speech & Hearing Association.

Perkins, W. H. (1986). Functions and malfunctions of theories in therapies. *ASHA, 28*, 31–33.

Prutting, C. A. (1983). Scientific inquiry and communicative disorders: An emerging paradigm across six decades. In T. A. Gallagher, & C. A. Prutting (Eds.), *Pragmatic assessment and intervention issues in language* (pp. 247–266). San Diego, CA: College-Hill Press.

Siegel, G. M. & Ingham, R. J. (1987). Theory and science in communication disorders. *Journal of Speech and Hearing Disorders, 52*, 99–104.

Vygotsky, L. S. (1962). *Thought and language.* Cambridge, MA: MIT Press.

Neuropsychological Theory

Arbib, M. A. (1982). From artificial intelligence to neurolinguistics. In M. A. Arbib, D. Caplan, & J. C. Marshall (Eds.), *Neural models of language processes* (pp. 77–94). New York: Academic Press.

Bellugi, U., Poizner, H., & Zurif, E. B. (1982). Prospects for the study of aphasia in a visual-gestural language. In M. A. Arbib, D. Caplan, & C. Marshall (Eds.), *Neural models of language processes* (pp. 271–292). New York: Academic Press.

Berry, M. F. (1969). *Language disorders of children: The bases and diagnosis.* New York: Appleton-Century-Crofts.

Eisenson, J. (1968). Developmental aphasia (dyslogia): A postulation of a unitary concept of the disorder. *Cortex, 4*, 184–200.

Eisenson, J. (1972). *Aphasia in children.* New York: Harper and Row.

Gruber, F. A., & Segalowitz, S. J. (1977). Some issues and methods in the neuropsychology of language. In S. J. Segalowitz, & F. A. Gruber (Eds.), *Language development and neurological theory* (pp. 3–19). New York: Academic Press.

Horner, J. (1981). *A model of language emergences from a neuropsychological perspective.* Paper presented at the North Carolina Speech-Language-Hearing Association, Asheville, NC.

Lenneberg, E. H. (Ed.). (1966). *New directions in the study of language.* Cambridge, MA: The MIT Press.

Lenneberg, E. H. (1967). *Biological foundations of language.* New York: John Wiley and Sons, Inc.

Lenneberg, E. H., & Lenneburg, E. (1975). *Foundations of language development. A multidisciplinary approach* (Vol. 2). New York: Academic Press.

Millar, J. M., & Whitaker, H. A. (1981). The right hemisphere's contribution to language. In S. J. Segalowitz (Ed.), *Language functions and brain organization* (pp. 87–113). New York: Academic Press.

Myklebust, H. (1954). *Auditory disorders in children.* New York: Grune & Stratton.

Rapin, I., & Allen, D. A. (1983). Developmental language disorders: Nosologic considerations. In U. Kirk (Ed.), *Neuropsychology of language, reading, and spelling* (pp. 155–184). New York: Academic Press.

Waryas, C. L., & Crowe, T. A. (1982). Language delay. In N. Lass, L. McReynolds, J. Northern, & D. Yoder (Eds.), *Speech, language and hearing* (Vol. II) (pp. 761–779). Pathologies of Speech and Language. Philadelphia: W. B. Saunders.

Behavioral Theory

Bricker, W. A., & Bricker, D. D. (1970). A program for language training for the severely retarded handicapped child. *Exceptional Children, 37*, 101–111.

Bricker, W., & Bricker, D. (1974). An early language training strategy. In R. Schiefelbusch, & L. Lloyd (Eds.), *Language perspectives—Acquisition, retardation and intervention* (pp. 431–468). Baltimore: University Park Press.

Gray, B., & Ryan, B. (1973). *A language program for the nonlanguage child*. Champaign, IL: Research Press.

Guess, D., Sailor, W., & Baer, D. M. (1978). Children with limited language. In R. L. Schiefelbusch (Ed.), *Language intervention strategies* (pp. 101–144). Baltimore: University Park Press.

Kent, L., Klein, D., Falk, A., & Guenther, H. (1972). A language acquisition program for the retarded. In J. McLean, D. Yoder, & R. Schiefelbusch (Eds.), *Language intervention with the retarded* (pp. 151–190). Baltimore: University Park Press.

McDonald, J. (1975). Environmental language intervention: Program for establishing initial communication in handicapped children. In F. Withron, & C. Nygren (Eds.), *Language and the handicapped learner: Curricula, programs, and media*. Columbus, OH: Charles E. Wesnel.

Miller, J. F., & Yoder, D. E. (1974). An ontogenic language teaching strategy for retarded children. In R. L. Schiefelbusch, & L. L. Lloyd (Eds.), *Language perspectives—Acquisition, retardation and intervention* (pp. 505–528). Baltimore: University Park Press.

Mowrer, O. H. (1958). Hearing and speaking: An analysis of language learning. *Journal of Speech and Hearing Disorders, 23*, 143–152.

Mowrer, O. H. (1960). *Learning theory and the symbolic processes*. New York: Wiley.

Sloane, H. N., & MacAulay, B. (1968). *Operant procedures in remedial speech and language*. Boston: Houghton Mifflin.

Skinner, B. F. (1957). *Verbal behavior*. New York: Appleton-Century-Crofts.

Staats, A. (1971). Linguistic-mentalistic theory versus an explanatory S-R learning theory of language development. In D. Slobin (Ed.), *The ontogenesis of grammar* (pp. 103–150). New York: Academic Press.

Stremel, K., & Waryas, C. (1974). A behavioral-psycholinguistic approach to language training. In L. V. McReynolds (Ed.), *Developing systematic procedures for training children's language* (pp. 96–130). ASHA Monographs, 18.

Warren, S. F., & Kaiser, A. P. (1986b). Incidental language teaching: A critical review. *Journal of Speech and Hearing Disorders, 51*, 291–299.

Warren, S. F., McQuarter, R. J., & Rogers-Warren, A. K. (1984). The effects of mands and models on the speech of unresponsive language-delayed preschool children. *Journal of Speech and Hearing Disorders, 49*, 43–52.

Information Processing Theory

Aram, D. M., & Nation, J. E. (1975). Patterns of language behavior in children with developmental language disorders. *Journal of Speech and Hearing Research, 18*, 229–241.

Carrow, E. (1972). Assessment of speech and language in children. In J. E. McLean, D. E. Yoder, & R. L. Schiefelbusch (Eds.), *Language intervention with the retarded* (pp. 52–88). Baltimore: University Park Press.

Johnson, D. J. (1981). Factors to consider in programming for children with language disorders. *Topics in Learning and Learning Disabilities, 1*, 13–27.

Kirk, S. A., McCarthy, J. J., & Kirk, W. D. (1968). *Illinois test of psycholinguistic abilities*. Urbana, IL: University of Illinois Press.

Osgood, C. E. (1967). The nature of meaning. In J. P. DeCecco (Ed.), *The psychology of language thought and instruction* (pp. 156–164). New York: Holt, Rinehart & Winston.

Osgood, C. E. (1968). Toward a wedding of insufficiencies. In T. R. Dixon, & D. L. Horton (Eds.), *Verbal behavior and general behavior theory* (pp. 495–519). Englewood Cliffs, NJ: Prentice-Hall.

Osgood, C. E., & Miron, M. S. (1963). *Approaches to the study of aphasia*. Urbana, IL: University of Illinois Press.

Wepman, J. M., Jones, L. V., Bock, R. D., & van Pelt, D. (1960). Studies in aphasia: Background and theoretical formulations. *Journal of Speech and Hearing Disorders, 25*, 323–332.

Linguistic Theory

Bloom, L. (1970). *Language development: Form and function in emerging grammars*. Cambridge, MA: MIT Press.

Bloom, L., & Lahey, M. (1978). *Language development and language disorders*. New York: John Wiley and Sons.

Bloom, L., Merkin, S., & Wooten, J. (1982). Wh- questions: Linguistic factors that contribute to the sequence of acquisition. *Child Development, 53*, 1084–1092.

Bloom, L., Rocissano, L., & Hood, L. (1976). Adult-child discourse: Developmental interaction between information processing and linguistic knowledge. *Cognitive Psychology, 8*, 521–552.

Brown, R. (1973). *A first language: The early stages*. Cambridge, MA: Harvard University Press.

Chomsky, N. (1957). *Syntactic structures*. The Hague: Mouton.

Chomsky, N. (1965). *Aspects of the theory of syntax*. Cambridge, MA: MIT Press.

Crowder, R. G. (1978). Language and memory. In J. F. Kavanagh, & W. Strange (Eds.), *Speech and language in the laboratory, school and clinic* (pp. 331–376). Cambridge, MA: MIT Press.

Leonard, L. B. (1984). Semantic considerations in early language training. In K. F. Ruder, & M. D. Smith (Eds.), *Development language intervention: Psycholinguistic applications* (pp. 141–170). Baltimore: University Park Press.

Leonard, L. B., Steckol, K. F., & Panther, K. M. (1983). Returning meaning to semantic relations: Some clinical applications. *Journal of Speech and Hearing Disorders, 48*, 25–36.

McNeill, D. (1971). The capacity for the ontogenesis of grammar. In D. I. Slobin (Ed.), *The ontogenesis of grammar* (pp. 17–40). New York: Academic Press.

Cognitive Organization Theory

Brown, A. L., & Palencsar, A. S. (1982). Inducing strategic learning from texts by means of informed, self-control training. *Topics in Learning and Learning Disabilities, 2*, 1–17.

Bruner, J. S. (1974). The integration of early skilled action. In M. P. M. Richards (Ed.), *The integration of a child into a social world* (pp. 167–184). Cambridge: Cambridge University Press.

Camarata, S., Newhoff, M., & Rugg, B. (1981). Perspective taking in normal and language-disordered children. *Proceedings of the Symposium on Research in Child Language Disorders*. Madison: University of Wisconsin.

Dinsmore, J. (1987). Mental spaces from a functional perspective. *Cognitive Science, 11*, 1–21.

Fauconnier, G. (1985). *Mental spaces: Aspects of meaning construction in natural language*. Cambridge, MA: Bradford/MIT Press.

Kamhi, A. G. (1981). Nonlinguistic symbolic and conceptual abilities of language impaired and normally developing children. *Journal of Speech and Hearing Research, 24*, 446–453.

Kamhi, A. G., Catts, H. W., Koenig, L. A., & Lewis, B. A. (1984). Hypothesis testing and non-linguistic symbolic abilities in language-impaired children. *Journal of Speech and Hearing Disorders, 49*, 169–176.

Kirk, U. (1983). Introduction: Toward an understanding of the neuropsychology of language, reading, and spelling. In U. Kirk (Ed.), *Neuropsychology of language, reading and spelling* (pp. 3–31). New York: Academic Press.

Miller, J. F. (1981). *Assessing language production in children*. Baltimore: University Park Press.

Miller, S. A. (1982). Cognitive development: A Piagetian perspective. In R. Vasta (Ed.), *Strategies and techniques of child study* (pp. 161–205). New York: Academic Press.

Nelson, L. K., Kamhi, A. G., & Apel, K. (1987). Cognitive strengths and weaknesses in language-impaired children: One more look. *Journal of Speech and Hearing Disorders, 52*, 36–43.

Piaget, J. (1952). *The origins of intelligence in children*. New York: W. W. Norton.

Piaget, J. (1955). *Language and thought of the child*. Cleveland: World.

Piaget, J., & Inhelder, B. (1958). *The growth of local thinking from childhood to adolescence*. New York: Basic Books.

Sinclair-de Zwart, H. (1969). Developmental psycholinguistics. In D. Elkind, & J. H. Flavell (Eds.), *Cognitive development: Essays in honor of Jean Piaget* (pp. 315–336). New York: Oxford University Press.

Sinclair-de Zwart, H. (1973). Language acquisition and cognitive development. In T. E. Moore (Ed.), *Cognitive development and the acquisition of language* (pp. 9–26). New York: Academic Press.

Pragmatic Theory

Bates, E. (1976a). *Language and context: The acquisition of pragmatics*. New York: Academic Press.

Bates, E. (1976b). Pragmatics and sociolinguistics in child language. In D. M. Morehead, & A. E. Morehead (Eds.), *Normal and deficient child language* (pp. 411–463). Baltimore: University Park Press.

Bates, E., Benigni, L., Bretherton, I, Camaioni, L., & Volterra, V. (1977). From gesture to first word: On cognitive and social prerequisites. In M. Lewis, & L. A. Rosenblum (Eds.), *Interaction, conversation and the development of language* (pp. 247–307). New York: John Wiley and Sons.

Dore, J. (1976). Children's illocutionary acts. In R. Freedle (Ed.), *Discourse production and comprehension* (Vol. 1). Hillsdale, NJ: Lawrence Erlbaum Associates.

Duncan, J. C., & Perozzi, J. A. (1987). Concurrent validity of a pragmatic protocol. *Language, Speech, and Hearing Services in Schools, 18*, 80–85.

Fey, M. (1986). *Language intervention with young children*. San Diego: College Hill Press.

Geffner, D. (1981). Assessment of language disorders: Linguistic and cognitive functions. *Topics in Language Disorders, 1*, 1–9.

Klecan-Aker, J., & Swank, P. (1988). The use of a pragmatic protocol with normal pre-school children. *Journal of Communication Disorders, 21*, 1–15.

Lasky, E. Z. (1983). Facilitating comprehension, recall, and production of language. In H. Winitz (Ed.), *Treating language disorders* (pp. 43–56). Baltimore: University Park Press.

Liles, B. Z. (1985). Cohesion in the narratives of normal and language-disordered children. *Journal of Speech and Hearing Research, 123–133.*

Lucas, E. V. (1980). *Semantic and pragmatic language disorders: Assessment and remediation.* Rockville, MD: Aspen.

Lund, N. J., & Duchan, J. F. (1983). *Assessing children's language in naturalistic contexts.* Englewood Cliffs, NJ: Prentice-Hall.

McLean, J., & Snyder, L. K. (1978). *A transactional approach to early language training.* Columbus, OH: Charles E. Merrill.

Muma, J. R. (1986). *Language acquisition. A functional approach.* Austin, TX: Pro-Ed.

Prutting, C. A. (1982a). Pragmatics as social competence. *Journal of Speech and Hearing Disorders, 47*, 123–134.

Prutting, C. A. (1982b). Observational protocol for pragmatic behaviors [Clinic Manual]. Developed for the University of California Speech and Hearing Clinic, Santa Barbara, CA.

Prutting, C. A., & Kirchner, D. M. (1987). A clinical appraisal of the pragmatic aspects of language. *Journal of Speech and Hearing Disorders, 52*, 105–119.

Rice, M. L. (1986). Mismatched premises of the communicative competence model and language intervention. In R. L. Schiefelbusch (Ed.), *Language competence: Assessment and intervention* (pp. 261–280). San Diego: College-Hill Press.

Roth, F. P., & Spekman, N. J. (1984a). Assessing the pragmatic abilities of children: Part 1. Organizational framework and assessment parameters. *Journal of Speech and Hearing Disorders, 49*, 2–11.

Roth, F. P., & Spekman, N. J. (1984b). Assessing the pragmatic abilities of children: Part 2. Guidelines, considerations, and specific evaluation procedures. *Journal of Speech and Hearing Disorders, 49*, 12–17.

Searle, J. R. (1975). Speech acts and recent linguistics. In D. Aaronson, & R. W. Rieber (Eds.), *Developmental psycholinguistics and communication disorders* (pp. 27–38). New York: New York Academy of Sciences.

Taenzer, S. F., Cermak, M. S., & Hanlon, R. C. (1981). Outside the therapy room: A naturalistic approach to language intervention. *Topics in Learning and Learning Disabilities, 1*, 41–46.

PERFORMANCE/KNOWLEDGE DISTINCTION

Ackerman, P. T., & Dykman, R. A. (1982). Automatic and effortful information-processing deficits in children with learning and attention disorders. *Topics in Learning and Learning Disabilities, 2*, 12–23.

Bellugi, U., Poizner, H., & Zurif, E. B. (1982). Prospects for the study of aphasia in a visual-gestural language. In M. A. Arbib, D. Caplan, & C. Marshall (Eds.), *Neural models of language processes* (pp. 271–292). New York: Academic Press.

Bever, T. G. (1970). The cognitive basis for linguistic structures. In J. R. Hayes (Ed.), *Cognition and the development of language* (pp. 279–352). New York: John Wiley and Sons.

Bloom. L., & Lahey, M. (1978). *Language development and language disorders.* New York: John Wiley and Sons.

Brown, A. L., & Palencsar, A. S. (1982). Inducing strategic learning from texts by means of informed, self-control training. *Topics in Learning and Learning Disabilities, 2*, 1–17.

Bruner, J. S. (1974). The integration of early skilled action. In M. P. M. Richards (Ed.), *The integration of a child into a social world* (pp. 167–184). Cambridge: Cambridge University Press.

Caplan, D. (1982). Reconciling the categories: Representation in neurology and in linguistics. In M. A. Arbib, D. Caplan, & C. Marshall (Eds.), *Neural models of language processes* (pp. 411–427). New York: Academic Press.

Carrow-Woolfolk, E. (1985). *TACL-R examiner's manual* (rev. ed.). Allen, TX: DLM Teaching Resources.

Cedergren, H. E., & Sankoff, D. (1974). Variable rules: Performance as a statistical reflection of competence. *Language, 50*, 333–355.

Chapanis, L. (1977). Language deficits and cross-modal sensory perception. In S. J. Segalowitz, & F. A. Gruber (Eds.), *Language development and neurological theory* (pp. 107–120). New York: Academic Press.

Chomsky, N. (1980). *Rules and representations*. New York: Columbia University Press.

Clark, R. (1974). Performing without competence. *Journal of Child Language, 1*, 1–10.

Fodor, J. D., & Frazier, L. (1980). Is the human sentence parsing mechanism an ATN? *Cognition, 8*, 417–459.

Frazier, L. (1982). Shared components of production and perception. In M. A. Arbib, D. Caplan, & C. Marshall (Eds.), *Neural models of language processes* (pp. 225–236). New York: Academic Press.

Fromkin, V. A. (1972). Discussion paper on speech physiology. In J. H. Gilbert (Ed.), *Speech and cortical functioning* (pp. 73–105). New York: Academic Press.

Garrett, M. F. (1982). Remarks on the relation between language production and language comprehension systems. In M. A. Arbib, D. Caplan, & J. C. Marshall (Eds.), *Neural models of language processes* (pp. 209–224). New York: Academic Press.

Goodenough, C., Zurif, E. B., & Weintraub, S. (1977). Aphasic's attention to grammatical morphemes. *Language and Speech, 20*, 11–19.

Goodglass, H., Barton, M. I., & Kaplan, E. F. (1968). Sensory modality and object-naming in aphasia. *Journal of Speech and Hearing Research, 11*, 488–496.

Halle, M. (1978). Preface. In M. Halle, J. Bresnan, & G. A. Miller (Eds.), *Linguistic theory and psychological reality* (pp. xi–xv). Cambridge, MA: The MIT Press.

Kamhi, A. G., Catts, H. W., Koenig, L. A., & Lewis, B. A. (1984). Hypothesis testing and non-linguistic symbolic abilities in language-impaired children. *Journal of Speech and Hearing Disorders, 49*, 169–176.

Kean, M. L. (1982). Three perspectives for the analysis of aphasia syndromes. In M. A. Arbib, D. Caplan, & C. Marshall (Eds.), *Neural models of language processes* (pp. 173–201). New York: Academic Press.

Kempen, G., & Hoenkamp, E. (1987). Incremental procedural grammar for sentence formulation. *Cognitive Science, 11*, 201–258.

Kirchner, D. M., & Skarakis-Doyle, E. A. (1983). Developmental language disorders: A theoretical perspective. In T. M. Gallagher, & C. A. Prutting (Eds.), *Pragmatic assessment and intervention issues in language* (pp. 215–246). San Diego, CA: College-Hill Press, Inc.

Kirk, U. (1983). Introduction: Toward an understanding of the neuropsychology of language, reading, and spelling. In U. Kirk (Ed.), *Neuropsychology of language, reading and spelling* (pp. 3–31). New York: Academic Press.

Labov, W. (1969). Contraction, deletion and inherent variability of the English copula. *Language, 45*, 715–762.

McNeil, M. R., & Kimelman, M. D. Z. (1986). Toward an integrative information-processing structure of auditory comprehension and processing in adult aphasia. *Seminars in Speech and Language, 7*, 123–146.

Miller, G. A. (1975). Some comments on competence and performance. In D. Aaronson, & R. W. Rieber (Eds.), *Developmental psycholinguistics and communication disorders* (pp. 201–204). New York: The New York Academy of Sciences.

Prizant, B. M. (1983). Language acquisition and communicative behavior in autism: Toward an understanding of the "whole" of it. *Journal of Speech and Hearing Disorders, 48*, 296–307.

Salzinger, K. (1975). Are theories of competence necessary? In D. Aaronson, & R. W. Rieber (Eds.), *Developmental psycholinguistics and communication disorders* (pp. 178–196). New York: The New York Academy of Sciences.

Samuels, S. J., & Eisenberg, P. (1981). A framework for understanding the reading process. In F. J. Pirozzolo, & M. C. Wittrock (Eds.), *Neuropsychological and cognitive processes in reading* (pp. 31–67). New York: Academic Press.

Sternberg, R. J., & Wagner, R. K. (1982). Automatization failure in learning disabilities. *Topics in Learning and Learning Disabilities, 2*, 1–12.

Tallal, P., & Stark, R. (1983). Perceptual prerequisites for language development. In U. Kirk (Ed.), *Neuropsychology of language, reading, and spelling* (pp. 97–106). New York: Academic Press.

Wechsler, D. (1974). *Wechsler Intelligence Scale for Children*. New York: Psychological Corp.

MODULARITY OF THE LANGUAGE SYSTEM

Bates, E. (1976a). *Language and context: The acquisition of pragmatics*. New York: Academic Press.

Berndt, R. S., Caramazza, A., & Zurif, E. (1981). Language function: Syntax and semantics. In S. J. Segalowitz (Ed.), *Language functions and brain organization* (pp. 5–28). New York: Academic Press.

Bever, T. G. (1970). The cognitive basis for linguistic structures. In J. R. Hayes (Ed.), *Cognition and the development of language* (pp. 279–352). New York: John Wiley and Sons.

Blank, M. (1975a). Mastering the intangible through language. In D. Aaronson, & R. W. Reiber (Eds.), *Developmental psycholinguistics and communication disorders* (pp. 44–58). New York: The New York Academy of Sciences.

Bradley, D. C., Garrett, M., & Zurif, F. B. (1980). Syntactic deficits in Broca's aphasia. In D. Caplan (Ed.), *Biological studies of mental processes* (pp. 269–286). Cambridge, MA: MIT Press.

Chiat, S., & Hirson, A. (1987). From conceptual intention to utterance: A study of impaired language output in a child with developmental dysphasia. *British Journal of Disorders of Communication, 22*, 37–64.

Chomsky, N. (1980). *Rules and representations.* New York: Columbia University Press.

Dinsmore, J. (1987). Mental spaces from a functional perspective. *Cognitive Science, 11*, 1–21.

Dodd, D., & White, R. M. (1980). *Cognition: Mental structures and processes.* Boston: Allyn & Bacon.

Fey, M. Leonard, L., & Wilcox, K. (1981). Speech style modifications of language-impaired children. *Journal of Speech and Hearing Disorders, 46*, 91–96.

Fodor, J. A. (1983). *The modularity of mind.* Cambridge, MA: The MIT Press.

Foster, S. H. (1984a). *Modularity and language acquisition: Distinguishing syntax and pragmatics.* Paper presented at the meeting of the International Association for the Study of Child Language, Austin, TX.

Fraser, C., Bellugi, U., & Brown, R. (1963). Control of grammar in imitation, comprehension and production. *Journal of Verbal Learning and Verbal Behavior, 2*, 121–135.

Garrett, M. F. (1982). Remarks on the relation between language production and language comprehension systems. In M. A. Arbib, D. Caplan, & J. C. Marshall (Eds.), *Neural models of language processes* (pp. 209–224). New York: Academic Press.

Geschwind, N., Quadfasel, F. A., & Segarra, J. M. (1968). Isolation of the speech area. *Neuropsychologia, 6*, 327–340.

Glucksberg, S. (1975). Discussion. Comments by Bever. In D. Aaronson, & R. W. Rieber (Eds.), *Developmental psycholinguistics and communication disorders* (pp. 39–43). New York: New York Academy of Sciences.

Hamburger, H., & Crain, S. (1987). Plans and semantics in human processing of language. *Cognitive Science, 11*, 103–136.

Katz, L., Boyce, S., Goldstein, L., & Lukatela, G. (1987). Grammatical information effects in auditory word recognition. *Cognition, 25*, 235–264.

Kirchner, D. M., & Klatzky, R. L. (1985). Verbal rehearsal and memory in language disordered children. *Journal of Speech and Hearing Research, 28*, 556–565.

Leonard, L. B. (1984). Semantic considerations in early language training. In K. F. Ruder, & M. D. Smith (Eds.), *Development language intervention: Psycholinguistic applications* (pp. 141–170). Baltimore: University Park Press.

Lucariello, J., Kyratzis, A., & Engel, S. (1986). Event representation, context, and language. In K. Nelson (Ed.), *Event knowledge: Structure and function in development* (pp. 137–160). Hillsdale, NJ: Lawrence Erlbaum Associates.

McCawley, J. D. (1971). Prelexical syntax. In R. J. O'Brien (Ed.), *Monograph series on language and linguistics.* 22nd Annual Round Table. Washington, D.C.: Georgetown University Press.

Nelson, K. (1986b). Event knowledge and cognitive development. In K. Nelson (Ed.), *Event knowledge: Structure and function in development* (pp. 1–20). Hillsdale, NJ: Lawrence Erlbaum Associates.

Nelson, K. E., & Nelson, K. (1978). Cognitive pendulums and their linguistic realization. In K. E. Nelson (Ed.), *Children's language* (Vol. 1) (pp. 223–285). New York: Gardner Press.

Nelson, L. K., Kamhi, A. G., & Apel, K. (1987). Cognitive strengths and weaknesses in language-impaired children: One more look. *Journal of Speech and Hearing Disorders, 52*, 36–43.

Piaget, J. (1955). *Language and thought of the child.* Cleveland: World.

Rapin, I., & Allen, D. A. (1983). Developmental language disorders: Nosologic considerations. In U. Kirk (Ed.), *Neuropsychology of language, reading, and spelling* (pp. 155–184). New York: Academic Press.

Rice, M. L. (1983). Contemporary accounts of the cognition/language relationship: Implication for speech-language clinicians. *Journal of Speech and Hearing Disorders, 48*, 347–359.

Rowan, L. E., Leonard, L. B., Chapman, K., & Weiss, A. L. (1983). Performative and presuppositional skills in language-disordered and normal children. *Journal of Speech and Hearing Research, 26*, 97–106.

Rumelhart, D. E., & Ortony, A. (1977). The representation of knowledge in memory. In R. C. Anderson, R. J. Spiro, & W. E. Montague (Eds.), *Schooling and the acquisition of knowledge* (pp. 99–135). Hillsdale, NJ: Erlbaum.

Saffran, E., Schwartz, M., & Marin, O. (1980). Evidence from aphasia: Isolating the components of a production model. In B. Butterworth (Ed.), *Language production* (Vol. 1) (pp. 221–241). London: Academic Press.

Schank, R. C., & Abelson, R. P. (1977). *Scripts, plans, goals and understanding: An inquiry into human knowledge structure.* New York: Halsted Press, John Wiley and Sons.

Schlesinger, I. (1977). The role of cognitive development and linguistic input in language acquisition. *Journal of Child Language, 4*, 153–170.

Schlesinger, I. M. (1981). Semantic assimilation in the development of relational categories. In W. Deutsch (Ed.), *The child's construction of language* (pp. 223–243). New York: Academic Press.

Whitaker, H. (1976). A case of the isolation of the language function. In H. Whitaker, & H. A. Whitaker (Eds.), *Studies in neurolinguistics* (pp. 1–58). New York: Academic Press.

Zurif, E. B. (1982). The use of data from aphasia in constructing a performance model of language. In M. A. Arbib, D. Caplan, & J. C. Marshall (Eds.), *Neural models of language processes* (pp. 203–207). New York: Academic Press.

AUDITORY PROCESSING: SPEECH PERCEPTION AND MEMORY

Bernstein, L. E., & Stark, R. E. (1985). Speech perception development in language-impaired children: A 4-year follow-up study. *Journal of Speech and Hearing Disorders, 50*, 21–30.

Bever, T. G. (1970). The cognitive basis for linguistic structures. In J. R. Hayes (Ed.), *Cognition and the development of language* (pp. 279–352). New York: John Wiley and Sons.

Carrow, M. A. (1968). Language disorders: A theory. In M. A. Carrow (Ed.), *A theoretical approach to the diagnosis and treatment of language disorders in children* (pp. 1–18). Harry Jersig Speech and Hearing Center, Our Lady of the Lake College, San Antonio, TX.

Crowder, R. G. (1978). Language and memory. In J. F. Kavanagh, & W. Strange (Eds.), *Speech and language in the laboratory, school and clinic* (pp. 331–376). Cambridge, MA: MIT Press.

Cutler, A., Mehler, J., Norris, D., & Segui, J. (1987). Phoneme identification and the lexicon. *Cognitive Psychology, 19*, 141–177.

Duchan, J. F. (1983). Language processing and geodesic domes. In T. M. Gallagher, & C. A. Prutting (Eds.), *Pragmatic assessment and intervention issues in language* (pp. 83–100). San Diego, CA: College-Hill Press.

Fodor, J. A. (1983). *The modularity of mind*. Cambridge, MA: The MIT Press.

Forster, K. I. (1976). Accessing the mental lexicon. In R. J. Wales, & E. Walker (Eds.), *New approaches to language mechanisms* (pp. 257–287). Amsterdam: North Holland.

Frauenfelder, U. H., & Tyler, L. K. (1987). The process of spoken word recognition: An introduction. *Cognition, 25*, 1–20.

Garret, M., & Fodor, J. (1968). Psychological theories and linguistic constructs. In T. R. Dixon, & D. L. Horton (Eds.), *Verbal behavior and general behavior theory* (pp. 451–477). Englewood Cliffs, NJ: Prentice-Hall.

Gibson, E. J. (1971). Perceptual learning and the theory of word perception. *Cognitive Psychology, 2*, 351–368.

Gough, P. B. (1972). One second of reading. In J. F. Kavanogh, & I. G. Mattingly (Eds.), *Language by eye and by ear* (pp. 331–358). Cambridge, MA: MIT Press.

Grossberg, S. (1987). Competitive learning: From interative activation to adaptive resonance. *Cognitive Science, 11*, 23–63.

Keir, E. H. (1977). Auditory information processing and learning disabilities. In L. Tarnopol, & M. Tarnopol (Eds.), *Brain function and reading disability* (pp. 147–176). Baltimore: University Park Press.

Lange, G. (1978). Organization-related processes in children's recall. In P. A. Ornstein (Ed.), *Memory development in children* (pp. 101–128). Hillsdale, NJ: Lawrence Erlbaum Associates.

Leonard, L. B., Nippold, M. A., Kail, R., & Hale, C. A. (1983). Picture naming in language-impaired children. *Journal of Speech and Hearing Research, 26*, 609–615.

Liberman, A. M., Cooper, F. S., Shankweiter, D. P., & Studdert-Kennedy, M. (1967). Perception of the speech code. *Psychological Review, 74*, 431–461.

Lubert, N. (1981). Auditory perceptual impairments in children with specific language disorders: A review of the literature. *Journal of Speech and Hearing Disorders, 46*, 3–9.

Marin, O. S. M. (1982). Brain and language: The rules of the game. In M. A. Arbib, D. Caplan, & J. C. Marshall (Eds.), *Neural models of language processes* (pp. 45–69). New York: Academic Press.

McClelland, J. L., & Rumelhart, D. E. (1986). *Parallel distributed processing: Explorations in the microstructure of cognition*. Cambridge, MA: Bradford Books.

McNeil, M. R., & Kimelman, M. D. Z. (1986). Toward an integrative information-processing structure of auditory comprehension and processing in adult aphasia. *Seminars in Speech and Language, 7*, 123–146.

Myers, N. A., & Perlmutter, M. (1978). Memory in the years from two to five. In P. A. Ornstein (Ed.), *Memory development in children* (pp. 243–258). Hillsdale, NJ: Lawrence Erlbaum Associates.

Nelson, K. (1978). Semantic development and the development of semantic memory. In K. E. Nelson (Ed.), *Children's language* (Vol. 1) (pp. 39–80). New York: Gardner Press, Inc.

Nelson, K. (1986a). *Event knowledge: Structure and function in development.* Hillsdale, NJ: Lawrence Erlbaum Associates.

Nelson, K., & Brown, A. L. (1978). The semantic-episodic distinction in memory development. In P. A. Ornstein (Ed.), *Memory development in children* (pp. 233–241). Hillsdale, NJ: Lawrence Erlbaum Associates.

Paris, S. G. (1978). The development of inference and transformation as memory operations. In P. A. Ornstein (Ed.), *Memory development in children* (pp. 129–156). Hillsdale, NJ: Lawrence Erlbaum Associates.

Paris, S., Lindauer, B., & Cox, G. (1977). The development of inferential comprehension. *Child Development, 48,* 1728–1733.

Pisoni, D. B., & Luce, P. A. (1987). Acoustic representations in word recognition. *Cognition, 25,* 21–52.

Rees, N. S. (1973). Auditory processing factors in language disorders: The view from Procrustes' bed. *Journal of Speech and Hearing Disorders, 3,* 304– 315.

Rice, M. L. (1983). Contemporary accounts of the cognition/language relationship: Implication for speech-language clinicians. *Journal of Speech and Hearing Disorders, 48,* 347–359.

Samuels, S. J., & Eisenberg, P. (1981). A framework for understanding the reading process. In F. J. Pirozzolo, & M. C. Wittrock (Eds.), *Neuropsychological and cognitive processes in reading* (pp. 31–67). New York: Academic Press.

Satz, P. (1968). Laterality effects in dichotic listening. *Nature, 218,* 277–278.

Schank, R. C. (1975). The structure of episodes in memory. In D. G. Bobrow, & A. M. Collins (Eds.), *Representation and understanding* (pp. 237–272). New York: Academic Press.

Studdert-Kennedy, M., & Shankweiler, D. (1970). Hemispheric specialization for speech perception. *Journal of the Acoustical Society of America, 48,* 579–594.

Tallal, P. (1980). Auditory temporal processing, phonics, and reading disabilities in children. *Brain and Language, 9,* 182–198.

Tallal, P., & Piercy, M. (1978). Defects of auditory perception in children with developmental dysphasia. In N. A. Wyke (Ed.), *Developmental dysphasia* (pp. 63–84). New York: Academic Press.

Tallal, P., & Stark, R. (1976). Relation between speech perception and speech production impairment in children with developmental dysphasia. *Brain and Language, 3,* 305–317.

Tallal, P., & Stark, R. (1983). Perceptual prerequisites for language development. In U. Kirk (Ed.), *Neuropsychology of language, reading, and spelling* (pp. 97–106). New York: Academic Press.

Torgesen, J. K., & Greenstein, J. J. (1982). Why do some learning disabled children have problems remembering? Does it make a difference? *Topics in Learning and Learning Disabilities, 2,* 54–61.

Trevarthen, C. (1983). Development of the cerebral mechanisms for language. In U. Kirk (Ed.), *Neuropsychology of language, reading, and spelling* (pp. 45–80). New York: Academic Press.

Tulving, E. (1972). Episodic and semantic memory. In E. Tulving, & W. Donaldson (Eds.), *Organization of memory* (pp. 382–403). New York: Academic Press.

Vellutino, F. R. (1979). *Dyslexia: Theory and research.* Cambridge, MA: MIT Press.

COMPREHENSION OF LANGUAGE

Bowerman, M. (1978). The acquisition of word meaning: An investigation of some current concepts. In N. Waterson, & C. Snow (Eds.), *Development of communication: Social and pragmatic factors in language acquisition* (pp. 263–287). New York: John Wiley and Sons.

Bradley, D. C., & Forster, K. I. (1987). A reader's view of listening. *Cognition, 25,* 103–134.

Bridges, A., Sinha, C., & Walkerdine, V. (1981). The development of comprehension. In G. Wells (Ed.), *Learning through interaction* (pp. 116–156). Cambridge: Cambridge University Press.

Brinton, B., & Fujiki, M. (1982). A comparison of request-response sentences in the discourse of normal and language disordered children. *Journal of Speech and Hearing Disorders, 47,* 57–62.

Carrow-Woolfolk, E. (1985). *TACL-R examiner's manual* (rev. ed.). Allen, TX: DLM Teaching Resources.

Chapman, R. S. (1978). Comprehension strategies in children. In J. F. Kavanaugh, & W. Strange (Eds.), *Speech and language in the laboratory, school, and clinic* (pp. 308–327). Cambridge, MA: MIT Press.

Clark, E. V. (1982). The young word-maker: A case study of innovation in the child's lexicon. In E. Wanner, & L. R. Gleitman (Eds.), *Language acquisition: The state of the art* (pp. 390–428). Cambridge: Cambridge University Press.

Cutler, A. (1976). Beyond parsing and lexical hook-up: An enriched description of auditory sentence comprehension. In R. J. Wales, & E. Walker (Eds.), *New approaches to language mechanisms* (pp. 133–150). Amsterdam: North Holland Publishing Co.

Cutler, A. (1976). Beyond parsing and lexical hook-up: An enriched description of auditory sentence comprehension. In R. J. Wales, & E. Walker (Eds.), *New approaches to language mechanisms* (pp. 133–150). Amsterdam: North Holland Publishing Co.

Cutler, A., Mehler, J., Norris, D., & Segui, J. (1987). Phoneme identification and the lexicon. *Cognitive Psychology, 19*, 141–177.

Dollaghan, C., & Kaston, N. (1986). A comprehension monitoring program for language-impaired children. *Journal of Speech and Hearing Disorders, 51*, 264–271.

Ellis Weismer, S. (1985). Constructive comprehension abilities exhibited by language-disabled children. *Journal of Speech and Hearing Research, 28*, 175–184.

Fey, M. E., & Leonard, L. B. (1983). Pragmatic skills of children with specific language impairment. In T. M. Gallagher, & C. A. Prutting (Eds.), *Pragmatic assessment and intervention issues in language* (pp. 65–82). San Diego, CA: College-Hill Press.

Fischler, I., & Bloom, P. (1979). Automatic and attentional process in the effects of sentence contexts on word recognition. *Journal of Verbal Learning and Verbal Behavior, 18*, 1–20.

Frauenfelder, U. H., & Tyler, L. K. (1987). The process of spoken word recognition: An introduction. *Cognition, 25*, 1–20.

Johnson-Laird, P. N. (1987). The mental representation of the meanings of words. *Cognition, 25*, 189–212.

Kamhi, A. G., & Catts, H. W. (1986). Toward an understanding of developmental language and reading disorders. *Journal of Speech and Hearing Disorders, 51*, 337–347.

Marcus, M. P. (1982). Consequences of functional deficits in a parsing model: Implications for Broca's aphasia. In M. A. Arbib, D. Caplan, & J. C. Marshall (Eds.), *Neural models of language processes* (pp. 115–133). New York: Academic Press.

Marslen-Wilson, W. D. (1984). Function and process in spoken word recognition. In H. Bouma, & O. C. Bouwhuis (Eds.), *Attention and performance X*: Control of language processes. Hillsdale, NJ: Erlbaum.

Marslen-Wilson, W. D., & Tyler, L. K. (1980). The temporal structure of spoken language understanding. *Cognition, 8*, 1–71.

Ryan, E. B., Ledger, G. W., Short, E. J., & Weed, K. A. (1982). Promoting the use of active comprehension strategies by poor readers. *Topics in Learning and Learning Disabilities, 2*, 53–60.

Schlesinger, I. (1977). The role of cognitive development and linguistic input in language acquisition. *Journal of Child Language, 4*, 153–170.

Tyler, L. K. (1981). Syntactic and interpretive factors in the development of language comprehension. In W. Deutsch (Ed.), *The child's construction of language* (pp. 149–181). New York: Academic Press.

Van der Lely, H., & Dewart, H. (1986). Sentence comprehension strategies in specifically language impaired children. *The British Journal of Disorders of Communication, 21*, 291–306.

Weismer, S. E. (1985). Constructive comprehension abilities exhibited by language-disordered children. *Journal of Speech and Hearing Research, 28*, 175–184.

Winitz, H. (1973). Problem solving and the delaying of speech as strategies in the teaching of language. *ASHA, 15*, 583–586.

Winitz, H. (1976). Full time experience. *ASHA, 18*, 404.

Wittrock, M. C. (1981). Reading comprehension. In F. J. Pirozzolo, & M. C. Wittrock (Eds.), *Neurological and cognitive processes in reading* (pp. 229–259). New York: Academic Press.

Wolfus, B., Moskovitch, M., & Kinsbourne, M. (1980). Subgroups of developmental language impairment. *Brain and Language, 10*, 152–171.

Woods, W. A. (1982). HWIM: A speech understanding system on a computer. In M. A. Arbib, D. Caplan, & J. C. Marshall (Eds.), *Neural models of language processes* (pp. 95–113). New York: Academic Press.

LANGUAGE DEVELOPMENT THEORIES

Bates, E., Benigni, L., Bretherton, I, Camaioni, L., & Volterra, V. (1977). From gesture to first word: On cognitive and social prerequisites. In M. Lewis, & L. A. Rosenblum (Eds.), *Interaction, conversation and the development of language* (pp. 247–307). New York: John Wiley and Sons.

Berko-Gleason, J., & Weintraub, S. (1978). Input language and the acquisition of communicative competence. In K. E. Nelson (Ed.), *Children's language* (pp. 171–222). New York: Gardner Press.

Bloom, L. (1970). *Language development: Form and function in emerging grammars*. Cambridge, MA: MIT Press.

Bruner, J. S. (1975). The ontogenesis of speech acts. *Journal of Child Language, 2*, 1–19.

Bruner, J. S. (1981). The social context of language acquisition. *Language and Cognition, 1*, 155–178.

Cazden, C. B. (1968). The acquisition of noun and verb inflections. *Child Development, 39*, 433–438.

Clark, R. (1974). Performing without competence. *Journal of Child Language, 1*, 1–10.

Cook-Gumperz, J. (1977). Situated instructions: Language socialization of school age children. In S. Ervin-Tripp, & C. Mitchell-Kernan (Eds.), *Child discourse* (pp. 103–121). New York: Academic Press.

Cromer, R. F. (1976). The cognitive hypothesis of language acquisition and its implications for child language deficiency. In D. M. Morehead, & A. E. Morehead (Eds.), *Normal and deficient child language* (pp. 283–335). Baltimore: University Park Press.

Dale, P. S. (1976). *Language development, structure and function.* New York: Holt, Rinehart and Winston.

De Maio, L. J. (1982). Conversational turn taking: A salient dimension of children's language learning. In N. J. Lass (Ed.), *Speech and language: Advances in basic research and practice* (pp. 159–190). New York: Academic Press.

De Maio, L. J. (1984). Establishing communication networks through interactive play: A method for language programming in the clinic setting. *Seminars in Speech and Language, 5*, 199–210.

Deutsch, W. (1981). Introduction. In I. W. Deutsch (Ed.), *The child's construction of language* (pp. 1–13). New York: Academic Press.

Foster, S. H. (1984b). The development of discourse topic skills by infants and young children. Unpublished manuscript.

Freedle, R., & Lewis, M. (1977). Prelinguistic conversations. In M. Lewis, & L. A. Rosenblum (Eds.), *Interaction, conversation, and the development of language* (pp. 157–186). New York: John Wiley & Sons.

Gleitman, L. R., Newport, E. L., & Gleitman, H. (1984). The current status of the motherese hypothesis. *Journal of Child Language, 11*, 43–79.

Halliday, M. A. K. (1975). *Learning how to mean: Explorations in the development of language.* New York: Elsevier North-Holland.

Jenkins, J. J. (1969). Language and thought. In J. F. Voss (Ed.), *Approaches to thought* (pp. 211–237). Columbus, OH: Merrill.

Karmiloff-Smith, A. (1981). The grammatical marking of thematic structure in the development of language production. In W. Deutch (Ed.), *The child's construction of language* (pp. 121–147). New York: Academic Press.

Kaye, K., & Chainey, R. (1981). Conversational asymmetry between mothers and children. *Journal of Child Language, 8*, 35–50.

Lewis, M., & Cherry, L. (1977). Social behavior and language acquisition. In M. Lewis, & L. A. Rosenblum (Eds.), *Interaction, conversation, and the development of language* (pp. 227–245). New York: John Wiley and Sons.

Lucariello, J., Kyratzis, A., & Engel, S. (1986). Event representation, context, and language. In K. Nelson (Ed.), *Event knowledge: Structure and function in development* (pp. 137–160). Hillsdale, NJ: Lawrence Erlbaum Associates.

Rees, N. S. (1978). Pragmatics of language: Applications to normal and disordered language development. In R. L. Schiefelbusch (Ed.), *Bases of language intervention* (pp. 196–268). Baltimore: University Park Press.

Rice, M. L. (1983). Contemporary accounts of the cognition/language relationship: Implication for speech-language clinicians. *Journal of Speech and Hearing Disorders, 48*, 347–359.

Salzinger, K. (1975). Are theories of competence necessary? In D. Aaronson, & R. W. Rieber (Eds.), *Developmental psycholinguistics and communication disorders* (pp. 178–196). New York: The New York Academy of Sciences.

Schlesinger, I. (1977). The role of cognitive development and linguistic input in language acquisition. *Journal of Child Language, 4*, 153–170.

Shatz, M. (1981). Learning the rules of the game: Four views of the relation between grammar acquisition and social interaction. In W. Deutsch (Ed.), *The child's construction of language* (pp. 17–38). New York: Academic Press.

Shatz, M. (1987). Bootstrapping operations in child language. In K. Nelson, & A. Van Kleeck (Eds.), *Children's language* (Vol. VI). Hillsdale, NJ: Lawrence Erlbaum Associates.

Slobin, D. I. (1973). Cognitive prerequisites for the development of grammar. In C. A. Ferguson, & D. I. Slobin (Eds.), *Studies of child development* (pp. 175–208). New York: Holt, Rinehart & Winston.

Slobin, D. (1982). Universal and particular in the acquisition of language. In L. Gleitman, & E. Wanner (Eds.), *Language acquisition: The state of the art.* Cambridge: Cambridge University Press.

Snow, C. E. (1972). Mothers' speech to children learning language. *Child Development, 43*, 549–565.

Wardhaugh, R. (1976). Theories of language acquisition in relation to beginning reading instruction. In H. Singer, & R. B. Ruddell (Eds.), *Theoretical models and processes of reading* (pp. 42–66). Newark, DE: International Reading Association.

Waryas, C. L., & Crowe, T. A. (1982). Language delay. In N. Lass, L. McReynolds, J. Northern, & D. Yoder (Eds.), *Speech, language and hearing* (Vol. II) (pp. 761–779). Pathologies of Speech and Language. Philadelphia: W. B. Saunders.

Wells, G. (1981). Language as interaction. In G. Wells (Ed.), *Learning through interaction* (pp. 22–72). Cambridge: Cambridge University Press.

Wulz, S. V., Hall, M. K., & Klein, M. D. (1983). A home-centered instructional communication strategy for severely handicapped children. *Journal of Speech and Hearing Disorders, 48*, 2–10.

ORAL AND WRITTEN LANGUAGE

Beach, R., & Bridwell, L. (1984). Learning through writing: A rationale for writing across the curriculum. In A. D. Pellegrini, & T. D. Yawkey (Eds.), *The development of oral and written language in social contexts* (pp. 183–200). Norwood, NJ: Ablex.

Bradley, D. C., & Forster, K. I. (1987). A reader's view of listening. *Cognition, 25*, 103–134.

Haber, L. R., & Haber, R. N. (1981). Perceptual processes in reading: An analysis-by-synthesis model. In F. J. Pirozzolo, & M. C. Wittrock (Eds.), *Neuropsychological and cognitive processes in reading* (pp. 167–200). New York: Academic Press.

Kamhi, A. G., & Catts, H. W. (1986). Toward an understanding of developmental language and reading disorders. *Journal of Speech and Hearing Disorders, 51*, 337–347.

Katz, L., Boyce, S., Goldstein, L., & Lukatela, G. (1987). Grammatical information effects in auditory word recognition. *Cognition, 25*, 235–264.

Kinsbourne, M. (1982). The role of selective attention in reading disability. In R. N. Malatesha, & P. G. Aaron (Eds.), *Reading disorders: Varieties and treatments* (pp. 199–214). New York: Academic Press.

Masson, M. E. J. (1982). A framework of cognitive and metacognitive determinants of reading skill. *Topics in Learning and Learning Disabilities, 2*, 37–43.

Mehegan, C. C., & Dreifuss, M. B. (1972). Hyperlexia. *Neurology, 22*, 1105–1111.

Ryan, E. B., Ledger, G. W., Short, E. J., & Weed, K. A. (1982). Promoting the use of active comprehension strategies by poor readers. *Topics in Learning and Learning Disabilities, 2*, 53–60.

Samuels, S. J., & Eisenberg, P. (1981). A framework for understanding the reading process. In F. J. Pirozzolo, & M. C. Wittrock (Eds.), *Neuropsychological and cognitive processes in reading* (pp. 31–67). New York: Academic Press.

Wallach, G., & Lee, D. (1980). So you want to know what to do with language disabled children above the age of six. *Topics in Language Disorders, 1*, 99–113.

Wanat, S. F. (1976). Relations between language and visual processing. In H. Singer, & R. B. Ruddell (Eds.), *Theoretical models and processes of reading* (pp. 108–136). Newark, DE: International Reading Association.

Wardhaugh, R. (1976). Theories of language acquisition in relation to beginning reading instruction. In H. Singer, & R. B. Ruddell (Eds.), *Theoretical models and processes of reading* (pp. 42–66). Newark, DE: International Reading Association.

Wittrock, M. C. (1981). Reading comprehension. In F. J. Pirozzolo, & M. C. Wittrock (Eds.), *Neurological and cognitive processes in reading* (pp. 229–259). New York: Academic Press.

LANGUAGE DISORDERS

Ackerman, P. T., & Dykman, R. A. (1982). Automatic and effortful information-processing deficits in children with learning and attention disorders. *Topics in Learning and Learning Disabilities, 2*, 12–23.

Aram, D. M., & Nation, J. E. (1975). Patterns of language behavior in children with developmental language disorders. *Journal of Speech and Hearing Research, 18*, 229–241.

Aram, D. M., Ekelman, B. L., & Nation, J. E. (1984). Pre-schoolers with language disorders: 10 years later. *Journal of Speech and Hearing Research, 27*, 232–244.

Bernstein, L. E., & Stark, R. E. (1985). Speech perception development in language-impaired children: A 4-year follow-up study. *Journal of Speech and Hearing Disorders, 50*, 21–30.

Bishop, D. V. M., & Edmundson, A. (1987). Language-impaired 4-year olds: Distinguishing transient from persistent impairment. *Journal of Speech and Hearing Disorders, 52*, 156–173.

Brinton, B., & Fujiki, M. (1982). A comparison of request-response sequences in the discourse of normal and language disordered children. *Journal of Speech and Hearing Disorders, 47*, 57–62.

Brinton, B., Fujiki, M., Winkler, E., & Loeb, D. F. (1986). Responses to requests for clarification in linguistically normal and language-impaired children. *Journal of Speech and Hearing Disorders, 51*, 370–378.

Camarata, S., Newhoff, M., & Rugg, B. (1981). Perspective taking in normal and language-disordered children. *Proceedings of the Symposium on Research in Child Language Disorders*. Madison: University of Wisconsin.

Carrow-Woolfolk, E. (1975). Disordered language and its management. In D. B. Tower (Ed.), *The nervous system* (Vol. 3) (pp. 429–436). New York: Raven Press.

Chapanis, L. (1977). Language deficits and cross-modal sensory perception. In S. J. Segalowitz, & F. A. Gruber (Eds.), *Language development and neurological theory* (pp. 107–120). New York: Academic Press.

Crais, E. R., & Chapman, R. S. (1987). Story recall and inferencing skills in language/learning-disabled and nondisabled children. *Journal of Speech and Hearing Disorders, 52*, 50–55.

Donahue, M., Pearl, R., & Bryan, T. (1980). Learning disabled children's conversational competence: Responses to inadequate messages. *Applied Psycholinguistics, 1*, 387–403.

Fey, M. E., & Leonard, L. B. (1983). Pragmatic skills of children with specific language impairment. In T. M. Gallagher, & C. A. Prutting (Eds.), *Pragmatic assessment and intervention issues in language* (pp. 65–82). San Diego, CA: College-Hill Press.

Gillam, R., & Johnston, J. (1985). Development of print awareness in language disordered preschoolers. *Journal of Speech and Hearing Research, 28*, 521–526.

Inhelder, B. (1976). Observations on the operational and figurative aspects of thought in dysphasic children. In D. M. Morehead, & A. E. Morehead (Eds.), *Normal and deficient language* (pp. 335–344). Baltimore: University Park Press.

Johnston, J., & Weismer, S. (1983). Mental rotation abilities in language-disordered children. *Journal of Speech and Hearing Research, 26*, 397–404.

Kail, R., & Leonard, L. (1986). Word finding abilities in language-impaired children. *ASHA Monographs, 25*, Rockville, MD: The American Speech, Language and Hearing Association.

Kamhi, A. G. (1981). Nonlinguistic symbolic and conceptual abilities of language impaired and normally developing children. *Journal of Speech and Hearing Research, 24*, 446–453.

Kamhi, A. G., Catts, H. W., Koenig, L. A., & Lewis, B. A. (1984). Hypothesis testing and non-linguistic symbolic abilities in language-impaired children. *Journal of Speech and Hearing Disorders, 49*, 169–176.

Kamhi, A. G., Lee, R., & Nelson, L. (1985). Word, syllable, and sound awareness in language disordered children. *Journal of Speech and Hearing Disorders, 50*, 207–213.

Kirchner, D. M., & Klatzky, R. L. (1985). Verbal rehearsal and memory in language disordered children. *Journal of Speech and Hearing Research, 28*, 556–565.

Kirchner, D. M., & Skarakis-Doyle, E. A. (1983). Developmental language disorders: A theoretical perspective. In T. M. Gallagher, & C. A. Prutting (Eds.), *Pragmatic assessment and intervention issues in language* (pp. 215–246). San Diego, CA: College-Hill Press.

Lasky, E. Z., & Klopp, K. (1982). Parent-child interaction in normal and language-disordered children. *Journal of Speech and Hearing Disorders, 47*, 7–18.

Leonard, L., Bolders, J., & Miller, J. (1976). An examination of the semantic relations reflected in the language usage of normal and language disordered children. *Journal of Speech and Hearing Research, 45*, 336–345.

Leonard, L. B., Schwartz, R. G., Chapman, K., Rowan, L. E., Prelock, P. A., Terrell, B., Weiss, A. L., & Messick, C. (1982). Early lexical acquisition in children with specific language impairment. *Journal of Speech and Hearing Research, 25*, 554–564.

Menyuk, P. (1964). Comparison of grammar of children with functionally deviant and normal speech. *Journal of Speech and Hearing Research, 7*, 109–121.

Menyuk, P., & Looney, P. L. (1972). A problem of language disorder: Length versus structure. *Journal of Speech and Hearing Research, 15*, 264–279.

Morehead, D. M., & Ingram, D. (1973). The development of base syntax in normal and linguistically deviant children. *Journal of Speech and Hearing Research, 16*, 330–352.

Nelson, L. K., Kamhi, A. G.,, & Apel, K. (1987). Cognitive strengths and weaknesses in language-impaired children: One more look. *Journal of Speech and Hearing Disorders, 52*, 36–43.

Savich, P. (1984). Anticipatory imagery ability in normal and language-disabled children. *Journal of Speech and Hearing Research, 27*, 494–502.

Tallal, P., & Piercy, M. (1978). Defects of auditory perception in children with developmental dysphasia. In N. A. Wyke (Ed.), *Developmental dysphasia* (pp. 63–84). New York: Academic Press.

Tallal, P., & Stark, R. (1976). Relation between speech perception and speech production impairment in children with developmental dysphasia. *Brain and Language, 3*, 305–317.

Van der Lely, H., & Dewart, H. (1986). Sentence comprehension strategies in specifically language impaired children. *The British Journal of Disorders of Communication, 21*, 291–306.

Wolfus, B., Moskovitch, M., & Kinsbourne, M. (1980). Subgroups of developmental language impairment. *Brain and Language, 10*, 152–171.

ASSESSMENT

Allen, D. V., Bliss, L. S., & Timmons, J. (1981). Language evaluation: Science or art? *Journal of Speech and Hearing Disorders, 46*, 66–68.

Blank, M. (1975a). Mastering the intangible through language. In D. Aaronson, & R. W. Reiber (Eds.), *Developmental psycholinguistics and communication disorders* (pp. 44–58). New York: The New York Academy of Sciences.

Blank, M. (1975b). A methodology for fostering abstract thinking in deprived children. Unpublished manuscript.

Carrow, E. (1972). Assessment of speech and language in children. In J. E. McLean, D. E. Yoder, & R. L. Schiefelbusch (Eds.), *Language intervention with the retarded* (pp. 52–88). Baltimore: University Park Press.

Dollaghan, C., & Miller, J. (1986). Observational methods in the study of communicative competence. In R. L. Schiefelbusch (Ed.), *Language competence: Assessment and intervention* (pp. 99–130). San Diego, CA: College-Hill Press.

Geffner, D. (1981). Assessment of language disorders: Linguistic and cognitive functions. *Topics in Language Disorders, 1*, 1–9.

Hubbell, R. D. (1981). *Children's language disorders: An integrated approach.* Englewood Cliffs, NJ: Prentice-Hall.

Johnson, D. J. (1981). Factors to consider in programming for children with language disorders. *Topics in Learning and Learning Disabilities, 1*, 13–27.

Klecan-Aker, J. (1985). Syntactic abilities in normal and language deficient middle school children. *Topics in Langage Disorders, 5*, 46–54.

Klecan-Aker, J., & Swank, P. R. (1987). The narrative styles of normal first and third grade children. *Language and Speech, 30*, 251–262.

Klein, M. D., Wulz, S. N., Hall, M. K., Waldo, L. K., Carpenter, S. A., Rathan, D. A., Myers, S. P., Fox, F., & Marshall, A. M. (1981). *Comprehensive curriculum communication guide* (pp. 185–197). Lawrence: Early Childhood Institute, University of Kansas.

Kretschmer, R. E. (1984). Metacognition, metalinguistics, and intervention. In K. F. Ruder, & M. D. Smith (Eds.), *Developmental language intervention: Psycholinguistic applications* (pp. 209–230). Baltimore: University Park Press.

Kuczaj, S. T. (1983). *Crib speech and language play.* New York: Springer-Verlag.

Kunge, L. H., Lockhart, S. K., Didow, S. M., & Caterson, M. (1983). Interactive assessment and treatment model. In H. Winitz (Ed.), *Treating language disorders* (pp. 79–96). Baltimore: University Park Press.

Lasky, E. Z. (1983). Facilitating comprehension, recall, and production of language. In H. Winitz (Ed.), *Treating language disorders* (pp. 43–56). Baltimore: University Park Press.

Lee, L. (1966). Developmental sentence types: A method for comparing normal and deviant syntactic development. *Journal of Speech and Hearing Disorders, 31*, 311–330.

Lee, L., Koenigsknecht, R., & Mulhern, S. (1975). *Interactive language development teaching: The clinical presentation of grammatical structure.* Evanston, IL: Northwestern University Press.

Leonard, L. (1975). Modeling as a clinical procedure in language. *Speech and Hearing Services in Schools, 6*, 72–85.

Miller, J. F. (1981). *Assessing language production in children.* Baltimore: University Park Press.

Prutting, C. A. (1982a). Pragmatics as social competence. *Journal of Speech and Hearing Disorders, 47*, 123–134.

Prutting, C. A. (1982b). Observational protocol for pragmatic behaviors [Clinic Manual]. Developed for the University of California Speech and Hearing Clinic, Santa Barbara, CA.

Prutting, C. A., & Kirchner, D. M. (1987). A clinical appraisal of the pragmatic aspects of language. *Journal of Speech and Hearing Disorders, 52*, 105–119.

Roth, F. P., & Spekman, N. J. (1984a). Assessing the pragmatic abilities of children: Part 1. Organizational framework and assessment parameters. *Journal of Speech and Hearing Disorders, 49*, 2–11.

Roth, F. P., & Spekman, N. J. (1984b). Assessing the pragmatic abilities of children: Part 2. Guidelines, considerations, and specific evaluation procedures. *Journal of Speech and Hearing Disorders, 49*, 12–17.

Turton, L. J. (1983). Curriculum concepts for language treatment of children. In H. Winitz (Ed.), *Treating language disorders* (pp. 57–78). Baltimore: University Park Press.

INTERVENTION

Allen, R. R., & Brown, K. L. (1977). Developing communication competence in children. A report of the Speech Communication Association's National Project on Speech Communication Competencies. Skokie, Il: National Textbook Company.

Applebee, A. N. (1978). *The child's concept of story.* Chicago: Chicago University Press.

Bandura, A., & Harris, M. A. (1966). Modification of syntactic style. *Journal of Experimental Child Psychology, 4*, 341–352.

Carrow-Woolfolk, E. (1980). *Teaching reading through an auditory method.* Houston: Communication Press.

Cazden, C. B. (1973). Problems in education: Language as curriculum content and learning environment. *Daedalus, Journal of the American Academy of Arts and Sciences, 102*, 135–148.

Cole, K. N., & Dale, P. S. (1986). Direct language instruction and interactive language instruction with language delayed preschool children: A comparison study. *Journal of Speech and Hearing Research, 29*, 206–217.

Connell, P. J. (1987). An effect of modeling and imitation teaching procedures on children with and without specific language impairment. *Journal of Speech and Hearing Research, 30*, 105–113.

Conti-Ramsden, G., & Friel-Patti, S. (1986). Mother-child dialogues: Considerations of cognitive complexity for young language learning children. *The British Journal of Disorders of Communication, 21*, 245–255.

Courtright, J., & Courtright, I. (1976). Imitative modeling as a theoretical base for instructing language-disordered children. *Journal of Speech and Hearing Research, 19*, 655–663.

Courtright, J., & Courtright, I. (1979). Imitative modeling as a language intervention strategy. *Journal of Speech and Hearing Research, 22*, 389–402.

Craig, H. K. (1983). Applications of pragmatic language models for intervention. In T. M. Gallagher, & C. A. Prutting (Eds.), *Pragmatic assessment and intervention issues in language* (pp. 101–127). San Diego, CA: College-Hill Press.

Culatta, B., & Horn, D. (1982). A program for achieving generalization of grammatic rules to spontaneous discourse. *Journal of Speech and Hearing Disorders, 47*, 174–180.

Dollaghan, C., & Kaston, N. (1986). A comprehension monitoring program for language-impaired children. *Journal of Speech and Hearing Disorders, 51*, 264–271.

Duchan, J. F. (1986a). Language intervention through sensemaking and fine tuning. In R. L. Schiefelbusch (Ed.), *Language competence: Assessment and intervention* (pp. 187–212). San Diego, CA: College-Hill Press.

Duchan, J. F. (1986b). Learning to describe events. *Topics in Language Disorders, 6*, 27–36.

Duchan, J. F., & Weitzner-Lin, B. (1987). Nurturant-naturalistic intervention for language-impaired children: Implications for planning lessons and tracking progress. *ASHA, 29*, 45–50.

Fey, M. (1986). *Language intervention with young children.* San Diego: College-Hill Press.

Fivush, R., & Slackman, E. A. (1986). The acquisition and development of scripts. In K. Nelson (Ed.), *Event knowledge: Structures and functions in development* (pp. 71–96). New Jersey: Lawrence Erlbaum Associates.

Flores D'Arcais, G. B. (1981). The acquisition of meaning of the connectives. In W. Deutsch (Ed.), *The child's construction of language* (pp. 265–298). New York: Academic Press.

Friel-Patti, S., & Lougeay-Mottinger, J. (1986). Preschool language intervention: Some key concerns. *Topics in Language Disorders, 6*, 46–57.

Galda, L. (1984). Narrative competence: Play, storytelling, and story comprehension. In A. D. Pellegrini, & T. D. Yawkey (Eds.), *The development of oral and written language in social contexts* (pp. 105–117). Norwood, NJ: Ablex.

Gardner, H. E. (1980). Children's literary development: The realms of metaphors and stories. In P. McGhee, & A. Chapman (Eds.), *Children's humor.* New York: John Wiley and Sons.

Garvey, C. (1974). Some properties of social play. *Merrill-Palmer Quarterly, 20*, 163–180.

Gleitman, L. R., Newport, E. L., & Gleitman, H. (1984). The current status of the motherese hypothesis. *Journal of Child Language, 11*, 43–79.

Gordon, C., & Braun, C. (1983). Using story schema as an aid to reading and writing. *The Reading Teacher, 37*, 116–121.

Halle, J. W. (1984). Arranging the natural environment to occasion language: Giving severely language-delayed children reasons to communicate. *Seminars in Speech and Language, 5*, 185–197.

Halliday, M. A. K. (1975). *Learning how to mean: Explorations in the development of language.* New York: Elsevier North-Holland.

Hart, B., & Risley, T. R. (1975). Incidental teaching of language in the preschool. *Journal of Applied Behavior Analysis, 8*, 411–420.

Hart, B., & Risley, T. (1986). Incidental strategies. In R. L. Schiefelbusch (Ed.), *Language competence: Assessment and intervention* (pp. 213–226). San Diego, CA: College-Hill.

Hetenyi, K. B. (1974). Interactions between language-delayed children and their parents—A case study. Paper presented at the Annual Convention of the American Speech and Hearing Association, Las Vegas.

Highnam, C., & Morris, V. (1987). Linguistic stress judgments of language learning disabled students. *Journal of Communication Disorders, 20*, 93–103.

Howe, C. (1981). *Acquiring language in a conversational context.* New York: Academic Press.

Hubbell, R. D. (1977). On facilitating spontaneous talking in young children. *Journal of Speech and Hearing Disorders, 42*, 216–231.

Hubbell, R. D. (1981). *Children's language disorders: An integrated approach.* Englewood Cliffs, NJ: Prentice-Hall.

Johnson, D. J. (1981). Factors to consider in programming for children with language disorders. *Topics in Learning and Learning Disabilities, 1,* 13–27.

Johnston, J. R. (1983). What is language intervention: The role of theory. In J. Miller, D. E. Yoder, & R. Schiefelbusch (Eds.), *Contemporary issues in language intervention. ASHA Reports, 12,* 52–57. Rockville, MD: The American Speech and Hearing Association.

Karmiloff-Smith, A. (1979). *A functional approach to child language: A study of determiners and reference.* Cambridge: Cambridge University Press.

Karmiloff-Smith, A. (1981). The grammatical marking of thematic structure in the development of language production. In W. Deutch (Ed.), *The child's construction of language* (pp. 121–147). New York: Academic Press.

Linder, T. W. (1983). *Early childhood special education: Program development and administration.* Baltimore: Paul H. Brookes.

Lovell, K., Hoyle, H., & Sidall, M. (1968). A study of some aspects of the play and language of young children. *Journal of Child Psychology and Psychiatry, 9,* 41–50.

MacDonald, J. D., & Gillette, Y. (1984). Conversation engineering: A pragmatic approach to early social competence. *Seminars in Speech and Language, 5,* 171–184.

McDonald, L., & Pien, D. (1982). Mother conversational behavior as a function of interactional intent. *Journal of Child Language, 9,* 337–358.

McLean, J., & Snyder-McLean, L. (1984). Strategies of facilitating language development in clinics, schools, and homes. *Seminars in Speech and Language, 5.*

Moeller, M. P., Osberger, M. J., & Eccarius, M. (1986). Cognitively based strategies for use with hearing-impaired students with comprehension deficits. *Topics in Language Disorders, 6,* 37–50.

Muma, J. R. (1978). *Language handbook: Concepts, assessment, intervention.* New York: Prentice-Hall.

Muma, J. R. (1983). Speech-language pathology: Emerging clinical expertise in language. In T. M. Gallagher, & C. A. Prutting (Eds.), *Pragmatic assessment and intervention issues in language* (pp. 195–214). San Diego: College-Hill Press.

Muma, J. R., & Pierce, S. (1981). Language intervention: Data or evidence? *Topics in Language and Learning Disabilities, 1,* 1–11.

Nelson, K. (1977). Facilitating children's syntax acquisition. *Developmental Psychology, 13,* 101–107.

Nelson, K. (1986a). *Event knowledge: Structure and function in development.* Hillsdale, NJ: Lawrence Erlbaum Associates.

Nelson, K. (1986b). Event knowledge and cognitive development. In K. Nelson (Ed.), *Event knowledge: Structure and function in development* (pp. 1–20). Hillsdale, NJ: Lawrence Erlbaum Associates.

Nelson, K., & Gruendel, J. (1986). Children's scripts. In K. Nelson (Ed.), *Event knowledge: Structure and function in development* (pp. 21–46). Hillsdale, NJ: Lawrence Erlbaum Associates.

Nelson, K. E. (1975). Facilitating syntax acquisition. Paper presented to the Eastern Psychological Association. New York, NY.

Ninio, A., & Brunner, J. (1977). The achievement and antecedents of labelling. *Journal of Child Language, 5,* 1–15.

Olswang, L., Bain, B., Dunn, C., & Cooper, J. (1983). The effects of stimulus variation on lexical learning. *Journal of Speech and Hearing Disorders, 48,* 192–201.

Olswang, L. B., Kriegsman, E., & Mastergeorge, A. (1982). Facilitating functional requesting in pragmatically impaired children. *Language, Speech, and Hearing Services in Schools, 13,* 202–217.

Page, J. L., & Stewart, S. R. (1985). Story grammar skills in school-age children. *Topics in Language Disorders, 5,* 16–30.

Patterson, G., & Cobb, J. (1971). A dyadic analysis of "aggressive" behaviors. In J. Hill (Ed.), *Minnesota symposia on child psychology* (Vol. 5). Minneapolis: University of Minnesota Press.

Patterson, G., & Cobb, J. (1973). Stimulus control for noxious behaviors. In J. Knutson (Ed.), *The control of aggression: Implications from basic research* (pp. 145–199). Chicago: Aldine.

Prutting, C. A. (1982b). Observational protocol for pragmatic behaviors [Clinic Manual]. Developed for the University of California Speech and Hearing Clinic, Santa Barbara, CA.

Ratner, M., & Bruner, J. S. (1978). Games, social exchanges and the acquisition of language. *Journal of Child Language, 5,* 391–402.

Rice, M. L. (1986). Mismatched premises of the communicative competence model and language intervention. In R. L. Schiefelbusch (Ed.), *Language competence: Assessment and intervention* (pp. 261–280). San Diego: College-Hill Press.

Rice, M. L., & Haight, P. L. (1986). Motherese, of Mr. Rogers: A description of the dialogue of educational television programs. *Journal of Speech and Hearing Disorders, 51,* 282–287.

Roth, F. P., & Clark, D. M. (1987). Symbolic play and social participation abilities of language-impaired and normally developing children. *Journal of Speech and Hearing Disorders, 52,* 17–29.

Sachs, J., Goldman, J., & Chaille, C. (1984). Planning in pretend play: Using language to coordinate narrative development. In A. D. Pellegrini, & T. D. Yawkey (Eds.), *The development of oral and written language in social contexts* (pp. 119–128). Norwood, NJ: Ablex.

Schwartz, R. G., Chapman, K., Terrell, B. Y., Prelock, P., & Rowan, L. (1985). Facilitating word combination in language-impaired children through discourse structure. *Journal of Speech and Hearing Disorders, 50*, 31–39.

Seitz, S. (1975). Language intervention—Changing the language environment of the retarded child. In R. Kock, F. de la Cruz, & F. Menolascino (Eds.), *Down's syndrome: Research, prevention and management*. New York: Brunes/Magel.

Siegel, G. M., & Vogt, M. C. (1984). Pluralization instruction in comprehension and production. *Journal of Speech and Hearing Disorders, 49*, 128–135.

Sigel, I. E., & McGillicuddy-Delise, A. V. (1984). Parents as teachers of their children: A distancing behavior. In A. D. Pellegrini, & T. D. Yawkey (Eds.), *The development of oral and written language in social contexts* (pp. 71–94). Norwood, NJ: Ablex.

Slackman, E. A., Hudson, J. A., & Fivush, R. (1986). Actions, actors, links and goals: The structure of children's event representations. In K. Nelson (Ed.), *Event knowledge: Structure and function in development* (pp. 47–69). Hillsdale, NJ: Lawrence Erlbaum Associates.

Sleight, C. C., & Prinz, P. M. (1985). Use of abstracts, orientations and codas in narration by language-disordered and nondisordered children. *Journal of Speech and Hearing Disorders, 50*, 361, 371.

Snyder-McLean, L. K., & McLean, J. (1978). Verbal information gathering strategies: The child's use of language to acquire language. *Journal of Speech and Hearing Disorders, 43*, 306–325.

Snyder-McLean, L. K., Solomonson, B., McLean, J. E., & Sack, S. (1984). Structuring joint action routines: A strategy for facilitating communication and language development in the classroom. In J. McLean, & L. K. Snyder-McLean (Eds.), Strategies of facilitating language development in clinics, schools, and homes. *Seminars in Speech and Language, 5*, 213–225.

Spradlin, J. E., & Siegel, G. M. (1982). Language training in natural and clinical environments. *Journal of Speech and Hearing Disorders, 47*, 2–6.

Staab, C. F. (1983). Language functions elicited by meaningful activities: A new dimension in language programs. *Language, Speech, and Hearing Services in Schools, 14*, 164–170.

Stewart, S. (1985). Development of written language proficiency: Methods for teaching text structure. In C. S. Simon (Ed.), *Communication skills and classroom success: Therapy methodologies for language-learning disabled children*. Austin: College-Hill Press.

Taenzer, S. F., Cermak, M. S., & Hanlon, R. C. (1981). Outside the therapy room: A naturalistic approach to language intervention. *Topics in Learning and Learning Disabilities, 1*, 41–46.

Terrell, B., Schwartz, R. G., Prelock, P. A., & Messick, C. K. (1984). Symbolic play in normal and language-impaired children. *Journal of Speech and Hearing Research, 27*, 424–429.

Turton, L. J. (1983). Curriculum concepts for language treatment of children. In H. Winitz (Ed.), *Treating language disorders* (pp. 57–78). Baltimore: University Park Press.

Van Kleeck, A., & Richardson, A. (in press). In N. Lass, L. McReynolds, J. Northern, & D. Yoder (Eds.), *Handbook of speech-language pathology and audiology*. New York: Appleton-Century-Crofts.

Warren, S. F., & Kaiser, A. P. (1986a). Generalization of treatment effects by young language delayed children: A longitudinal analysis. *Journal of Speech and Hearing Disorders, 51*, 239–251.

Weiner, F., & Ostrowski, A. (1979). Effects of listener uncertainty on articulatory inconsistency. *Journal of Speech and Hearing Disorders, 44*, 487–503.

Weiss, A. L., Leonard, L. B., Rowan, L. E., & Chapman, K. (1983). Linguistic and nonlinguistic features of style in normal and language-impaired children. *Journal of Speech and Hearing Disorders, 48*, 150–154.

Weitzner-Lin, B., & Duchan, J. (1982). What comes after pragmatic assessment? Assessing pragmatic therapy. Paper presented at the Annual Convention of the American Speech-Language-Hearing Association, Toronto.

Wells, G. (1981). Language as interaction. In G. Wells (Ed.), *Learning through interaction* (pp. 22–72). Cambridge: Cambridge University Press.

Whitaker, H. (1976). A case of the isolation of the language function. In H. Whitaker, & H. A. Whitaker (Eds.), *Studies in neurolinguistics* (pp. 1–58). New York: Academic Press.

Winitz, H. (1973). Problem solving and the delaying of speech as strategies in the teaching of language. *ASHA, 15*, 583–586.

Winitz, H. (1976). Full time experience. *ASHA, 18*, 404.

Winitz, H. (1983). Use and abuse of the developmental approach. In H. Winitz (Ed.), *Treating language disorders* (pp. 25–42). Baltimore: University Park Press.

Yawkey, T. D., & Miller, T. J. (1984). The language of social play in young children. In A. D. Pellegrini, & T. D. Yawkey (Eds.), *The development of oral and written language in social context* (pp. 95–104). Norwood, NJ: Ablex.

GENERAL LANGUAGE

Bloom. L., & Lahey, M. (1978). *Language development and language disorders*. New York: John Wiley and Sons.

Brown, R. (1973). *A first language: The early stages*. Cambridge, MA: Harvard University Press.

Carrow-Woolfolk, E., & Lynch, J. (1982). *An integrative approach to language disorders in children*. New York: Grune & Stratton.

Crowder, R. G. (1978). Language and memory. In J. F. Kavanagh, & W. Strange (Eds.), *Speech and language in the laboratory, school and clinic* (pp. 331–376). Cambridge, MA: MIT Press.

de Villiers, J., & de Villiers, P. (1978). *Language acquisition*. Cambridge, MA: Harvard University Press.

de Villiers, J. G., & de Villiers, P. A. (1982). Language development. In R. Vasta (Ed.), *Strategies and techniques of child study* (pp. 117–159). New York: Academic Press.

Fey, M. (1986). *Language intervention with young children*. San Diego: College-Hill Press.

Linder, T. W. (1983). *Early childhood special education: Program development and administration*. Baltimore: Paul H. Brookes.

Nelson, K. (1986a). *Event knowledge: Structure and function in development*. Hillsdale, NJ: Lawrence Erlbaum Associates.

Owens, R. E. (1984). *Language development: An introduction*. Columbus, OH: Merrill.

Schiefelbusch, R. L. (1986). *Language competence: Assessment and intervention*. San Diego, CA: College-Hill Press.

Tyler, L. K. (1981). Syntactic and interpretive factors in the development of language comprehension. In W. Deutsch (Ed.), *The child's construction of language* (pp. 149–181). New York: Academic Press.

Wells, G. (1985). *Language development in the pre-school years*. Cambridge: Cambridge University Press.

AUTHOR INDEX

SUBJECT INDEX

Note: the letter *f* following a page number indicates a figure; the letter *t* following a page number indicates a table.